Clinically Oriented Documentation of Laboratory Data

*Proceedings of a Conference on Clinically
Oriented Documentation of Laboratory Data
Held at the School of Medicine
State University of New York at Buffalo
Buffalo, New York, on May 10-12, 1971*

*A Symposium in Continuing Medical Education
Sponsored by the Department of Pathology and
Western New York Health Data Network, Inc.*

Clinically Oriented Documentation of Laboratory Data

Edited by

E. R. Gabrieli

Department of Pathology
School of Medicine
State University of New York at Buffalo

and

Clinical Information Center
E. J. Meyer Memorial Hospital
Buffalo, New York

Academic Press
New York and London
1972

COPYRIGHT © 1972, BY ACADEMIC PRESS, INC.
ALL RIGHTS RESERVED
NO PART OF THIS BOOK MAY BE REPRODUCED IN ANY FORM,
BY PHOTOSTAT, MICROFILM, RETRIEVAL SYSTEM, OR ANY
OTHER MEANS, WITHOUT WRITTEN PERMISSION FROM
THE PUBLISHERS.

ACADEMIC PRESS, INC.
111 Fifth Avenue, New York, New York 10003

United Kingdom Edition published by
ACADEMIC PRESS, INC. (LONDON) LTD.
24/28 Oval Road, London NW1 7DD

LIBRARY OF CONGRESS CATALOG CARD NUMBER: 74-182658

PRINTED IN THE UNITED STATES OF AMERICA

CONTENTS

CONTRIBUTORS ix
PREFACE xiii

The University and Comprehensive Care in the Community. . . . 1
    Robert L. Ketter

The Need for Coordinated Laboratory Communication 5
    John B. Sheffer

Information Content of Laboratory Data 9
    E. R. Gabrieli

Conceptual Problems in the Interpretation of Multitest Surveys . . 39
    F. William Sunderman, Jr.

Geochemical Ecology and Interpretation of Laboratory Data . . . 69
    Howard C. Hopps

Normal Ranges of Values Derived from Large Scale
Multitest Surveys 83
    David C. Hohnadel

A Discussion of Some Estimation Problems
Encountered in Establishing Normal Values 117
    Lila Elveback

Evaluation of Clinical Laboratory Computers: Introduction . . . 139
    Marion J. Ball

Off-Line Batch Processing 145
    Paul R. Finley

The Clinical Lab-12 Laboratory Computer System:
Its Evolution and Its Operation 175
    Sidney A. Goldblatt

CONTENTS

Evaluation of Clinical Laboratory Systems:
Infotronics CL-II System 201
   L. E. Loveless

The B-D Spear Clinical Laboratory Automation
System in a Community Hospital Laboratory:
A Case Report 209
   William W. McLendon

An Approach to Automated Data Collection and
Processing (1130 Systems) 241
   David Seligson and Donald McKay

Use of the IBM 1800: University of Kentucky
Medical Center Hospital Laboratories 257
   Wellington B. Stewart

Evaluation of Clinical Laboratory Computors:
Diversified Numeric Applications 267
   Thomas O. Swallen

Meaning and Potential Content Information of Laboratory Studies:
Problems of Clinical Microbiology 281
   Erwin Neter

Coordinated Communication between Clinician and Laboratory
for Diagnosis and Therapy of Urinary Tract Infections 285
   Alf M. Tannenberg

Bedside Aspects of Microbiology 301
   Martin E. Plaut

Computer-Oriented Thinking in Hematology 311
   Ralph L. Engle, Jr. and Betty J. Flehinger

The Hematology Chart 327
   Michael A. Sullivan

Context Free Results and Their Meaning in Biochemistry 341
   S. Raymond Gambino

Problems of Regional Uniformity in Biochemistry 347
   Charles Bishop, Max E. Chilcote, and Gustavo Reynoso

CONTENTS

Problems in Standardization of Immunological
Laboratory Results 359
    H. Hugh Fudenberg

Explicit Documentation of Laboratory Data: Introduction . . . 391
    Gerald R. Cooper

Principles of Usefully Reporting Laboratory Data 393
    Edward L. Burns

The Problem and Progress of Explicit Documentation
of Laboratory Data for Communications 395
    Gerald R. Cooper

Documentation as a Concern of Professional Societies
and Individual Laboratory Directors 411
    Roy N. Barnett

Documentation Interest of the National Bureau of Standards
and Collaborating Groups for Communication of Laboratory
Results in Clinical Analysis 419
    Robert Schaffer

Documentation Concerns of State and Community
for Communication of Laboratory Results 425
    William Kaufmann

Practical Plans Suggested by Panel for Explicit Documentation
of Clinical Laboratory Data in Communications 447

Planning the Future 451
    R. S. Melville

Planning the Future: A Panel Discussion 457
    Roy N. Barnett, E. R. Gabrieli, Robert S. Melville,
    and Wellington B. Stewart

CONTRIBUTORS

Marion J. Ball, M. A., Assistant Director, Medical Computer Activity, Temple University School of Medicine, Philadelphia, Pennsylvania

Roy N. Barnett, M. D., Associate Clinical Professor of Pathology, Yale University School of Medicine, New Haven, Connecticut, Vice Chairman, Standards Committee, College of American Pathologists, and Director of Laboratories, Norwalk Hospital, Norwalk, Connecticut

Charles Bishop, Ph.D., Buffalo General Hospital, E. J. Meyer Memorial Hospital, and Roswell Park Memorial Institute, Buffalo, New York

Edward L. Burns, M.D., Clinical Professor of Pathology, Medical College of Ohio at Toledo, Toledo, Ohio

Max E. Chilcote, Ph.D., Buffalo General Hospital, E. J. Meyer Memorial Hospital, and Roswell Park Memorial Institute, Buffalo, New York

Gerald R. Cooper, M.D., Ph.D., Medical Director, Chief, Clinical Chemistry and Hematology Branch, Center for Disease Control, Department of Health, Education and Welfare, Atlanta, Georgia

Lila Elveback, Ph.D., Professor of Biostatistics, Section of Medical Statistics, Mayo Graduate School of Medicine, Rochester, Minnesota

Ralph L. Engle, Jr., M.D., Professor of Medicine, Chief, Division of Medical Systems and Computer Science, Department of Medicine, Cornell University Medical College, New York, New York

Paul R. Finley, M.D., Director of Clinical Laboratories, Fairview Hospital, Minneapolis, Minnesota

Betty J. Flehinger, Ph.D., Visiting Associate Professor of Biomathematics, Graduate School of Medical Sciences, Cornell University, Ithaca, New York, and Research Staff Member, I.B.M., Thomas J. Watson Research Center, Yorktown Heights, New York

CONTRIBUTORS

H. Hugh Fudenberg, M.D., Professor of Medicine, University of California School of Medicine, San Francisco, and Professor of Bacteriology and Immunology, University of California at Berkeley, Berkeley, California

E. R. Gabrieli, M.D., Clinical Associate Professor of Pathology, Department of Pathology, School of Medicine, State University of New York at Buffalo, and Director, Clinical Information Center, E. J. Meyer Memorial Hospital, Buffalo, New York

S. Raymond Gambino, M.D., Professor of Pathology, College of Physicians and Surgeons of Columbia University, New York, New York

Sidney A. Goldblatt, M.D., Director of Laboratories, Conemaugh Valley Hospital, Johnstown, Pennsylvania

David C. Hohnadel, Ph.D., Assistant Director of Clinical Chemistry, Department of Laboratory Medicine, University of Connecticut School of Medicine, Hartford, Connecticut

Howard C. Hopps, M.D., Curators' Professor of Pathology, University of Missouri School of Medicine, Columbia, Missouri

William Kaufmann, M.D., Division of Laboratories and Research, New York State Department of Health, Albany, New York

Robert L. Ketter, Ph.D., President, State University of New York at Buffalo, Buffalo, New York

L. E. Loveless, Ph.D., Clinical Laboratories, Inc., St. Louis, Missouri

Donald McKay, Director of Automation and Computation of the Department of Laboratory Medicine, Yale-New Haven Hospital, New Haven, Connecticut

William W. McLendon, M.D., Director of Laboratories, The Moses H. Cone Memorial Hospital, Greensboro, North Carolina

R. S. Melville, Ph.D., Chief, Biochemical Sciences Section, General Medical Sciences, National Institutes of Health, Bethesda, Maryland

Erwin Neter, M.D., Professor of Microbiology in Department of Pediatrics, School of Medicine, State University of New York at Buffalo, Buffalo, New York

CONTRIBUTORS

Martin E. Plaut, M.D., Chief, Infectious Disease Service and Assistant Professor of Medicine, School of Medicine, State University of New York at Buffalo, Buffalo, New York

Gustavo Reynoso, M.D., Buffalo General Hospital, E. J. Meyer Memorial Hospital, and Roswell Park Memorial Institute, Buffalo, New York

Robert Schaffer, Ph.D., Chief, Organic Chemistry Section, National Bureau of Standards, Washington, D. C.

David Seligson, M.D., Professor and Chairman, Division of Clinical Pathology, Yale University School of Medicine, New Haven, Connecticut

John B. Sheffer, M.D., Clinical Associate Professor of Pathology, State University of New York at Buffalo, Buffalo, New York

Wellington B. Stewart, M.D., Professor of Pathology, School of Medicine, University of Missouri, and Director, Medical Computer Center, Columbia, Missouri

Michael A. Sullivan, M.D., Clinical Assistant Professor of Medicine, School of Medicine, State University of New York at Buffalo, Buffalo, New York

F. William Sunderman, Jr., M.D., Professor and Chairman, Department of Laboratory Medicine, University of Connecticut School of Medicine, Hartford, Connecticut

Thomas O. Swallen, M.D., Pathologist, North Memorial Hospital, Minneapolis, Minnesota

Alf M. Tannenberg, M.D., Clinical Assistant Professor of Medicine, School of Medicine, State University of New York at Buffalo, Buffalo, New York

PREFACE

The primary task of laboratory medicine is to assist in clinical decisions concerning diagnosis, therapy, and prognosis. One limiting element in this process is the ability of the clinician to interpret the laboratory report and to fit it into the context of the clinical data.

Only a few years ago most clinicians were familiar enough with the methodology to utilize laboratory reports. But explosive progress of the last few decades has eroded this overlapping competence. Mushrooming of new tests and methods forced the clinician to limit his interest to the bedside meaning of the tests. This has created a communication barrier, a grave concern of laboratory medicine.

The rapidly growing gap separating the laboratory world from bedside medicine is a particularly serious problem in computerization of clinical medicine. To resolve this problem laboratory medicine must deliberately build communication channels to conserve the potential information content of laboratory data. It is a new task of laboratory medicine to provide the qualifying documentation, i.e., "the contexting," along with the finding. Instead of expecting that each clinician know all about the technology and meaning of each test, laboratory medicine should formulate the statistical meaning of the results obtained at the bench.

To improve communication between laboratory medicine and clinical practice we must encourage the uniform use of terms, we must develop explicit data presentation and purposeful background documentation. The traditional transmission of results in the form of raw primary data must be replaced by full documentation.

This growing problem of communication was the basis for organizing a conference to examine the factors involved in a deteriorating interdisciplinary information transfer and to seek solutions for the problems identified. The answers presented to meet this challenge are compiled in this book. The reader will readily detect the great difficulties in this vital area and the need for much further effort. My feeling is that this conference succeeded only in defining the problems. The solutions offered reflect the present state of the art. We hope this book will stimulate further work in the areas of clinical information transfer to find better solutions.

PREFACE

This conference which was held in Buffalo, New York, was organized by the Continuing Medical Education, School of Medicine, State University of New York at Buffalo.

E. R. Gabrieli

Clinically Oriented
Documentation
of
Laboratory Data

THE UNIVERSITY AND COMPREHENSIVE CARE IN THE COMMUNITY

Robert L. Ketter, Ph.D.

The development of comprehensive health care is a legitimate and vital concern to the University, and it is by no means an unfamiliar concern. Our Faculty of Health Sciences, and specifically our School of Medicine, has been active in fulfillment of its teaching, research, and service roles in this area for many years. This symposium, sponsored by the Department of Pathology and the Western New York Health Data Network, is but one example of that activity. We will continue to act within our institutional purposes and resources to provide the comprehensive health care to which our citizens are entitled.

In some instances, this activity is shaded by two qualities (and two problems) which are inherent in higher education: specialization and communication. Universities have been so successful at creating new knowledge that, consciously or unconsciously, they have bred faculties of super specialists and, as a result, sub-specialists. The time of the generalist who could be competent in one or more broad disciplines has passed.

Yet there has arisen an immense paradox in that while we have achieved great advances at the frontiers of knowledge, we simultaneously have made it more difficult to communicate with one another. Each speciality and sub-speciality has developed its own terminology and methodology to the point where all too often we have become effective only as academic inbreeders.

This is not a desirable situation, especially in a university, for communication is the key to the advancement of knowledge. We lock ourselves into the restrictions of our own specialties, failing ourselves to see--or to allow others to see--the inter-relationships and extensions of all we have learned. Ultimately, we are denying to ourselves the broadest fulfillment of the educational process.

Once universities became fully aware of this situation of self-reinforcing isolation, they acted to emphasize inter-disciplinary studies. Sometimes they acted naively, seeming to think that by putting two or more persons from two or more disciplines together, communication would occur. It often did not, for the problem of communication was more difficult than some persons anticipated. Yet there have been numerous instances in which progress has been made on similar problems in different disciplines. Generally, and broadly, speaking, medicine and engineering have been among the vanguard in this progress.

Your presence at this symposium indicates that you are concerned about these problems as they relate to communication between persons in laboratory and clinical practice. Your concern should be vital, for you know better than I of the difficulties in transforming laboratory data into meaningful information for the clinician to apply to individual cases.

Obviously, standardization of language is one necessary step toward overcoming the barriers of specialization; and this need will become even more acute in medicine as the whole area of information science becomes applied with increasing refinement in the clinic and in the laboratory.

I can speak from my own experience in engineering and tell you that it is not going to be an easy task to bring the clinical and laboratory practitioner into agreement on a mutual language which will facilitate their efforts to help each other--and ultimately to help the patient. Nevertheless, it can be done; and there is no more appropriate place to undertake such a task than in a university.

As I indicated earlier, this University is concerned with the development of a comprehensive health care system, and we are more aware than ever that this development will require a broad multi-and inter-disciplinary approach. Meaningful communication will be a key to success.

In conclusion, I would like to speak as a consumer-- a medical consumer. I am especially interested in being assured that the practitioner fully understands the results and implications of the laboratory tests, and that the data retrieved be in a form most readily used. This conference should help in this regard--and I wish you well in this pursuit.

THE NEED FOR COORDINATED LABORATORY COMMUNICATION

John B. Sheffer, M. D.

One of the most sobering things about life is the awareness that we are being trusted by someone. This is true whether we think of our families, friends, employees, or any other area of life. In clinical medicine, this trust becomes necessary between physicians and patients. In laboratory medicine the highest form of physician's trust must exist- that between pathologist and clinician.

I would say that success is the achievement of a high degree of worthiness for whatever trust people afford you. To be overtrusted is to be unworthy, it is dangerous, and spells unsuccess.

If I were to describe our hospital laboratory in glowing language, as a modern, fully automated and computerized facility that is all anyone could ask for, and at the same time show you ancient photos of it in its Model T stage, you would quickly decide that you could not trust me. In doing this, I am not trying to destroy your faith in the profession, but am only making the point that where there is faith, there must be an element of doubt. Pathologists must always be in doubt about themselves and what they are doing.

The extent to which we call upon machines to work for us is the measure of how much we trust machines. And the more we do this, the more we must be in doubt about machines and what they are doing.

My description of our laboratory was brief and precise but highly inaccurate. And I could probably repeat it again and again with brevity and precision. But we can only trust that which is accurate. Dr. Seligson (who will be speaking tomorrow) makes a very cogent point about the distinction between precision and accuracy.

My description of the laboratory can be made accurate by either changing the description or changing the laboratory.

In other words, if we want to be worthy of trust in a laboratory, we should not only sound like a laboratory but be one. In order to succeed at this, we have to doubt, out of which will come the indications of truth and error in what we say. Much of this Conference is directed toward these indications.

But, suppose we are satisfied that we have achieved a state of trustworthiness in regard to what information comes out of our lab. We always find we are at variance with other labs where our pathologist colleagues may be just as confident.

Some clinicians may accept lab data without doubting, across the board. Others who are more lab oriented will tend to make judgements according to which hospital or lab the data come from. Thus, one physician may in effect practice different kinds of medicine all in one day. To use some common hospital names, he may have a general hospital practice, a Presbyterian practice, a Mt. Sinai practice, a St. Mary's practice or a city hospital practice. All of us have heard such statements as "they always find a few urine red cells in that lab", or "their calciums are always a little on the high side". Most of us have experienced having a piece of tissue brought in by a surgeon which he snipped off of a tumor he removed at another hospital.

DOCUMENTATION OF LABORATORY DATA

This audience is well aware of the many reasons for this variation from laboratory to laboratory--such as differences in methodology and terminology. The benefit of doing something about it from the standpoint of the clinical dilemma just described is obvious. Hence, the need for coordinated laboratory communication.

As I understand the concept of this Conference, the need for coordinated laboratory communication must be partially met before there is any sense to the computer storage of laboratory data as a part of comprehensive medical information to be available in a massive health data network. Gross inaccuracies and language confusion do not disappear by going through the computer.

It has already been shown by concerted efforts that complete uniformity and standardization of results from a group of laboratories operated at different institutions is impossible to achieve.

But, as I understand computers (and I am neither a computerologist nor a computerologian) the first thing necessary in developing the software for such a network would be a uniform laboratory language, which in itself is a giant step in coordinating laboratory communications.

Secondly, and most fortunately, the computer itself can be used to correct data and thus minimize the error and maximize the truth in what comes out on data retrieval. In other words, within limits, one can put in error and get back truth.

If these benefits can really be achieved, the system is trustworthy, and is therefore, in my judgement, a success.

This Conference is in no sense the fulfillment of my own design. Dr. Gabrieli is to be congratulated for the achievement of bringing together this group for conference. I say hopefully, however, that the Conference is a fulfillment of my own desire. To explain, let me say that one reason for the variability of laboratory structure, procedure, equipment, language, etc., is that laboratory directors are caught in the cross-fire of conflicting interests, both professional and commercial, in a day when procedures and products are almost obsolete by the time they are marketed. Management recommendations and administrative prerogatives must be a part of every decision. And now comes an economic switch which requires trying to keep up with the progress which emerged in an expanding economy but now demands tailoring to a contracting economy. If this Conference had been held last year, or even a couple of months ago, the mood would have been different in the minds of most of us, especially those from New York State.

What I'm saying is that the onus of wise decision-making in lab direction is heavier upon the individual pathologist now than at any other time. And in the jungle that he finds himself, he realizes that he has to be very much on his own, and is therefore vulnerable.

Hence, I would desire that as a spin-off to the main theme of this Conference, those like myself who are being trusted for the truth in laboratory medicine, will through exposure to the presentations and informal remarks of these many worthy participants, develop a more complete insight into their jungle environment and become more trustworthy in fulfilling their own role in finding truth. If this happens, I would repeat what Mark Twain replied when asked for a comment after his first long look at the Atlantic Ocean from the Boardwalk-"It looks like a success".

INFORMATION CONTENT OF LABORATORY DATA

E. R. Gabrieli, M. D.

(1) OBJECTIVE OF LABORATORY MEDICINE

Laboratory medicine is perhaps one of the more "scientific" fields of clinical medicine. Its task is to provide "hard data", thus enhancing the objective component of the art of healing. While we may be justfiably proud of this influence of laboratory data upon bedside medicine, we must remain sensitive to the fact that laboratory medicine is only one set of data upon which clinical medicine may build its diagnosis, therapy and prognosis. In essence, laboratory medicine is one type of supporting service with the explicit purpose of assisting the physician in his decisions. This definition excludes laboratory research which directs its thrust toward new knowledge, better understanding of physiologic or pathologic processes. In the customary sense, laboratory medicine is subordinated to the predominant clinical goal of better understanding of a patient and his illness so as to make better clinical decisions.

If we accept this definition as the sole objective of laboratory medicine, we may pursue this line of reasoning by stating that the measure of success of laboratory medicine is the utilization of laboratory data in the process of forming clinical opinions. The most accurate laboratory reports, if not used at the bedside, should be branded as economically unjustified. Conversely, even a rather unsophisticated laboratory statement, when fully utilized, serves the mission. In this introductory paragraph, let I_p represent POTENTIAL information content, and I_a the actual use of the same datum in forming the clinical opinion; hypothetically, the ratio is always

$$\frac{I_a}{I_p} > 1$$

but the challenge is to keep this ratio as close to one as possible, i.e., to approach "maximal" clinical use of the reported laboratory data.

It is further proposed by the author of this discussion that the value of this ratio is presently declining, an alarming phenomenon reflecting a growing gap between laboratory and clinical medicine. The purpose of this discussion is to seek out some of the major factors which lead to this situation, and to propose, in general terms, corrective measures to reverse the present trend and thus to fulfill the mission of laboratory medicine, viz., to assist in clinical decision making.

(2) HISTORIC BACKGROUND

In order to appreciate the present conditions, we should first examine briefly the "case history" of medical sciences. This evolutionary process was interestingly sketched out by Sterling in 1913 in Great Britain: "Nearly all the medical schools had their origin as informal arrangements between the physicians and surgeons employed in the service of the hospitals, the hospitals themselves being charities either dependent on private endowments or subsisting by communal appeals for subscription. The schools sprang from the apprenticeship and pupilage systems. Men who had served their apprenticeship under an apothecary came to London to "walk the hospitals" and to learn from the members of the hospital staffs. At the same time, they would study anatomy at one of the various anatomy schools existing in London. The governors of the hospitals allowed the members of the staff to take pupils and later assisted them by building dissecting rooms in which the pupils could study anatomy under the supervision of the surgeons of the hospital. In this way, medical schools sprang up in connection with the hospitals "(Deryck Taverner: The Impending Medical Revolution; Hodder and Stoughton, London, 1968, p. 147.) Taverner continues: "During the nineteenth century, the revolution in science spread gradually toward medicine with the development of 'clinical science'. This led to methods for the detection of physical evidence of disease by means of physical examination and to the rise of instrumental and laboratory techniques to elicit information. The old "walking the hospital" slowly changed into a planned activity in which the student under supervision became active rather than passive and instruction merged with education."

The first decades of this twentieth century provided a unique climate for contribution to medical education by great clinician-teachers. In this period, there was a healthy balance between "clinical sciences" and personal experience, and the lectures of the brilliant Viennese professors attracted from remote parts of the world, the ambitious young clinicians. This golden era of personal prominence became gradually eroded by those who stressed evidence over convincing, disarming dialectics, experimental findings over speculative theories, cold figures of success rates over isolated heroic therapeutic reports. Specialization seemed to lead to well-founded excellence in complex areas. Medicine began to fragment.

In the 1930's the practicing clinician still carried out urine analysis or hemoglobin determination as a part of his routine physical examination, and there was no difference in data utilization whether the information was obtained with the stethoscope or by testing for hemoglobin level. As laboratory examinations became more complex and technically demanding, a gradual segregation took place, resulting on both sides in decrease of overlapping competence: clinicians knew less and less laboratory

technology, and laboratory scientists began to reduce
their own sphere of interest to the basic science aspects
of laboratory medicine. This created gaps, first a main
gap between the mainstream of clinical medicine and laboratory sciences. Later, further gaps developed within
the field of laboratory medicine, owing to evolving subunits such as chromosome studies, steroid chromotography or fluorescent antibody laboratories. Each of
these subunits moved toward autonomy in thinking since
each new unit wanted to be distinguished from the "routine"
wanted autonomy to evolve its own subgoals to be able to
support specific clinical interests, wanted autonomy in
data reporting, and wanted to use a technical jargon understandable only to the few "chosen" elite working in that
particular area. The curse of Babel is currently a major
threat to laboratory medicine, particularly with regard
to bedside use of reports.

(3) NEED FOR QUANTITATIVE COMMUNICATION

In order to conserve the potential information content
of a laboratory study, it is crucial to transmit the finding
in such a way that it facilitates its clinical use. Our
present challenge is to communicate with our clinical colleagues. In the past years, this communication was
kept up by the pathologist. In the hospital setting, he
conducted clinical pathological conferences, attended
various clinical meetings, consulted interesting clinical
cases, and acted as a liaison between the laboratory
bench and bedside medicine. When a new test was introduced, the normal values, as well as the expected
changes in various pathologic states, were presented to
the clinical staff, and after some time the new test gained
the confidence of the clinician who began to relate laboratory findings to the clinical course. This arrangement
was quite effective in the 1950's and even in the early
1960's. Laboratory medicine could communicate with
clinical medicine in a satisfactory manner, by means of
the scientific literature, formalized meetings, informal

hospital conferences, and personal communications with pathologists. This system began to deteriorate in an alarmingly rapid way during the last 5-6 years. As the distance between two people increases, in order to continue communication, they must shout, and as the distance grows, even shouting will not help. They must switch communication media. To extend their human capabilities, they must use the telephone or other electronic devices. It is proposed that laboratory medicine must recognize the present failure of communication and must seek new ways of communication to assure quantitative information transfer in the future.

Even the pathologist can no longer remain competent in all fields of laboratory medicine, and the clinician is less and less able to interpret the avalanche of laboratory data, solicited and unsolicited, which reach the clinical chart for coordination and interpretation. We must plan for new media. Let us examine, now, still in general terms, the basic rules of human communication, so that we can fully appreciate the complexity of unambiguous, quantitative information transfer, a major task of laboratory medicine of the 1970's. Then let us critically assess the alternatives available.

(4) WHAT IS INFORMATION?

This term must be examined very closely, since the raison d'être for laboratory medicine is to provide information for clinical medicine. Therefore it is crucial to clarify this matter. The definition of information is:
"THE MEANING ASSIGNED TO DATA BY KNOWN CONVENTION (Weik, M.H.: Standard Dictionary of Computers and Information Processing, Hayden Co., N.Y., 1969). Thus data are the marks, such as characters, signs, or terms, whereas the KNOWLEDGE assigned to them is the information. Therefore, information is a relative term describing the END-RESULT of an intellectual activity: the end-product of human data

processing. Data, per se, are lifeless. They become information through interaction with the receiver's mind, with the preexisting storage in the receiver's memory. The receiver places the incoming data into CONTEXT, a unique process creating a specific receiver-information. The very process of information generation is unique, since the added meaning, i.e., the context, is a variable contribution depending on the receiver. Some feel that this aspect of the information bars any scientifically accurate information transfer, since each recipient is a unique entity who will generate his own personal information. Except in case of the identical twins, with identical life experience, the same datum will elicit different meanings in different recipients. This variability is an interesting chapter in psychology and one variable in communication.

It is also important to recognize that receiving data but not processing them results in complete INFORMATION LOSS. Further, insufficient processing of the data received results in partial loss of information. This leads us to the concept of information content, a theoretical potential maximum of information generated by the "best" (ideal) receiver, in possession of all presently available knowledge. This generation of maximal information postulated by considering all current knowledge, is the ultimate objective of scientific communication. In the real world, there is inevitably a certain variable loss of information:

$$I_m > I_a > I_o$$

Where I_m is the maximal information potential;
I_a is the actual information generation by a receiver I_o is data inflow without subsequent processing. Unprocessed data make little impact. The recipient considers tham as "noise". Actually, unprocessed or unprocessable data often irritate some recipients as incomprehensible garble, while others respond with a mental

block, boredom or go to sleep if data influx continues to fail to elicit processing. This is a sort of self-defense, but it indicates that the message failed to "turn on" the receiver. A message is interesting if the receiver is prepared to grasp the meaning.

The interaction between incoming data and the elicited mental response is a vast, fascinating field in communication sciences and all our relationship with the outer world is actually information-dependent. Inadequate information leads to speculations, intuitive actions, wars and hostilities, racism and other prejudices. In contrast, scientific reasoning is an attempt to process data strictly in a rational manner.

The current status and future fate of laboratory medicine depends on the success of data transfer (communication) to the clinician. If the laboratory produces only data which elicit no processing by the clinician, the laboratory's effort has been wasted. We must understand the ground rules of communication: otherwise our cherished assay results will only pollute clinical communication, and laboratory medicine will become self-destructive. Unless we follow the ground rules of communication, laboratory medicine will be considered by the economically minded clinician as an expensive noise. If I_a I_o i.e., if the actual information generated approaches zero value, laboratory testing should be terminated.

(5) THE THREE LEVELS OF COMMUNICATION IN MEDICINE

Fundamentally communication is an attempt to transfer information from one human to another. This is one of the basic elements of our civilization and a major determinant of our personal destiny. Communication is successful if the thought of the sender is grasped by the recipient. There are some interesting mathematical models describing the effectiveness of communication. For the sake of orderly discussion, we can divide the process of communication into three levels - the fidelity level, the semantic level, and the effectiveness level. Since the future of laboratory medicine may depend on the success of our communication, we should examine these three levels more closely.

(a) FIDELITY LEVEL

Initially, Shannon advanced his history-making information theory as a strictly technical concept, stating: "Semantic aspects of communication are irrelevant to the engineering problem" (Shannon, Claude E. and Weaver, W.: The Mathematical Theory of Communication, University Press, 1949). [3] This classical concept distinguishes the following elements:

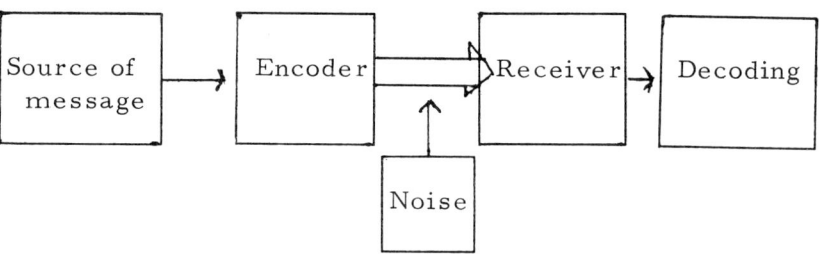

In the context of laboratory medicine,

SOURCE OF MESSAGE may be the output of the Autoanalyzer, the appearance of the immunoelectrophoretic plate or the growth on the sensitivity plate;

ENCODER is the technologist guided by the laboratory scientist, expressing the findings in qualitative, descriptive, or quantitative terms;

CHANNEL is the mechanical process of presenting the report on the appropriate chart, or the electronic process of computer terminals presenting the printout at the end point;

RECEIVER is the clinician using the message to form his clinical opinion;

DECODING is the mental process of generating the clinical information around the message, the aim of laboratory medicine.

Actually, the channle is the success-limiting area at the fidelity level. The engineering aspect of the information theory states that "It is possible to transmit information through a noisy channel at any rate less than the channel capacity with an arbitrarily samll probability of error". If we limit our thinking to the engineering aspects, information transfer can be measured in at least those different contexts (Wilson, I. G. and M. E. Wilson: <u>Information, Computers, and Systems Design</u>: J. Wiley, N. Y., 1966) [4] where each answers the <u>amount by what it does</u>:

(1) <u>Improbability</u> is the most popular aspect. Importantly, this does <u>not</u> refer to the semantic content of the message, only to its "expectedness". If a message contains no element of unexpectedness, the received message is fully predictable, hence there was no communication. If two alternatives, and only two alternatives, are present, and if the two alternatives are EQUIPROBABLE, we are dealing with the unit of information. The usual example is the light switch which may either be ON or OFF. If both switch positions are equally probable, i.e.

$$P_1 = P_2 \quad (1)$$

and if these two positions fully describe all possibilities,

i.e., $$P_1 + P_2 = 1.0 \quad (2)$$

then, $$P_1 = (\log_2).5 = 1.0$$

i.e., one binary digit or one BIT

Generally, INFORMATION = log (number of choices) (3)

The AMOUNT of information, or the "content of a message" is the number of bits contained in the message, again from an engineering aspect. The channel may have a capacity to transfer information. The ratio

$$\frac{\text{bits}}{\text{time}} = \text{information rate} \quad (4)$$

(2) Structural complexity is the expression of the number of LOGONS provided by an information source. From an engineering point of view if an instrument gives 10 per cent accuracy, it provides less information than another with 1% accuracy. It must be stressed again that this is at the fidelity level of communication, ignoring the semantic aspect, i.e., the significance of the gain in accuracy. The number of logons provided by a data source per unit of coordinate-space (e.g., cm, cm^2, cm^3, etc.) is referred to as logon capacity. For example, a microscope's logon capacity is the measure of resolving power in logons/cm. In the time domain, a channel whose band width permits X independent readings per second has a logon capacity of X.

(3) Metrical information supplies one element, a metron for a pattern. Each metrical unit is an elementary event unit of the sequence of physical or chemical events which the pattern represents. Then, the amount of metrical information is one logon, i.e., its metron content can be thought of as the number of elementary

events subsummed or "condensed" to form it. The number of logical elements in a group or pattern is termed its metrical information content.

The measure of success in information transfer at the TECHNICAL LEVEL is the level of fidelity the information reaches the receiver. The less distortion or noise occurs technically during the transmission process the better is the communication. There are ways to reinforce the fidelity of transmission by REDUNDANCY. Often used as an example that we write the amount of money on our check in two different ways, and in laboratory medicine we write behind the digital value, in parentheses, the number in English: 2 (two), if we want to avoid an error in transmission.

Although information theory was a technical approach to communication, its impact on our thinking is far greater. Once the technical aspects of information became defined, this provided tools for much deeper analysis of human thought transfer.

(b) SEMANTIC LEVEL OF COMMUNICATION

This aspect deserves our particular attention, since this is the central theme of this Conference. Semantic level of information transfer is affected by the effectiveness at the technical level, since a "noisy channel" will impair the semantic level of communication. However, this level is "meaning-oriented": HOW ACCURATELY IS THE MEANING OF THE MESSAGE CONVEYED? Wiener defined the semantic problem as a distinct aspect of communication "concerned with the identity, or satisfactory close approximation, in the interpretation of meaning by the receiver as compared with the intended meaning of the sender". (Norbert Wiener, The Human Use of Human Beings, Houghton Mifflin, Boston, 1950). [5] He deemphasized the two quantitative aspects of meaning using the two expressions "amount of information" and "amount of meaning" interchangeably. On the other hand, Ziff(P. Ziff: Semantic Analysis, Cornell University Press, Ithaca, New York, 1960),[6] proposed the following line of reasoning: Words(i.e., signs and terms) have meaning but not significance. Utterances, (phrases, sentences) have significance, but no meaning. However, the analysis of significance of a whole utterance cannot be completed without an analysis of the individual meaning of the words in the utterance. Ullman(S. Ullman: Words and Their Use: Philosophical Library, New York, 1951) [7], considers the word as the smallest unit with isolated specific, "content"; phrases and sentences express relations between the contents attached to the words. Here, meaning is defined as a reciprocal relationship between the name and the sense, which enables the one to call up the other. "Sense" is the thought or reference to an object or association which is represented by the words. A laboratory report is a word and it becomes a sentence in the clinical content.

WORD TYPES IN COMMUNICATION

In laboratory medicine we use two types of words:

(a) SIGNS
(b) TERMS

Signs are numerical expressions, the products of human intellect, and represent a highly "formalized language" for information transfer. Signs are due to successful adaptations of some matrix system, to sharpent the content information to be transferred. Blood pressure, serum albumin level, or urine output have been converted into numerical expressions. These signs are actually CONTEXT-FREE values, since they are independent of the content they temporarily represent. "The white cell count is 7,000" represents the message: in every cubic millimeter of blood there are 7,000 white cells . However, the number 7,000 contains no message. Further, such signs can be readily processed; regardless of their ad hoc content they can be added, subtracted correlated.

Once we succeed in applying a matrix to a natural phenomenon, we have "tamed the beast", we have created a closed system with finite elements. Time continuance has been forced into a closed system by expressing it in a matrix of days, seven days make a week, and 52 weeks make a year. A sender's message: "wait 5 minutes" is a formalized expression representing exactly his idea, and the receiver has little room for personal interpretation of "5 minutes". If we want to narrow it further, we may say, "wait 5.0 minutes" an instruction with greater precision. This formalized language permits all those complex processive manipulations with some signs that modern mathematics has developed, within such cloased systems, with a predetermined, finite number of components (e.g., 60 minutes in an hour). By closing a system the meaning becomes as sharply defined as scientifically possible.

Signs have denotation but no connotation. Therefore, the accuracy of idea transfer is not endangered by connotations.

Terms are the alternate means of information packaging. Evidently a term is a less accurate carrier of information, since neither its attributes nor its connotations are clearly defined. Connotations represent a particularly difficult area in communication. Attricutes and connotations in the mind of the sender govern the choice of the term, and the receiver's own set of attributes recalled by the term, and the prestored connotations will further modify the information generation process in the mind of the recipient. The attributes stored in the recipient's mind and the unknown quantity of connotations coloring the attricutes represent the product, the semantic information transfer, the net effect of the message presentation. In more explicit terms (a) the choice of the terms, (b) the attributes pictured by the recipient, and (c) the connotations further contributed by the recipient are all modifiers of the semantic level communication.

The content information of a term is definable by explicating a set of sub-terms, as attributes. When an area is truly conquered, science creates a closed system matrix. In such an area, still using terms instead of signs is a deliberate inaccuracy. The phrase "wait a little" immediately raises the question: "What is little to you?" Similarly, after extensive laboratory studies, the term: "liver involvement" is a deliberate inaccuracy.

Terms are the building block of our "natural language" communication, each term carrying its own often ill-defined content information. Many medical terms are shorthand symbols with a vast amount of attributes and often they are rich in connotation. The sender can accelerate his message verbalization by using higher terms, incorporating a number of ill-defined sub-terms and expecting the receiver to "decode" them. Instead of transmitting the more specific terms, one by one, the higher terms imply many of these primary terms. The rich content information in the "package" of a higher term results in a high rate of communication, but the risk of semantic inaccuracy is correspondingly high. For instance, the content information of the high term "alcoholic" depends on the criteria of the sender, and the communication effectiveness is further limited by the receiver. To the psychiatrist, the attributes of "alcoholism" include a deep seated neurosis, feeling of inadequacy, personality defects, conflicts, frustrations, etc., with clinical manifestations of deterioration of the intellect, impaired memory, deterioration of judgement and moral values, hallucinations, delirium, etc. The internist's "frame of reference" may be vitamin deficiency, palmar erythema, spiders, scanty hair, parotid swelling, hepatomegaly, etc. The biochemist recalls abnormal serum enzyme levels, and/or disturbed lipid metabolism, whereas the hematologist will bring up the changed morphology of erythrocytes and prolonged prothrombin time, leukopenia. Therefore, the set of attributes recalled by a particular receiver may be substantially different from the encoder's intention, a well studied defect in using terms for semantic level communication.

One obvious solution for this inaccuracy in medical communication would be the development of a dictionary with clear, unambiguous defintion of content information for each term used by clinical medicine. This idea is not new. Leibnitz proposed a closed system for terms, a "logical positivism" to achieve sharper, more accurate communication. For centuries, standardization of content information attached to terms is alternatingly either enthusiastically proposed and/or bitterly criticized. The opponents claim that any attempt to catalog attributes of a medical term would slam the door on progress. They argue that almost daily new attributes are added or removed; freezing of attributes would defy the dynamic aspects of medical sciences. Opponents say we should deliberately keep the meaning of our terms open, to encourage continual updating, since any dictionary would only reflect our current state of ignorance. Even otherwise rational scientists become unduly impatient when such standardization is proposed and they usually hasten to add that besides the perishable nature of such a dictionary of meanings, an emotional attachment to the dictionary would further obstruct progress. They predict that standardizers will not have the heart to discard their own brain child.

All these, and many related arguments, are well known to the taxonomists. This type of resistance is a natural expression of our fear of regimentation, perhaps directly traceable to the middle ages when scientific progress ran the risk of heresy. It is often claimed that constantly changing flexibility is essential for accurate expression of our thoughts. Actually, those sensitive to the inaccuracies of our language, the poets or writers, are the ones who particularly seek to expand the meaning of our trivial terms, and the generated literary expressions enrich our thinking by creating new associative pathways. However, if we consider the irreversible fragmentation of knowledge in medicine, and the grave danger of a separate jargon for each small area resulting in a labyrinth of communication barriers, we must realize that we must make a choice in communication between the freedom of the artist and the accuracy of the scientist.

QUANTITATIVE ASPECTS OF SEMANTIC COMMUNICATION

Probability theory supplied the basic vocabulary to the new field of communication theory. Probability theory is an attempt to predict the occurrence of an event X by placing P(X) between 0 and 1 inclusive. Before the data acquisition, the diagnosis of biliary obstruction is anywhere between 0 and 1. After examination, the diagnosis P(X) has a distinct level of uncertainty. If we bet on the correctness of our diagnosis, the payoff we would expect would be

$$\frac{1}{R(x)}$$ for each dollar wagered on X. If Px = 0.95, i.e., x is highly probable, the risk is small.

Communication theory expanded this thinking. Let us assume that a laboratory test y provides an amount of semantic information about the occurrence of an event x which is given by the formula

DOCUMENTATION OF LABORATORY DATA

$$l(X;y) = \log_2 \frac{P(X/y)}{Px}$$

where P(x/y) is the probability assigned to x <u>after y</u> has observed. The base of logarithm is 2, and therefore, the unit of information is the <u>bit,</u> the same unit used earlier at the fidelity level of commuication.

If the finding y doubles the probability of the diagnosis X, (that is, it halves the odds we would place on x_1) then y provides ONE BIT OF INFORMATION. This works of course in both directions. If finding y halves the probability of diagnosis X(that is, it doubles the odds we would place on X) then y provides <u>1 BIT</u> of information about X.

In order to make the diagnosis X <u>certain,</u> we must make P(X/y) = 1,

then y would provide $\log_2 \frac{1}{P(x)} = \log_2 P(X)$ bits of information about X.

Let us now assume that only two diagnoses are possible in a certain case, x_1 and x_2. Thus $P(x_1) + P(x_2) = 1$ and consequently

$$P(x_1) = 1 - P(x_2)$$

and this dichotomous situation can be fully characterized by the clinician's opinion: $P(x_1)$. Let us now suppose that the clinician considers x_1 highly probable and therefore $P(x_2)$ is very low, say 0.001; the "opinion" (Px_1) = 0.999, and the value of $P(x_2)$ is a measure of the clinician's doubt.

Let us now calculate the QUANTITY OF INFORMATION that is required to change the mind of the clinician with the strong clinical opinion on patient X with diagnosis

To strengthen an opinion requires less information than to weaken one. If the clinician closed his mind, i.e., $\varepsilon_1 = 0$, there is not chance for the laboratory to alter the value of $\varepsilon_1 = 0$.

C. THIRD LEVEL OF COMMUNICATION:

EFFECTIVENESS

The first or fidelity level of communication is <u>technical</u>: to reiterate the above, the objective is that the message should reach the receiver without distortion or noise. The second is the <u>semantic</u> level: <u>the meaning and significance</u> of the message should be conserved. The receiver should interpret the message the same way as the sender intended when formulating the message. The third level is focused on the <u>impact of the message upon the conduct of the receiver</u>. The primary purpose of a communication is to provide information which will affect the decision of the receiver. In terms of laboratory medicine, the justification of using laboratory procedures is to sharpen diagnostic, therapeutic, and/or prognostic decisions. Obviously, the first level alone, the technical aspects, can impair communication. Disturbance at the semantic level of the communication will injure the result even more. However, the third level, the effectiveness, is the real proof of the pudding.

Decision making is <u>automatic</u> at the lowest level. Therefore, this is the simplest form of behavior. As memory develops, learning by experience begins to replace automatic and intuitive decisions. The highest level of decisions, at least according to our present cultural belief, is the scientific decision, the product of rational thinking. The characteristic elements of scientific decisions are: (1) reason, (2) consistency, (3) logic, and (4) a predictive component. Consistency calls for similar decisions in similar situations. Recurring events call for optimized decisions. Clinical sciences face this task of recognizing patterns of similar cases. Further, a decision requires a decision situation (DS). There must be a "choice" : at least two alternatives must exist and the decision maker (DM) must be aware of the DS. "No decision" is also a type of decision: it is postponement of the decision.) Clinical medicine expresses this level of uncertainty as a "working diagnosis", or problem definition (Weed) [9]. Tentative reference points may function equally well. The important issue is to explicate the decision process. This is a merciless dissection of the elements entering the decision. The scientific decision requires rational processing of the pertinent information, to reach the "best" decision(s).

As the scientific component increases in medicine, at the expense of intuitive brilliance admired in the past, consistently "best" decisions gain respect and our value system keeps shifting. Diagnosis was the supreme goal of medicine when it reached its zenith as an art. The most rational therapy is the primary task of the new breed of the scientifically oriented generation of physicians, and diagnosis has become but an important tool for better communication. L. Weed is the pioneer of the purposeful logic in modern medicine.

In a DS, the DM needs all available PERTINENT DATA, for a rational decision making. Pertinent are those data which, if known prior to the decision, would alter the process of decision. This is the crucial area in the 1970's. As it will be discussed in quantitative terms below, the present volume of knowledge is so vast that our traditional memory-based decision system has reached a point of breakdown. Only a few decades ago, the typical clinical decision could be represented as follows:

x_1; i.e., to find the amount of information $l(X, y)$ attached to report y which would cause

$$P(x_1/y = 1 - P(x_1)$$

As Massey [8] demonstrated

$$l(X, y) = -\log_2 P(x_2)$$

which is rather small. If the clinician was willing to give a 1000 to 1 odds for the diagnosis of x_1, 10 <u>bits</u> of information from report y favoring the contrary opinion would suffice to state x_2 with equal confidence as x_1 before the report y. Even with a strong opinion of 1,000 to 1, as little as 20 bits of information would reverse the probability of the clinician.

It is equally interesting to calculate the amount of information needed to strengthen a clinical opinion. Suppose that the original opinion $P(x_1) = \varepsilon_1$, whereas finding y causes $P(x_1/y) = \varepsilon_2$ where ε_1 and ε_2 are both positive fractions. If ε_1 ε_2 the clinical opinion was stronger after the report y. Thus, the following equation describes the information content of y:

$$l(X, y) = 1.45 \,\varepsilon_1 + \varepsilon_2 \log_2 \frac{1}{\varepsilon_1}$$

This is a particularly important correlation: if $\varepsilon_1 = 0.001$ and $\varepsilon_2 = 0.000001$, it requires only one fourth the information as for the case $\varepsilon_1 = 0.000001$ and $\varepsilon_2 = 0.001$. As Massey states: "The point of this calculation is that the slide toward certainty is a very easy one indeed whereas the reverse trip is considerably more demanding" As a matter of fact, the above equation can be further expanded. Total conviction would be when $\varepsilon_1 = 0$. In this case, y must be an infinite amount of information, an impossible task. This was a handicap of laboratory medicine in the past, and it probably will be so in the future.

DOCUMENTATION OF LABORATORY DATA

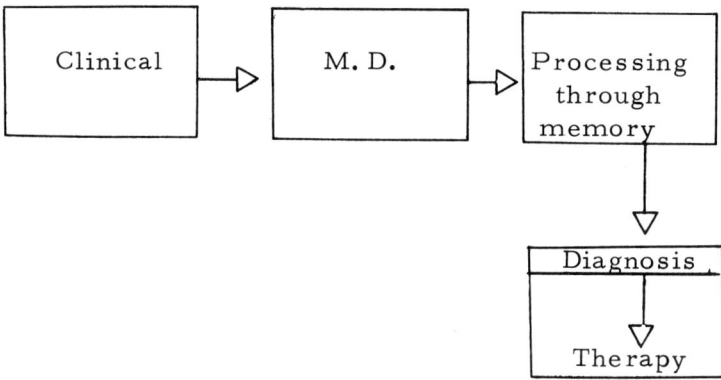

In this model, we assume that upon a comprehensive characterization of the clinical case, the physician can RECALL all pertinent data, stored in his memory with regard to the most likely diagnosis, most successful therapy and most probable prognosis.

FAILING HUMAN MEMORY

The pace of progress in clinical sciences during the last two to three decades is often quoted but rarely quantitated. The figure used mostly is 5 per cent compounded growth. Before accepting this figure, we have reviewed random areas of clinical medicine and have compared the number of specific terms available in 1930, 1950, and 1970. The first area explored was sickle cell anemia. Herrick reported in 1910 some "peculiar elongated and sickle shaped red corpuscles in a case of severe anemia" in the pages of Archives of Medicine, [20], as the first distinct idea recognizing sickle cell anemia. Differences in electrophoretic migrations of various hemoglobins became known only two decades ago. This was followed by an avalanche of new information. The dramatic fingerprinting provided the explanation for the differences in physical chemical behavior. The assembly errors were identified, and the related genetic data, geographic pathology and pertinent chrystallographic findings increased knowledge in this area. If we take 1930 as a reference point, our present volume of knowledge (1970) on normal and abnormal hemoglobin has increased about 18.2 times. Similar comparisons were made in opthalmology(retina), cardiology(subacute bacterial endocarditis), neurology (cord bladder), and hepatology(liver cirrhosis). The spread of knowledge increase was substantial, ranging from 11 to 20 times over the 1930 level. In possession of these data, let us examine the growth curve for the entire field of medicine using 5 per cent compounded growth as an apparently conservative figure. The following tabulation shows the consequences of this accelerating growth:

Year	Total valid clinical knowledge	Educational Pattern	Typical length of training	Amount of data to be memorized annually
1930	100*	Medical school	4 yrs.	25
1940	163	Informal specialcialization becomes formalized	4-6	27-41
1950	264	Residency becomes integrated with medical school training	5-10	26-53
1960	432	Super specialization proliferates, continuing education stressed	5-14	31-86
1970	703	Family practice concept. Group practice computers must become a media of data storage	8-15	47-88
1975	898	?	?	?

*The 1930 level is arbitrarily chosen as 100; subsequent values are calculated as 5% growth.

DOCUMENTATION OF LABORATORY DATA

This table has an important message for laboratory medicine. Only 10-15 years ago, for better utilization of laboratory data, the clinician needed more exposure to newer fields of laboratory medicine. If the physician fully comprehends the message of a BUN of 85mg% placing of this primary datum into the clinical content is assured. However, progress in all fields made a growing demand on the memory of the clinician. The above table should provide the inevitable conclusion. If we still insist on forcing <u>all</u> clinicians to understand and remember the meaning of every laboratory report, we ignore the maximum capability of human memory and recall.

MEANING VS. SIGNIFICANCE

A laboratory test can be treated as an isolated <u>TECHNICAL problem:</u> what is the "meaning" of a photometric reading of a color reaction, or of a precipitation in serologic system? Quality control aspects, comparison with a reference value, and similar considerations are well appreciated rules in "interpretating" the observations at the technical level.

At a higher level, a laboratory test also contains information at the <u>empirical level.</u> We have accumulated data on many apparently healthy people, so that we are quite familiar with the <u>usual</u> findings in the healthy population. Actually a great deal of information is available about the "normal values". As our precision and accuracy improve, we should keep up with it, to improve the definition of normal values.

A laboratory test is presented to the clinician in the form of a <u>primary datum,</u> e.g., "blood sugar of 127mg%" or "urine contained over 100,000 paracolon bacilli" or "the Monospot test was negative". This report of a primary datum is usually in a technical jargon, (e.g., level of CPK or A_2) stating exactly the observation at the bench.

The following diagram indicates the <u>expected logic,
the path or processing</u> of the laboratory data;

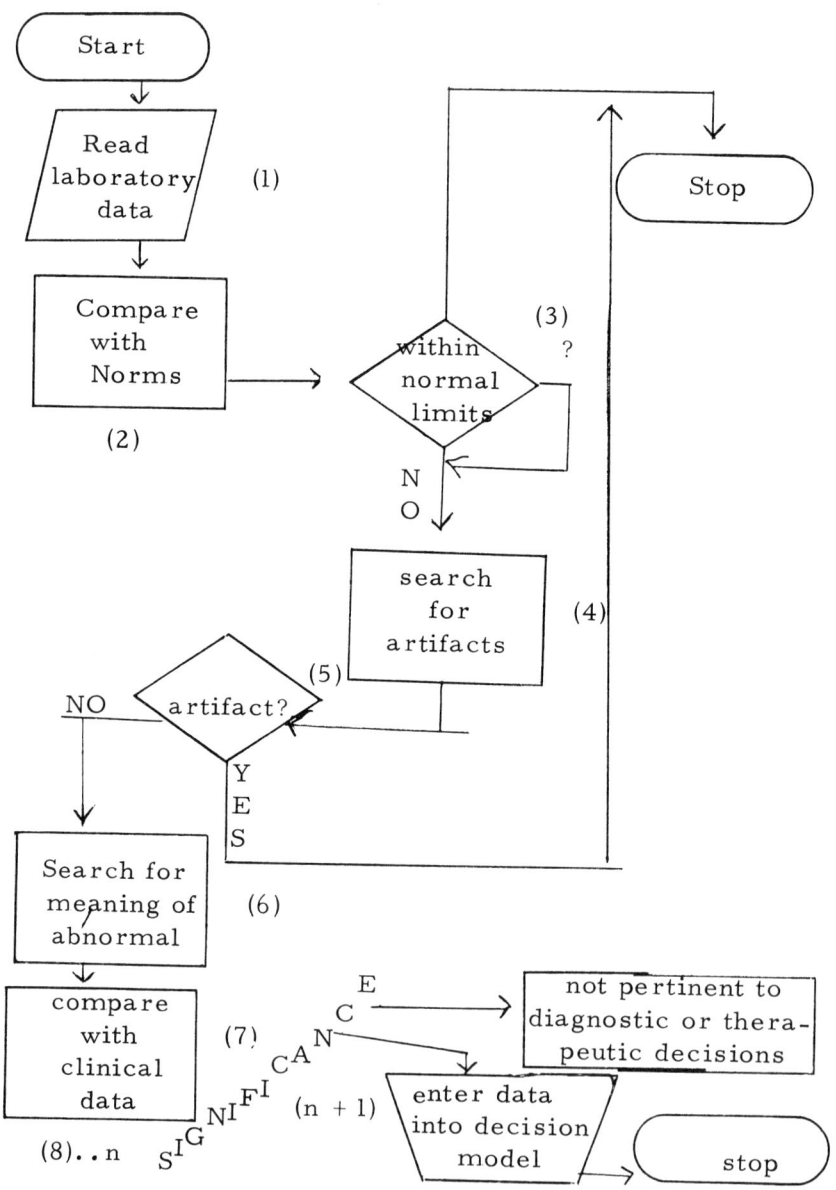

DOCUMENTATION OF LABORATORY DATA

In this grossly oversimplified processing model, there are steps traditionally done by the clinician, viz:

(1) comparison with norms

(2) finding possible reasons for abnormal results

(3) recall of association with diseases and conditions which are actually a matter of memorizing. The true clinical challenge is to fit the "meaning" of laboratory data into the clinical picture, to strengthen the evidence, to define the clinical significance with regard to a particular patient. The steps 2-3-4-5-6 on the above decision model represent past experience, i.e., how the aggregate of the findings in the past can be "packed" into a meaning. Accepting this logic, the challenge is to communicate to the clinician the finding + meaning, so that the interpretation is a comparison of the clinical data of a specific case with the general meaning of a test report. The true clinical task is to develop the significance of the laboratory finding, where significance is a single case-oriented interpretation.

The task of formulating the meaning of every laboratory test is rather large. If, however, we must make a choice between leaving it in the hands of all clinicians collectively, with the risk of a continued decline of utilization, or having the laboratory scientists develop the meaning and leaving the significance to the clinician, the choice is clear: I would propose that it should be the responsibility of laboratory medicine to accumulate a data base for each laboratory, and to create a regional data base, and a national data base, to determine the general meaning of each laboratory test. This meaning should consider:

(1) artifacts, e.g., high blood sugar due to I.V. therapy, prolonged prothrombin time due to anticoagulants, various drug effects, laboratory errors, etc.

(2) <u>non-signal</u> abnormal findings, e.g., high BUN following gastrectomy;

(3) local normal values in terms of age, sex, race, etc., and the technology of the laboratory;

(4) probabilistic correlations, reflecting clinical experience with the particular finding, including time, course, degree of clinical signs and symptoms, therapeutic, and prognostic meaning;

(5) <u>correlation with other laboratory data:</u> on same patient including sequential analysis and trend prediction, pattern recognition;

(6) <u>taxonomic interpretation</u>, perhaps the most sophisticated use of a laboratory's data, unthinkable until vast data banks become available. This development of the meaning must be preceded by a regional compatibility among laboratories, in order to pool experiences. This requires careful planning. Without meaningful coordination pooling of data would increase noise rather than sharpen the data.

CONCEPT OF A MAN-MACHINE SYSTEM

The outlined task of defining the meaning of various laboratory tests, and the change of meaning as the findings change, is a large-scale foundation of many formalized definitions. It calls for mass data handling including both laboratory and clinical data. This is feasible only if we can effectively exploit the capability of modern information technology. Computers can handle such a large task, if we can evolve a symbiosis between human thinking and computer technology. Theoretically, it should be possible to deposit the meaning of SGOT for "normal range", for mildly, moderately, and greatly increased SGOT, for mildly elevated SGOT with elevated SGPT or CPV, etc. It is quite feasible to deposit all these correlation rules so that the report can be in "context" containing the unprocessed observation as well as its "meaning". Thus, we shouldn't expect a clinician to recall the meaning of partial thromboplastin test or the meaning of IgG deficiency. We could create a computer-compatible language, to protect the potential context information of a laboratory assay. To achieve this, we must develop some standards in our communications so that the meaning can become uniformly acceptable.

If laboratory medicine is to remain a continuing expertise, the following information flow model should be realized:

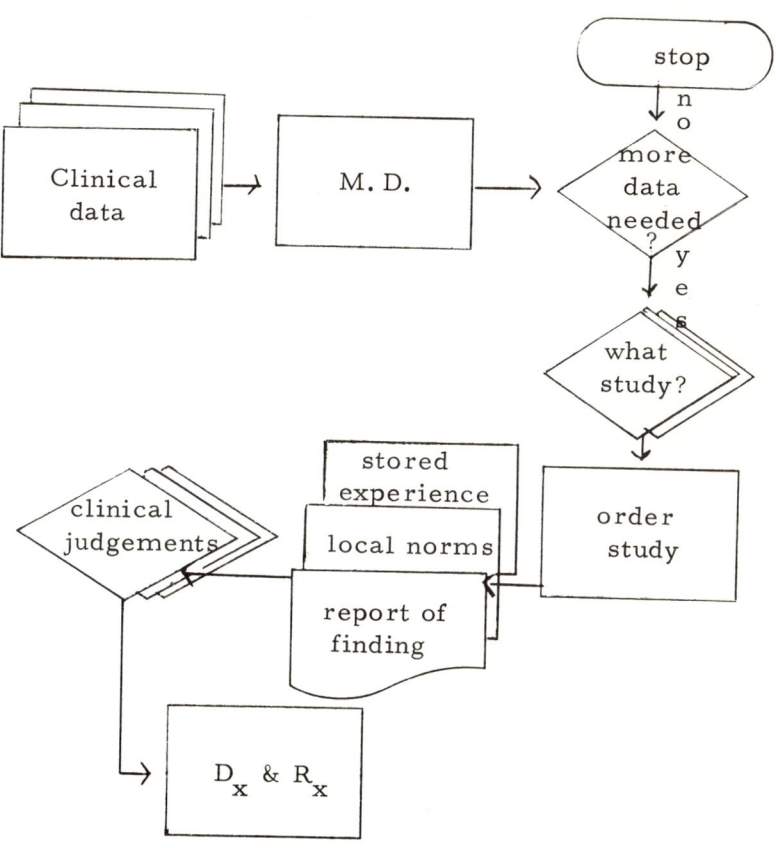

REFERENCE TERMS IN MEDICINE

Inherently, laboratory medicine assigns more uniform meaning to its technical terms, in contrast with clinical medicine. The difficulties in a man-machine system are much more serious in clinical medicine. The main reason for slow developments in medical computing is our inaccuracy in clinical communication. It is a most encouraging development of the last few months that the A. M. A. has formed a Steering Committee (and funded it) to develop a REFERENCE LANGUAGE for clinical medicine. This will be of great help to laboratory medicine. Clinical terms, e.g., problems, diagnoses, procedures will be defined for uniform usage, and algorithms will convert natural language terms into reference terms. All fields of medicine will be invited to participate in the development of a national reference language. The purpose of this Conference is in line with the evolving philosophy of the A. M. A.

The objective of this Conference is to focus on the various aspects of such a purposeful language for laboratory medicine. The content information must flow effectively between laboratory medicine and bedside use of the report, so that the clinician is no longer burdened with the vast number of data to be memorized for better use of laboratory reports.

At this stage, a single conference can't achieve much more than define the problem. The implementation of such a large task will require many experts, coordinated planning and effective use of information sciences. If, however, this effort is successful, a new dimension will open up for laboratory medicine.

References

1. The Impending Medical Revolution, Deryck Taverner, Hodder and Stoughton, London 1968, p. 147.
2. The Meaning Assigned to Data by Known Convention, Weik, M. H., Standard Dictionary of Computers and Information Processing, Hayden Col, N. Y., 1969.
3. The Mathematical Theory of Communication, Shannon, Claude E. and Weaver, W., University Press, 1949.
4. Information, Computers, and Systems Design, Wilson, I. G. and Wilson, M. E., J. Wiley, N. Y., 1966.
5. The Human Use of Human Beings, Wiener, Norbert, Houghton Mifflin, Boston, 1950.
6. Semantic Analysis, Ziff, P., Cornell University Press, Ithaca, New York, 1960.
7. Words and Their Use, Ullman, S., Philosophical Library, New York, 1951.
8. Information, Machines and Men, Massey, J. L., Philosophy and Cybernetics, Crosson, F. J. and Sayre, K. M., Simon & Schuster, New York 1967.
9. Medical Records, Medical Education and Patient Care, Weed, Lawrence L., M. D., C   -Western Reserve University.
10. Archives of Medicine, Herrick.

CONCEPTUAL PROBLEMS IN THE INTERPRETATION OF MULTITEST SURVEYS*

F. William Sunderman, Jr., M.D.

Recent editorials (5, 6, 34) and articles (1, 7, 12, 42, 44) indicate that clinicians are becoming aware of the limitations and pitfalls of multitest biochemical surveys which are being used either for the detection of disease in asymptomatic persons, or for the identification of unspected abnormalities in patients who are admitted to hospitals and clinics. There is growing concern that the diagnostic value of such multitest surveys might become obscured by the confusions, anxieties and misinterpretations which can ensue from a plethora of so-called "false-positive" results of analyses. The tenor of current skepticism regarding multitest surveys is illustrated by the following quotation from an editorial (34) by Dr. W. K. C. Morgan, Associate Professor of Medicine at West Virginia University School of Medicine: "Let us recognize that 'multiphasic screening' is just a euphemism for biochemical bingo..."

The dissatisfactions which are being expressed regarding multitest surveys are primarily engendered by fundamental conceptual problems, rather than by limitations in the analytical instrumentation or in the computer systems for storage and reporting of laboratory data. These conceptual problems include: first, the definition of "normal range of values;" second, the Bayesian relation-

*Supported by U.S. Atomic Energy Commission Grant No. AT(30-1)4051 and by a contract with the International Business Machine Corporation.

ship of so-called "false positive" results for a laboratory test to the incidence of the relevant disease in the tested population; and third, the binomial distribution of abnormal results in certain multitest surveys. These conceptual problems are interdependent, and they are profoundly influenced by clinical, epidemiological, technical, and economic factors. In this discussion, attention will be focused upon each of these topics, and an attempt will be made to formulate means of facilitating and enhancing the clinical interpretation of multitest surveys.

1. "Normal Ranges of Values"

As stated in an earlier paper from our laboratory (49): "the 'normal range' for a laboratory test is defined as an appropriate segment of the distribution curve of values obtained by measurements of a large group of healthy subjects." This definition involves at least two arbitrary assumptions: (a) criteria for identifying healthy subjects, and (b) criteria for establishing the appropriate segment of the frequency distribution curve. For practical purposes, healthy subjects may be described as individuals who are judged to be free from disease on the basis of medical history, physical examination, and laboratory tests other than the parameter which is being evaluated. For use in clinical diagnosis, the appropriate segment of the frequency distribution curve may be designated as that portion of the distribution curve of values in healthy subjects which provides the least overlap with values found in the relevant diseased populations. In other words, the appropriate segment is that portion of the distribution curve which yields minimal proportions of "false positive" and "false negative" results for the relevant diseases. Thus, by somewhat circuitous reasoning, the delineation of normal ranges of values is dependent upon the definition of disease, and upon the range of values which are observed in diseases (35, 46). The circuitous reasoning becomes apparent from consideration of Scadding's definition of disease (43): "A disease is the sum of the abnormal phenomena displayed by a group of living organisms in association with a specified characteristic or set of characteristics by which they differ from the norm for their species in such a way as to place them at a biological disadvantage."

Cognizance must be taken of numerous factors which can influence the normal ranges of values for laboratory tests (49). These variable factors include: (a) population sampling: e. g. age, sex, race, diet, drugs, and environment; (b) physiological state: e. g. diurnal, post-prandial, exertional, postural, menstrual, and seasonal variations; (c) sample collection: e. g. arterial, venous, or capillary blood; anticoagulants; random or 24-hour collection of urine; urine preservatives; (d) analytical method: e. g. accuracy, precision, and reliability of analysis; and finally, (e) the statistical methods which are employed for the delineation of normal ranges of values.

Some of the statistical techniques which have been employed for the derivation of normal ranges include: (a) mean $\pm$ multiples of the standard deviation, with log transformation if needed to approximate a Gaussian distribution (59); (b) "Pryce's convention", in which the mode of the frequency curve of patients' results is equated to the mean of the Gaussian distribution of results in healthy subjects (13, 39); (c) "Hoffman's convention", which is based upon the mean $\pm$ two standard deviations of patients' results, selected within truncation limits (27, 28, 29); (d) the non-parametric percentile limits technique, as described by Herrera (26); (e) the non-parametric tolerance interval technique, as described by Brunden, et al (10); and (f) the non-parametric critical values technique, based upon the intersection of distribution curves of normal and diseased populations, as described by Murphy and Abbey (36). The relative merits of these various statistical techniques have been evaluated in recent studies by Amador and Hsi (2), Elveback, et al (16, 17), Files, et al (18), Mainland (31, 32), O'Halloren, et al (38), Reed, et al (41), and Werner, et al (56, 57, 58). It is the concensus of these studies that the non-parametric percentiles method is the most generally applicable technique for delineation of normal ranges of values for clinical laboratory data. Numerous investigations (16, 17, 41, 49, 56, 57) have demonstrated that laboratory results obtained with healthy subjects frequently do not conform precisely to a Gaussian distribution, even after logarthmic or other transformations have been performed.

Figure 1 is a computer-generated frequency distribution graph for measurements of fasting serum glucose in 19,969 male employees of the IBM Corporation, aged 41 to 65 years. These measurements were performed by an automated ferricyanide reduction technique, and they constitute one component of the IBM Corporation's multiphasic examination program for employees (14). The mean and median glucose concentrations in this population were 102.4 and 101.6 mg/dl, respectively. At first inspection, it would appear that these measurements of serum glucose conform to a Gaussian distribution. However, as shown in Figure 2, there is deviation from the Gaussian distribution, as evidenced by non-linearity of these data when plotted in a probit graph. This computer-generated probit graph shows that the distribution of values for serum glucose is approximately Gaussian in the range from the 5th to 95th percentiles, (i.e. from 84 to 121 mg/dl), but that there is deviation from the Gaussian distribution, particularly at the upper extremity. The non-linearity is partially attributable to the incidence of diabetes mellitus in this population. The distribution curves for measurements of glucose and other constituents in serums from various cohorts of this population are presented by Dr. Hohnadel in another paper in this symposium. As he discusses in detail, an adaptation of the Herrera percentiles method (26) is currently being employed routinely in the Medical Data Center of the IBM Corporation for the delineation of normal ranges of values. Analytical results which fall beyond the central 95th percentiles in healthy sub-groups of the IBM population, categorized according to age and sex, are designated with one asterisk. Analytical results which exceed the central 99th percentiles in the healthy sub-groups of the population are designated with two asterisks. Thus, it has been possible to abandon the simplistic concept of a single "normal range."

Experience has shown that the percentiles technique for delineation of normal values has three principal disadvantages: (a) extraordinarily large samples are necessary in order to establish useful confidence limits for the 99th percentiles; (b) the percentiles are particularly sensitive to influence by so-called "outlier" values, and hence to the various stratagems which are employed to eliminate "outliers" from the healthy populations (21); and, (c) for certain biochemical tests (e.g. serum uric acid), reliance upon the central 95th or 99th percentiles results in misclassification of some individuals who are known to suffer from the relevant disease (e.g. gout). In the author's opinion, the percentiles method will not provide the ultimate solution to the delineation of normal ranges for multitest surveys. Instead, non-parametric techniques need to be employed for the establishment of "critical values."

An example of the use of critical values is given in Figure 3. This figure includes frequency distribution curves and statistical indices for urinary vanilmandelic acid excretion in 68 healthy adults, 1,489 hypertensive patients who did not harbor pheochromocytomas, and 22 hypertensive patients with pheochromocytomas which were confirmed histologically after surgical resection. The VMA analyses were performed by a method developed in our laboratory (48). The interrupted vertical line corresponds to the mid-point between the 95th percentile for healthy subjects (and hypertensive patients without pheochromocytoma) and the 5th percentile for pheochromocytoma patients. This critical value of 9.3 mg per day was selected as the upper limit of the normal range, inasmuch as it leads to positive results in all of the proven cases of pheochromocytoma, while producing less than 1% "false positive" results among the patients with hypertension from other causes.

Another example of the use of critical values is the establishment of limits for hemoglobin A_2 for the diagnosis of B-thalassemia. The measurements of hemoglobin A_2 were performed by a starch gel electrophoretic technique which was developed in our laboratory (47). In Figure 4 are shown frequency distributions and statistical indices for hemoglobin A_2 percentages in 25 healthy adults and in 25 patients with hemolytic anemia, in whom the diagnosis of B-thalassemia was based upon family history and clinical findings which included typical erythrocyte morphology. In this example, the sample sizes are too small to permit application of the percentiles technique. The critical value of 3.1% is the midpoint between the highest percentage of hemoglobin A_2 in the healthy subjects and the lowest percentage of hemoglobin A_2 in the thalassemic patients. The critical value of 3.1% was selected as the upper limit of the normal range for hemoglobin A_2, since it appears to be the best index for separating the healthy and relevant diseased populations. It should be obvious that the relatively clear-cut results obtained by use of the critical values technique to establish norms for measurements of VMA and hemoglobin A_2 illustrate exceptional rather than customary clinical situations. Most laboratory tests are less specific, and there is frequently serious overlap of values between the healthy and diseased populations. As will be discussed later, this problem may potentially be circumvented by use of multiple-test panels, in conjunction with multivariate discriminant analysis.

II. Applications of Bayes' Theorem

The second problem which will be considered is the

relationship of the proportion of so-called "false-positive" and "false negative" results for a laboratory test to the incidence of the relevant disease in the tested population (22, 23, 51, 54). This relationship is responsible for the fact that diagnostic tests which are performed upon unselected populations have greater probabilities of yielding "false positive" results than do the same tests when performed in the usual clinical situations. To illustrate this problem, let it be supposed that there is a new diagnostic test "Tx" for a specific disease "X", and that "X" disease can be diagnosed by independent criteria, so that it is possible to measure the true incidence of "X" disease in populations to be tested. In terminology derived from Vecchio's study (54), the "sensitivity" and "nonspecificity" of test "Tx" and the "incidence" of "X" disease can be expressed as follows:

$$\text{Sensitivity (Se)} = \frac{\text{persons with ''X'' disease giving positive test}}{\text{all persons with ''X'' disease in tested population}}$$

$$\text{Nonspecificity (Ns)} = \frac{\text{persons without ''X'' disease giving positive test}}{\text{all persons without ''X'' disease in tested population}}$$

$$\text{Incidence of ''X'' disease (In)} = \frac{\text{persons with ''X'' disease}}{\text{all persons in tested population}}$$

It should be emphasized that the indices of incidence and sensitivity are dependent upon precise delineation of the earliest stage in the pathogenesis of "X" disease which is to be considered as the threshold for clinical diagnosis.

Let it be postulated that when the test "Tx" is applied to persons who are known to have "X" disease, the

test is positive in 98% of cases and is negative in 2%,
(i.e. - the sensitivity is 0.98). Similarly, when the test
"Tx" is applied to persons who are known not to have "X"
disease, the test is negative in 95% of cases and is positive in 5%, (i.e. - the non-specificity is 0.05). Then,
let us consider 2 examples, related to the customary
clinical situation in the first instance, and related to
screening of asymptomatic subjects in the second instance. In example #1, that of ordinary medical practice,
a physician is unlikely to order the diagnostic test "Tx"
for "X" disease unless he seriously suspects the disease
to be present on the basis of medical history and physical
examination. Therefore, in the population which is actually tested, the incidence of "X" disease is, say, 20%.
In example #2, that of multiphasic screening, the diagnostic test is performed upon an unselected population in
which the incidence of "X" is, say, 2%. Let us now estimate for each of the two examples, the probabilities
that "X" disease is actually present when the test result
is positive. The examples are depicted diagrammatically
in Figure 5 by compartmental models derived from Hem's
report (24).

In example #1, illustrated at the top of Figure 5, the
incidence of "X" disease is 20%. The hatched areas "ad"
anc "cf" represent the two subgroups which give positive
results for test "Tx". It is apparent that the proportion
of "true positive" results (area "cf") is much greater
than that of "false positive" results (area "ad"), and any
positive result hence has a high probability (p = 0.83) of
being a true indication of the presence of "X" disease.
In example #2, illustrated at the bottom of Figure 5, the
incidence of "X" disease is 2%. It may be seen that the
proportion of "true positive" results (area "cf") is less
than that of "false positive" results (area "ad"), and any
positive result hence has a relatively low probability
(p = 0.29) of indicating the presence of "X" disease. Thus,
Figure 5 illustrates graphically why a diagnostic test
which is performed upon an unselected population has a

DOCUMENTATION OF LABORATORY DATA

greater probability of yielding "false positive" results than does the same test when performed in the usual clinical situation.

The following are Bayesian probability equations for the interpretation of diagnostic tests:

Probability of "X" disease when test "Tx" is positive =

$$= \frac{In \cdot Se}{(1 - In)Ns + In \cdot Se}$$

Probability that "X" disease is absent when test "Tx" is negative

$$= \frac{(1 - In)(1 - Ns)}{(1 - In)(1 - Ns) + (In)(1 - Se)}$$

The derivation of these equations has been considered in an earlier paper from our laboratory (51). If values are available for the approximate incidence (In) of disease "X", and for the sensitivity (Se) and nonspecificity (Ns) of test "Tx", these equations may be used to compute the probability that "X" disease is present when test "Tx" is positive, and the converse probability that "X" disease is absent when test "Tx" is negative. These equations have been used to compute Tables 1 and 2 for use in the clinical interpretation of laboratory data.

In Table 1 is given the probability that "X" disease is present when test "Tx" is positive, covering incidences of "X" disease ranging from 50% of the tested population to 1 in 10,000 persons; for sensitivity indices from 0.95 to 0.99, and for non-specificity indices from 0.05 to 0.001. The possible applications of Table 1 to the design implementation, and interpretation of multitest screening programs should be evident. For example, in screening for a condition, (e.g. sickle cell trait) with an incidence of 5% in a given population, if the diagnostic test has a

sensitivity index of 0.99 and a non-specificity index of
0.01, then positive result has 84% probability of being
associated with the condition. As another example, in
screening for a disease such as phenlketonuria with an
approximate incidence of 1 per 10,000 live births (30),
it the diagnostic test has a sensitivity of 0.99 and non-
specificity of 0.001, then a positive test has a 9% probability of being associated with the disease.

In Table 2 are listed the converse probabilities that
"X" disease is absent when test "Tx" is negative. It is
apparent that the probability of excluding a disease by a
negative test is usually much greater than the probability
of diagnosing a disease by a positive test. For instance,
a negative test for Australia antigen in the serum of a
potential blood donor is associated with a relatively high
probability of excluding viral hepatitis. Conversely, a
positive test for Australia antigen is associated with a
considerable lower probability that viral hepatitis is actually present. It should be emphasized that there may be
greater hazard to a patient if a disease is actually
present and is overlooked as a result of a "false negative"
test, than if the patient is erroneously suspected of suffering from a disease on the basis of a "false positive"
test.

The examples which have been discussed up to this
point have been concerned with diagnostic tests in which
the results are simply categorized as "positive" or "negative". Let us now consider the usual situation of a disease "Y" which is diagnosed by a test"Ty" which measures the concentration of a specific constituent in blood
or other biological fluid. In this situation, clinical interpretation of any test result depends upon its degree of
"positivity" or "negativity". For example a higher concentration of constituent "Ty" is associated with a higher
probability that disease "Y" is actually present. Inasmuch as test results in normal and diseased populations
frequently do not conform to the Gaussian distribution,

it was proposed in a previous paper from our laboratory (51) that computations of the diagnostic probability of any quantitative test result "R" may be accomplished by using probit transformations of the percentile distribution of values obtained in persons with and without "Y" disease. These values may be stored in a computer, or they may be read from the ordinate of a probit graph, such as illustrated in Figure 6. Provided that the approximate incidence of "Y" disease is known for the population being tested, the probability that a specific result "R" is indicative of the presence of "Y" disease can be computed by the use of the following equation:

If the Probability of result R in presence of "Y" disease $=P[R/Y]$ and the Probability of result R in absence of "Y" disease $= P[R/\bar{Y}]$ then, the Probability of "Y" disease, given any result R=

$$\frac{\ln \cdot P[R/Y]}{(-\ln)\ P[R/\bar{Y}] + \ln\ P[R/Y]}$$

This non-parametric technique has general applicability for the interpretation of clinical laboratory data. The example in Figure 6 illustrates an exceptionally good diagnostic test. Let us consider a test which is neither so sensitive nor specific, and in which the two probit curves are closer together. For example, let us suppose that a fasting serum glucose concentration of 150 mg/dl represents the 99th percentile of values in a healthy population and the 50th percentile of values in patients with untreated diabetes mellitus, and let us assume that the approximate incidence of diabetes mellitus in the tested population is 5%. Then it may be calculated that a fasting glucose concentration of 150 mg/dl has a 72% probability of indicating the presence of diabetes mellitus. In the long range development of computer-assisted multitest screening, the author proposes that the report of each quantitative analytical result should include the probability level that the result is indicative of the presence of the disease which is being sought.

III. Applications of the Binomial Theorem

The third fundamental problem in multitest surveys is that clinicians seldom appreciate the proportion of "abnormal" results which would be expected to occur by chance in healthy subjects, assuming that the results of the component tests are all independent variables (9, 45). In a previous paper from our laboratory (50), the binomial theorem was used to compute the theoretical distributions of "normal" and "abnormal" results which would be anticipated to occur in multitest profiles of completely healthy persons. Table 3 is based upon these computations.

To illustrate the use of Table 3, let it be supposed than an 18 test survey is performed upon 100 healthy subjects from the same population which had previously been sampled in order to establish the "normal ranges". It may be seen that, if all of the tests are independent variables, and if the central 95th percentile limits are taken as the "normal ranges" of the component tests, approximately 40 healthy subjects would be expected to have no abnormal result; 38 healthy subjects would be expected to have one result outside the defined normal limits and 17 healthy subjects would have two results outside the normal limits. On the other hand, if the 99th percentile limits are taken as the "normal ranges," approximately 84 healthy subjects would have no abnormal results, 15 healthy subjects would be expected to have one abnormal result, and one healthy subject would be expected to have two abnormal results.

Table 3 should be useful to clinicians who are attempting to interpret the results of multitest surveys. The clinical implications of such computations are discussed in the following quotation from a paper by Best and co-workers (9): "The question of a 'normal profile' is multiphasic screening has not been adequately aired from the probability point of view. Concern has been expressed because of the great number of 'normals' who show one or more 'abnormalities' in a screening examination. It is apparent from our computations and considerations that if sufficient tests are made in a truly normal population it will be the rare person who has a completely normal profile as here defined. This is a matter of mathematics, not public health!"

It should be emphasized that Table 3 involves the basic assumption that the results of the component tests in a multitest survey are all independent variables. The table should not be applied to measurements which are mutually dependent, (e.g. hemoglobin, hematocrit, and erythrocyte count).

IV. Approaches to the Interpretation of Multiple Laboratory Tests.

A. "Decision-Tree" Approach. The time-honored strategy for the diagnosis of diseases by laboratory tests is illustrated by Best's "decision-tree" schema for the diagnosis of hemolytic anemias (8) (Figure 7). As one climbs such a tree, advancing stepwise from the lower limbs to the higher limbs, the incidence of a specific disease becomes progressively enhanced in the population which is actually being tested. Thereby, as has been discussed, the proportion of "false positive" results becomes progressively reduced, until finally a diagnosis can be reached with practical certainty. It is upon such branching "decision-trees" that most of our schemas for clinical and laboratory diagnosis are currently based.

B. Multivariate Discriminant Analysis. A fundamentally different approach is the use of "batteries" of diagnostic tests for the detection of specific diseases. When it is necessary to use tests with relatively low specificity, or when diseases with low incidence are being sought, there is advantage in performing simultaneously multiple screening tests for each specific disease or group of diseases (25). The interpretation of such batteries may entail the use of multivariate discriminant analysis (4). The application of this technique to laboratory diagnosis was introduced by Zieve and co-workers in 1955 (60-63), but it was not widely adopted until computer programs for multivariate discriminant analysis recently became available. Within the past two years, the technique has been applied to the interpretation of serum lipid profiles (53), LDH is isoenzymes (20), urinary steroid patterns (55), diagnostic tests for hyperparathyroidism (3), and to batteries of liver function tests (11, 40).

In multivariate discriminant analysis, the computer is used to compute equations which are linear functions of multiple test values, so derived as to separate two or more groups of subjects in an optimal manner (15). Figure 8, from a recent study of liver function tests by Ramsoe and associates (40), illustrates the application of multivariate discriminant analysis to the differentiation of healthy control subjects from patients with hepatic cirrhosis. Section I of Figure 8 shows the separation of the cirrhotic and control subjects on the basis of a single test (i.e. hepatic transport maximum for BSP). In this case, the discriminant equation consists of "Z" (the discriminator) equal to a factor, times the test result, plus a constant. Section II of Figure 8 shows the separation of the cirrhotic and control subjects on the basis of two tests (i.e. (a) hepatic transport maximum for BSP, and (b) serum gamma globulin concentration after log transformation). In this case, the discriminant equation consists of three terms. The discriminator "Z" is equal to a factor times the result of test (a) BSP-Tmax), plus a factor times the result of test (b) (log gamma globulin), plus a constant. Section III of Figure 8 shows the separation of the groups of cirrhotic and control subjects when nine tests were used. In this case, the discriminant equation consists of ten terms (i.e. nine factors times test results, plus a constant). It may be noted that the discrimination achieved by use of nine tests was not significantly greater than that obtained with the two tests.

Figure 9, also taken from the study by Ramsoe and associates (40), shows how the discriminator "Z" can be used to compute the "critical value" or "discrimination point" for separation of two groups, such as cirrhotic patients and control subjects, talking into account the relative proportions of the two groups in the population being tested. When the proportion of control subjects (Group A) is the same as that of cirrhotic subjects (Group B), the a priori probability that an observation belong to either group is 0.5, and the "discrimination point" is obtained at $Z=0$. On the other hand, when the cirrhotic subjects comprise only 10% of the population being tested, the a priori probability that an observation belongs to the cirrhotic group is 0.1, and the "discrimination point" is obtained at $Z=2$.

There are major limitations, restrictions and objections to the use of multivariate discriminant analysis in its present form for the interpretation of results of multitest batteries. In addition to the basic assumptions of parametric distribution curves for each of the variables being tested, it is assumed (a) that the tests are all lineraly related, and (b) that they have identical covariance matrices. These are gross oversimplifications of the problems as they occur with clinical laboratory data. In order to circumvent these obstacles, it will be necessary to utilize non-parametric strategies for multivariate discriminant analysis. Preliminary applications of non-parametric techniques for multivariate discrimination in analyses of medical data have been discussed by Fix and Hodge (19), Nilsson (37), and Miller (33).

C. Multidimensional Spatial Analysis. Thompson

and Woodbury (52) have recently described a computer technique for the representation of results of multiple laboratory and clinical measurements as points in a multidimensional space. This modified approach to cluster analysis differs markedly from the classical methodology of multivariate discriminant analysis, and it provides a technique for quantitating similarity and dissimilarity between groups of individuals on the basis of multiple interrelated parameters. The multidimensional spatial analysis method of Thompson and Woodbury (52) may potentially be applicable to the interpretation of results of multitest surveys.

Summary and Conclusions

In summary, attention has been focused upon conceptual problems which are involved in (a) the delineation of "normal ranges of values" for laboratory tests: (b) the Bayesian relationship of the incidence of disease to the proportion of "false positive" test results: and (c) the binomial distribution of results in multitest surveys. Consideration has been directed to logical approaches to the interpretation of multiple laboratory tests. It has been concluded that (a) the non-parametric "critical values" technique is the most reliable method for demarcation of normal ranges of values for the interpretation of results of laboratory tests; (b) that laboratory reports should ultimately include the diagnostic probabilities that a given test result is indicative of the presence of the disease under suspicion; and (c) that the use of batteries of interrelated tests for diagnosis of specific diseases may hold great promise, provided appropriate strategies can be evolved for the application of multivariate discriminant analysis or multidimensional spatial analysis.

References

1. Ahlvin, R. C., Biochemical screening- a critique. New Engl. J. Med 281:1084-1086 (1971)
2. Amador, E. and Hsi, B. P., Indirect methods for estimating the normal range. Amer. J. Clin. Path. 52:538:-546 (1969)
3. Amenta, J. S. and Harkins, M. L., The use of discriminant functions in laboratory medicine: Evaluation of phosphate clearance studies in the diagnosis of hyperparathyroidism. Amer. J. Clin. Path. 55:330-341 (1971)
4. Anderson, J. A. and Boyle, J. A., Computer diagnosis: statistical aspects. Brit. Med. Bull. 24:230-235 (1968)
5. Anon: (Editorial), Routine chemical screening. California Med. 108:476-477 (1968)
6. Anon: (Editorial), Internists see holes in mass screening. Medical World News, May 30, 1969, pp 15-17
7. Barnett, R. N., Civin, W. H., and Schoen, J., Multiphasic screening by laboratory tests - An overview of the problem. Amer. J. Clin. Path. 54:483-492 (1970)
8. Best, W. R., Differential diagnosis of hemolytic anemias. In: "Hemoglobin, Its Precursors and Metabolites," pp 307-317. Lippincott Co., (Sunderman, F. W. and Sunderman, F. W. Jr., Eds), Philadelphia, (1964)
9. Best, W. R., Mason, C. C., Barron, S. S., and Sheperd, H. G., Automated twelve-channel serum screening. I. What is normal? Med. Clin. N. Amer. 53:175-188 (1969)
10. Brunden, M. N., Clark, J. J., and Sutter, M. L., A general method of determining normal ranges applied to blood values for dogs. Amer. J. Clin. Path. 53:332-339 (1970)

11. Burbank, F., A computer diagnostic system for the diagnosis of prolonged undifferentiating liver disease. Amer. J. Med. 46:401-415 (1969)
12. Cochrane, A. L. and Holland, W. W., Validation of screening procedures. Brit. Med. Bull. 27:3-8 (1971)
13. Cook, M. G., Levell, M. J., and Payne, R. B., A method for deriving normal ranges from laboratory specimens applied to uric acid in males. J. Clin. Path. 23:778-780 (1970)
14. Duffy, J. C. and Moonan, K. F., Applying the computer to an international health screening program. Indust. Med. 39:35-39 (1970)
15. Ellund, G., (Editorial), Discriminant analysis. Scand. J. Clin. Lab. Invest. 26:305-306 (1970)
16. Elveback, L. R., Guillier, C. L., and Keating, F. R., Jr., Health, normality and the ghost of Gauss. J. Amer. Med. Assn. 211:69-75 (1970)
17. Elveback, L. R. and Taylor, W. F., Statistical methods of estimating percentiles. Ann. N.Y. Acad. Sci. 161:538-548 (1969)
18. Files, J. B., Van Peenen, H. J., and Lindberg, D. A. B., Use of "normal range" in multiphasic testing. J. Amer. Med. Assn. 205:684-688
19. Fix, E. and Hodges, J. L., Jr., Discriminatory analysis; nonparametric discrimination: consistency properties. University of California Report 4 on Project 21-49-004, USAF School of Aviation Medicine, Randolph Field, Texas (1951). (This document may be obtained as Report AT1-110633 from the Defense Document Center for Scientific and Technical Information, Cameron Station, Alexandria, Va.)
20. Glick, J. H., Jr., Serum lactate dehydrogenase isoenzyme and total lactate dehydrogenase values in health and disease, and clinical evaluation of these tests by means of discriminant analysis. Amer. J. Clin. Path. 52:320-328 (1969)
21. Grubbs, F. E., Procedures for detecting outlying observations in samples. Technometrics 11:1-21 (1969)
22. Hall, G. D., The clinical application of Bayes'

theorem. Lancet 2:555-557 (1967)
23. Hall, G. H., Laboratory data and diagnosis. Lancet 1:531 (1969)
24. Hems, G., Laboratory data and diagnosis. Lancet 1:267 (1969)
25. Henry, J. B. and Arras, M. S., Organ panels - an innovation in health care delivery. Texas Med. 66: 66-76 (1970)
26. Herrera, L., The precision of percentiles in establishing normal limits in medicine. J. Lab. Clin. Med. 52:34-43 (1958)
27. Hoffman, R. J., Statistics in the practice of medicine. J. Amer. Med. Assn. 185:864-873 (1963)
28. Hoffman, R. G., Establishing normal ranges. Clin. Chem. 17:456-457 (1971)
29. Hoffman, R. G. and Waid, M. E., A new scale of normal values for physicians. G. P. 30:112-121 (1964)
30. Hsia, D. Y.-Y., A critical evaluation of PKU screening. Hosp. Practice pp 101-112, April 1971
31. Mainland, D., Normal values in medicine. Ann. N. Y. Acad. Sci. 161:527-537 (1969)
32. Mainland, D., (Editorial) Remarks on clinical "norms". Clin. Chem 17:267-274 (1971)
33. Miller, R. G., Multivariate statistical techniques for medical data analysis. Ann. N. Y. Acad. Sci. 161:626-631 (1969)
34. Morgan, W. K. C., (Editorial) The annual physical: factitious farce or futile fetish? Medical Tribune, p 12, March 17, 1971
35. Murphy, E. A., A scientific viewpoint on normality. Perspectives Biol. Med. 9:333-348 (1965-66)
36. Murphy, E. A. and Abbey, H., The normal range - a common misuse. J. Chronic Dis. 20: 79-88 (1967)
37. Nilsson, N. J. Survey of pattern recognition. Ann. N. Y. Acad. Sci. 161:380-401 (1969)
38. O'Halloran, M. W., Studley-Ruxton, J., and Wellby, M., A comparison of conventionally derived normal ranges with those obtained from patients' results. Clin. Chim. Acta 27:35-46 (1970)

39. Pryce, J. D., Level of haemoglobin in whole blood and red blood cells, and proposed convention for defining normality. Lancet 2:333-335 (1960)
40. Ramsoe, K., Tygstrup, N., and Winkel, P., The redundancy of liver tests in the diagnosis of cirrhosis estimated by multivariate statistics. Scand. J. Clin. Lab. Invest. 26:307-312 (1970)
41. Reed, A. H., Henry, R. J., and Mason, W. B., Influence of statistical method used on the resulting estimate of normal range. Clin. Chem 17:275-284 (1971)
42. Reinke, W. A., Decisions about screening programs Can we develop a rational basis? Arch. Environ. Health 19:403-411) (1969)
43. Scadding, J. G., Diagnosis: The clinician and the computer. Lancet 2:877-882 (1967)
44. Schoen, I., Clinical chemistry: A retrospective look at routine screening. California Med. 108:430-436 (1968)
45. Schoen, I. and Brooks, S. H., Judgement based on 95% confidence limits: A statistical dilemma involving multitest screening and proficiency testing of multiple specimens. Amer. J. Clin. Path. 53:190-193 (1970)
46. Simonson, E., The concept and definition of normality. Ann. N. Y. Acad. Sci. 134:541-558 (1966)
47. Sunderman, F. W., Jr., Procedure for quantitation of hemoglobins separated by means of starch gel electrophoresis. Amer. J. Clin. Path. 40:227-238 (1963)
48. Sunderman, F. W., Jr., Measurements of vanilmandelic acid for the diagnosis of pheochromocytoma and nueroblastoma. Amer. J. Clin. Path. 42:481-497 (1964)
49. Sunderman, F. W., Jr., Computer applications in laboratory medicine: The delineation of normal values. Ann. N. Y. Acad. Sci. 161:549:571 (1969)
50. Sunderman, F. W., Jr., Expected distributions of normal and abnormal results in multitest surveys of healthy subjects. Amer. J. Clin. Path. 53:288-291 (1970)

51. Sunderman, F.W., Jr. and Van Soestbergen, A.A. Probability computations for clinical interpretations of screening tests. Amer. J. Clin. Path. 55:105-111 (1971)
52. Thompson, H.K., Jr. and Woodbury, M.A., Clinical data representation in multidimensional space. Computers Biomed. Res. 3:58-73 (1970)
53. Truett, J., Cornfield, J., and Kannel, W., A multivariate analysis of the risk of coronary heart disease in Framingham. J. Chron. Dis. 20:511-524 (1967)
54. Vecchio, T.J., Predictive value of a single diagnostic test in unselected populations. New Engl. J. Med. 274:1171-1173 (1966)
55. Weiner, J.M. and Marmorston, J., Statistical techniques of difference. Ann. N.Y. Acad. Sci. 161: 641-668 (1969)
56. Werner, M., Heilbron, D.C., Maruhn, D., and Atoba, M., Patterns of urinary enzyme excretion in healthy subjects. Clin. Chim. Acta 29:437-449 (1970)
57. Werner, M., Tolls, R.E., Hultin, J.V., and Mellecker, J., Influence of sex and age on the normal range of eleven serum constituents. Z. klin. Chem. u. klin. Biochem. 8:105-115 (1970)
58. Werner, M., Young, D.S., Heilbron, D.C., and Dixon, W.J., Normal ranges and Gaussian distribution. Clin. Chem. 16:809 (1970)
59. Zender, R., Valeurs normales on valeurs frequentes. Ann. Biol. Clin. Chem. 16:809 (1970)
60. Zieve, L., On interpreting variations in laboratory tests as illustrated by an analysis of liver function tests. Postgrad. Med. 35:A46-A56 (1964)
61. Zieve, L. and Hill, E., An evaluation of factors influencing the discriminative effectiveness of liver function tests. I. The utilization of multiple measurements in medicine. Gastroenterol. 28:759-765 (1955)
62. Zieve, L. and Hill, E., An evaluation of factors influencing the discriminative effectiveness of liver function tests. II. Normal limits of eleven representative hepatic tests. Gastroenterol. 28:766-784 (1955)

63. Zieve, L. and Hill, E., An evaluation of factors influencing the discriminative effectiveness of liver function tests. III Relative effectiveness of hepatic tests in cirrhosis. Gastroenterol. 28:785-802 (1955)

Table I

Probability That Disease "X" Is Present When Test "Tx" Is Positive

Incidence of Disease	Sensitivity = 0.95 Non-specificity =			Sensitivity = 0.99 Non-specificity =		
	0.050	0.010	0.001	0.050	0.010	0.001
0.5000	0.950	0.990	0.999	0.952	0.990	0.999
0.1000	0.679	0.913	0.991	0.688	0.917	0.991
0.0500	0.500	0.833	0.980	0.510	0.839	0.981
0.0100	0.161	0.490	0.906	0.167	0.500	0.909
0.0050	0.087	0.323	0.827	0.090	0.332	0.833
0.0010	0.019	0.087	0.487	0.019	0.090	0.498
0.0005	0.009	0.045	0.322	0.010	0.047	0.331
0.0001	0.002	0.009	0.087	0.002	0.010	0.090

Table 2

Probability That Disease "X" Is Absent When Test "Tx" Is Negative

Incidence of Disease	Sensitivity = 0.95 Non-specificity =			Sensitivity = 0.99 Non-specificity =		
	0.050	0.010	0.001	0.050	0.010	0.001
0.5000	0.950	0.952	0.952	0.990	0.990	0.990
0.2000	0.987	0.988	0.988	0.997	0.997	0.998
0.1000	0.994	0.994	0.994	0.999	0.999	0.999
0.0500	0.997	0.997	0.997	idem		
0.0200	0.999	0.999	0.999			
0.0100	idem					

Table 3

Distributions of Normal and Abnormal Results in

Multitest Profiles of Healthy Subjects

Number of Tests in Each Multitest Profile	Number of Abnormal Results in Each Multitest Profile								
	0	1	2	3	4	0	1	2	3
	(95th Percentile Limits)					(99th Percentile Limits)			
4	81.4	17.1	1.4	--	--	96.1	3.9	0.1	--
6	73.5	23.2	3.0	0.2	--	94.1	5.7	0.1	--
8	66.2	27.9	5.1	0.5	--	92.3	7.5	0.3	--
10	59.9	31.5	7.5	1.0	0.1	90.4	9.1	0.4	--
12	54.0	34.1	9.9	1.7	0.2	88.6	10.7	0.6	--
14	48.8	35.9	12.3	2.6	0.4	86.9	12.3	0.8	--
16	44.0	37.1	14.6	3.6	0.6	85.1	13.8	1.0	--
18	39.7	37.6	16.8	4.7	0.9	83.5	15.2	1.3	0.1
20	35.8	37.7	18.9	6.0	1.3	81.8	16.5	1.6	0.1
22	32.4	37.5	20.7	7.3	1.8	80.2	17.8	1.9	0.1

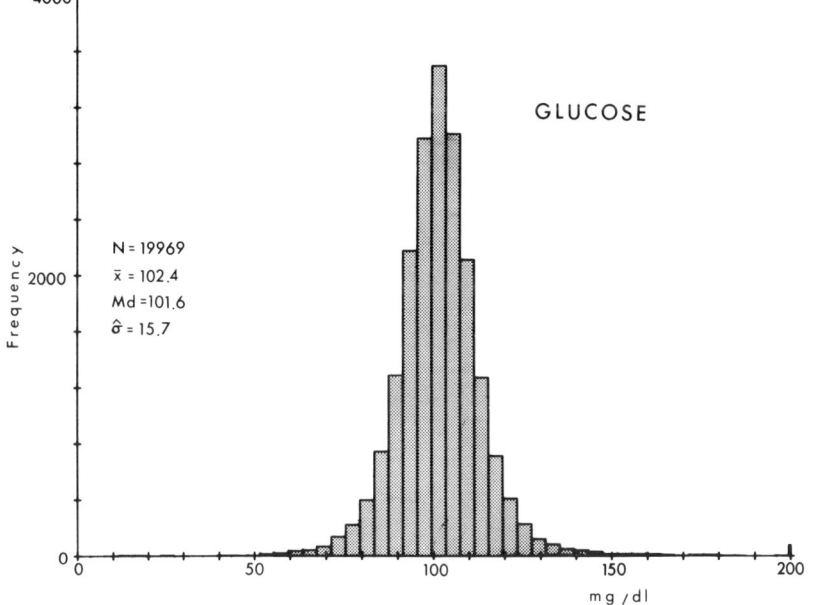

Figure 1: Frequency distribution graph of concentrations of fasting serum glucose in 19,969 male employees of the IBM Corporation, age 41 to 65 years.

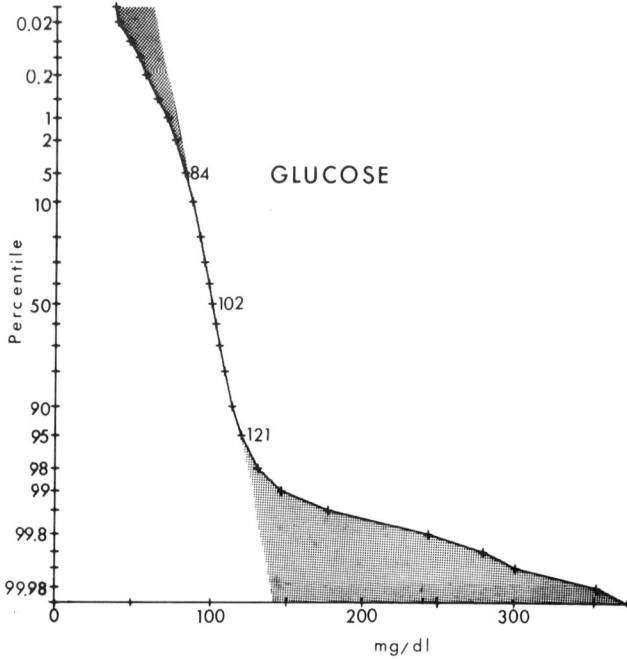

Figure 2: Probit graph of concentrations of fasting serum glucose in 19,969 male employees of the IBM Corporation, age 41 to 65 years.

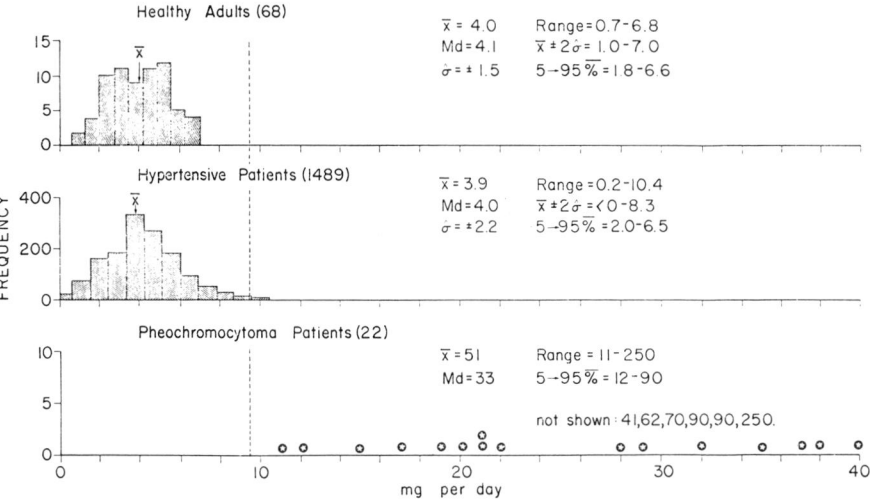

Figure 3: Excretion of urinary vanilmandelic acid in healthy adults, hypertensive patients and patients with pheochromocytoma. (Reproduced from Sunderman (49), with permission).

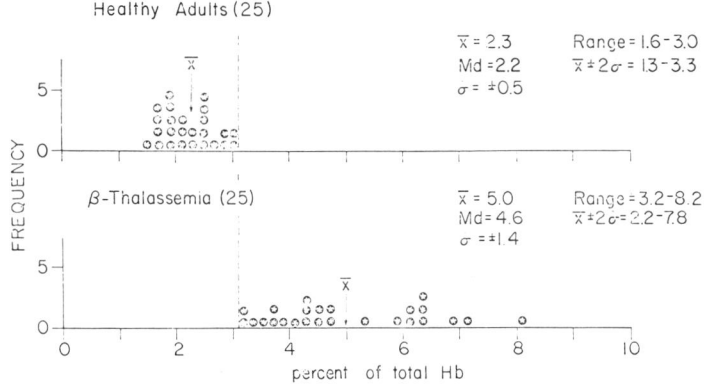

Figure 4: Percentages of hemoglobin A_2 in blood from healthy adults and patients with β-thalassemia. (Reproduced from Sunderman (49), with permission).

HYPOTHETICAL TEST ("Tx") FOR "X" DISEASE

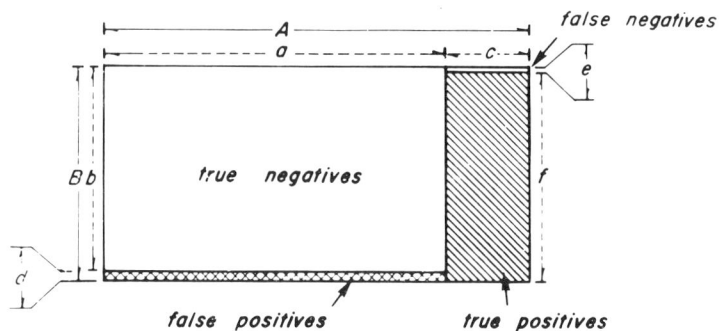

Example # 1: Incidence of "X" disease = 20 %

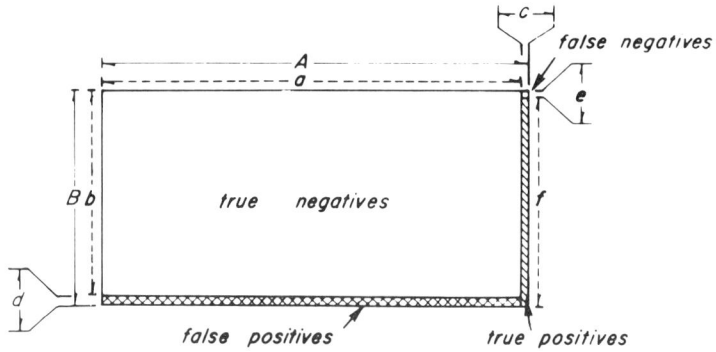

Example # 2: Incidence of "X" disease = 2 %

Figure 5: Compartmental models which illustrate how the interpretation of the results of a screening test for a specific disease is dependent upon the incidence of that disease in the tested population (see text). (Reproduced from Sunderman and Van Soestbergen (51), with permission).

DOCUMENTATION OF LABORATORY DATA

HYPOTHETICAL TEST ("TY") FOR "Y" DISEASE

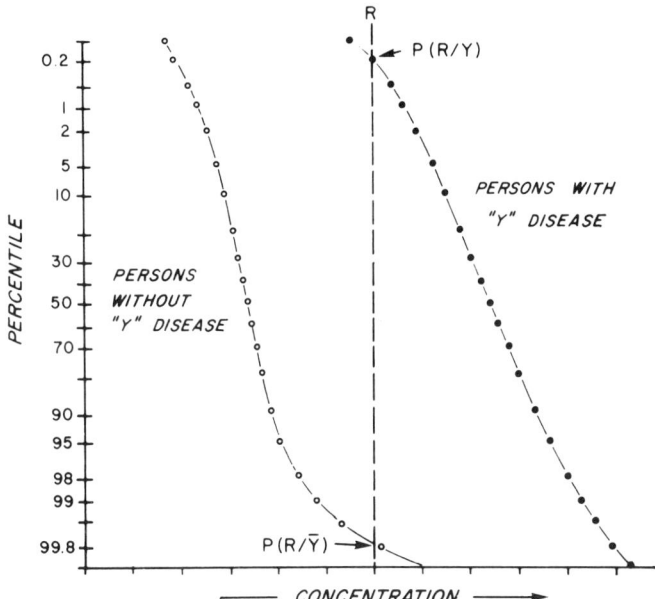

Figure 6: Probit graph of frequency distributions of results of a quantitative screening test in persons with and without a specific disease. Such a graph can be used for computations of the diagnostic probability of test results (see text). (Reproduced from Sunderman and Van Soestbergen (51), with permission).

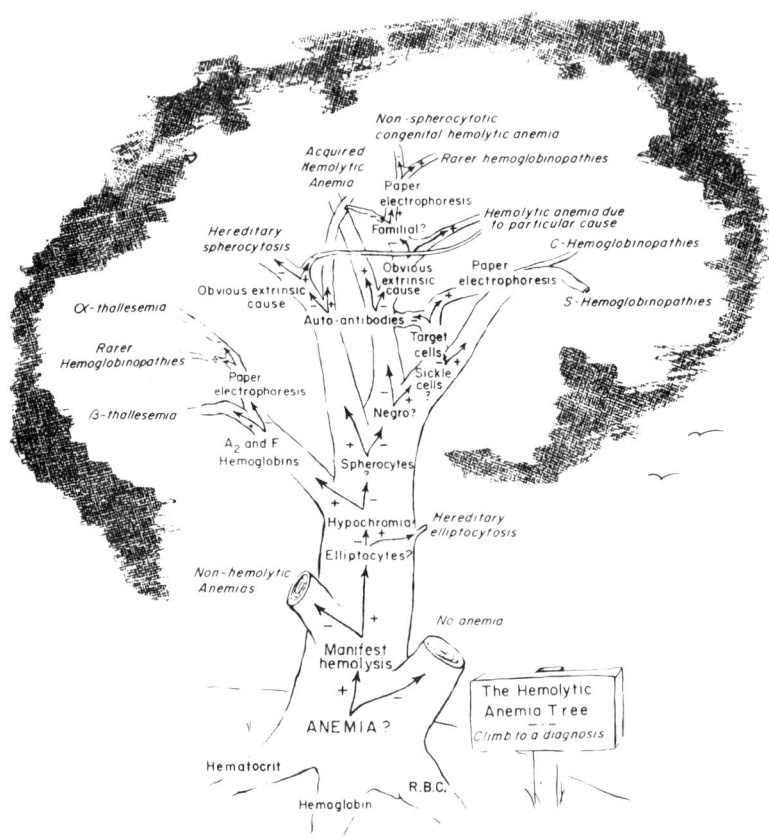

Figure 7: The "hemolytic anemia decision-tree." A schematic representation of the logical branching which leads to a specific diagnosis in the hemolytic anemias. (Reproduced from Best (8), with permission).

DOCUMENTATION OF LABORATORY DATA

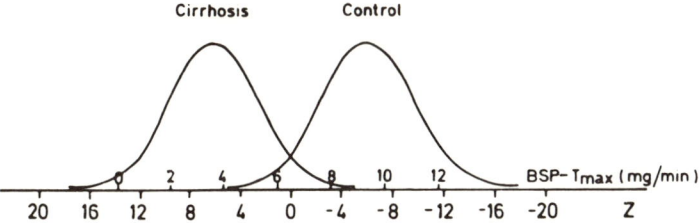

II

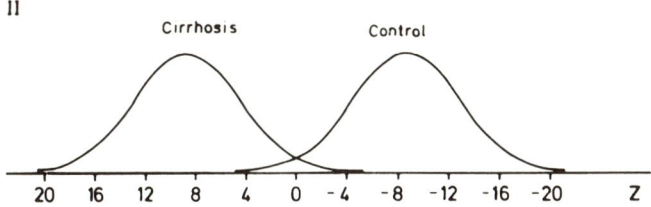

III

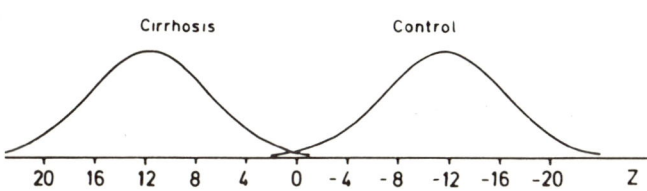

Figure 8: Application of multivariate discriminant analysis to liver function tests. The cumulative overlap area illustrates the reduction in misclassification of control and cirrhotic subjects obtained by increasing the number of liver function tests from one to nine (see text). (Reproduced from Ramsoe et al (40), with permission).

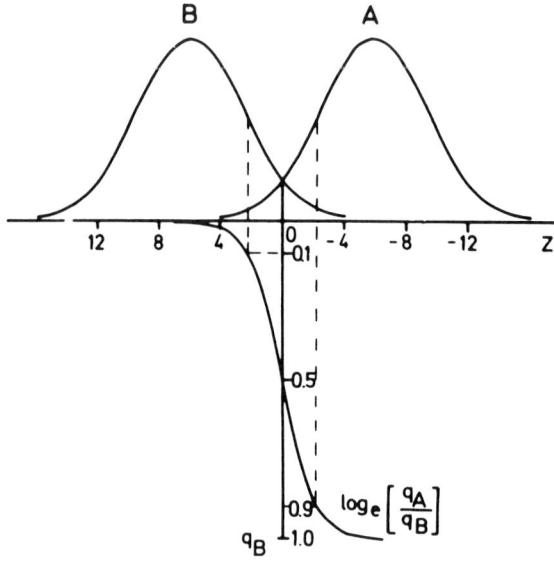

Figure 9: Applications of multivariate discriminant analysis to liver function tests. If the probability (q_A) that an observation belongs to population A is equal to the probability ($q_B = 1 - q_A$) that it belongs to population B, maximum discrimination corresponds to the point where Z, the discriminant function, + a constant is zero (i.e. to the intercept of the probability distribution curves). If $q_A > q_B$, maximum discrimination corresponds to $Z > 0$. The figure shows the probability distribution of Z (BSP-Tmax), and the discrimination point ($\log_e q_A/q_B = \log_e 1-q_B/q_B$) depicted as a function of the a priori probability q_B. (Reproduced from Ramsoe et al (40), with permission).

GEOCHEMICAL ECOLOGY AND INTERPRETATION OF LABORATORY DATA

Howard C. Hopps, M.D., Ph.D.

The greatest single obstacle to full exploitation of what computer technology has to offer medicine is the lack of data-structuring system that allows effective input. A second major obstacle is our inability to develop a format for displaying output that will communicate pertinent information effectively in the context of the particular problem. Sometimes we forget that data are simply a means to the end, which is not merely knowledge, per se, but UNDERSTANDING THE PROBLEM.

It was the second of these obstacles, the one related to output, that lead us to work for four years on the project we call MOD, an acronym for Mapping of Disease. (The long title of our project was Computerized Mapping of Disease and Environmental Data.) I will not involve you with the cartographic aspects of this study; I will, however, draw upon our experiences in converting narrative and tabular data to information suitable for presentation in a spatio-temporal contest. I will also discuss particular advantages of displaying data in map form. You may gather from this that my bias is a spatio-temporal one. I have been more interested in what diseases occur where, and when and why, than in the tests that detect these diseases though, of course, the two areas cannot be sharply separated.

As an aside, I should tell you that I have been most fortunate in four respects that are pertinent to the purposes of this Conference. One was my association with the Armed Forces Institute of Pathology for seven years, during which time my colleagues: Roger Cuffey, Jerome Morenoff, Wayne Richmond, Joseph Sidley, and I worked together on the MOD project. Another was--and is-- my continuing association with Helen Cannon, of the U.S. Geological Survey, through whom I have been lead into very rewarding relationships with geologists, hydrologists, agronomists, and the like. This relationship has been responsible, just recently, for the formation of a Subcommittee on the Geochemical Environment in Relation to Health and Disease, of the Earth Sciences Division of the National Academy of Sciences. The third was--and is-- my association with the Health Surveillance Center of the University of Missouri, under the direction of Dr. Carl Marienfeld, and I shall be showing you some of the data gathered by this group. Finally, it has been my very good fortune to have known Elemér Gabrieli as a colleague and as a friend for some 20 years, and to have learned much from him about data and information, their essential differences, and how to convert the one to the other.

Getting back to maps, our concern with mapping is because we feel that this is the best way to present large amounts of complex data in a form that permits one to visualize the distribution of disease with respect to a wide variety of possible causal environmental factors such as climate, geochemical environment, land usage, social behavior, etc., etc. In other words, the output of information in map form provides a direct and intimate association of primary variables in the context of the particular problem.

Basically, a map is simply a graph, but a special form of graph in which X and Y coordinates represent latitude and longtitude, or some equivalent. The principal point is that data are plotted with respect to their location according to a rigorous, logical, consistent grid pattern and scale that avoids non-systematic distortions of size, shape, or distance. Strictly speaking, a map is a representation of spatial relationships on the earth's surface, but shapes and locations on any kind of surface can be depicted using the techniques of mapping. I stress this because spatial location of things is an important area of weakness among pathologists. It took too long for us to realize that the variations in shape and location of cardiac infarcts are important with respect to the size, number and pattern of distribution of coronary arteries-- and that the shape and location of fibrous tissue masses occurring in cirrhosis of the liver is important with respect to cause of the disease--and that the precise location of intraglomerular lesions in glomerulonephritis is important in determining specific etiology. And many of us are just beginning to appreciate that the shape and location of intra-cellular lesions is also very important in understanding the etiology and pathogenesis of disease.

These considerations may seem a bit far afield, but they do bear on geographic pathology and mapping of disease since they consider spatio-temporal factors in their approach toward understanding cause/effect relationships in disease.

Computer techniques have progressed to the point, that today, the basic types of maps: dot-type, shading-type, even contour-type, can be produced by a computer/ printer or computer/plotter complex, quickly and accurately, assuming, of course, that one has an adequate data base. Maps produced in this way can be printed on transparent materials and overlaid on base maps that show topographic, political, or population data, etc. Moreover, multiple transparent overlays, each presenting different kinds of information, can be layered together to show relationships, i.e., the extent of pattern match.

Overlaying and visual comparison of patterns is a very powerful process because it permits human detection of relationships so complex that standard mathematical methods may be unable to detect them. Thus, the kinds of maps that we are describing allow one to detect correlations quickly and clearly. Since the computer/plotter can produce maps rapidly and relatively inexpensively (once the data base and appropriate programs have been established), this allows the geographic pathologist, epidemiologist, etc., to use maps as a research tool as well as a means of displaying the final results of his work. Obviously, another important advantage of computer-produced maps is that it allows one to maintain up-to-date presentations. In the past, the relatively few geographic atlases of disease that have been available have had to stand for many years, because the time and expense required to produce new editions was so great.

There is a long way to go before disease data in narrative or tabular form can be converted into maps. Except for certain dot-type ones, disease maps represent abstract statistical surfaces that must be calculated from field observational data, quite unlike road maps, political maps, topographic maps, type-of-bedrock geologicl maps, etc., which show the actual locations of things. It was this aspect of the problem that lead us head on into the difficulty that I mentioned at the beginning: the lack of a data-structuring system which would allow effective input into a computer system.

After considerable work, we developed our concept of a DATA POINT, i.e., a bit of mapable data, and defined the minimum limits of its content:

1. a precise LOCATION
2. a defined disease or environmental FACTOR
3. a specific VALUE for that factor
4. a particular TIME reference

We also included one other bit of data as minimum

information content in our system, and that was:

5. the DATA SOURCE

Characterization of location, value, time and data source gave relatively little trouble; factor proved to be very difficult indeed, but I don't wish to belabor this aspect of our study. Suffice to say that, after a great deal of work, we developed a hierarchical system which allowed sharp characterization of the factor that we wished to measure and locate. Once we had a system for production of data points, we were ready to determine which map form would offer the best format for the display of our information.

Maps are commonly classified according to the kinds of symbols used to show how the data are distributed, as I have implied. By this classification there are dot-type (data point), shading-type (chloropleth), and contour-type (isopleth) maps. DOT-TYPE MAPS are simplest to use, and show very well whether a particular factor is present or not at a particular point. The major difficulty with this approach is that only a yes-or-no answer can be given for a given place. SHADING-TYPE MAPS do much the same thing, but relate the occurence of a particular characteristic to an area. These two kinds of maps have been used most extensively to show distribution of disease, because of their simplicity. Their great weakness lies in the fact that only limited amounts of quantitative information can be presented. Varying dot size, shape, and color, or varying the texture or color of shaded areas helps somewhat, but not enough. CONTOUR-TYPE MAPS offer tremendous advantages because they can depict qualitative and quantitative aspects of the data simultaneously, at the same time, of course, giving precise arel distribution. Since each contour line (isopleth) connects a series of points of equal value, groups of contour lines form a series of distribution patterns that show amounts of involvement. It was because of this great advantage that we concentrated on developing methods for the computer/plotter production of contour maps that would show the distribution of disease and related environmental factors (see figure 1).

This is a much more complicated task than presenting disease data by dot-type or shading-type maps because of difficulties in interpolation and extrapolation. The latter was especially difficult, and lead to some embarrasing results during the early stages of work; one of our earliest maps indicated that schistosomiasis extended off the east coast of Brazil, well out into the Atlantic Ocean!

Contour maps are certainly most useful in searching for environmental causes of disease because of their unique capacity to relate what and where with how much. Moreover, by comparing different factors that have been plotted in this way, one can get an excellent idea of gradients--often it is a particular balance of (quantitative) levels of ecologic factors, coupled with particular levels of exposure, susceptibility, etc., that is required to yield a particular end point of disease. Properly prepared contour maps, especially those than can be overlaid, one on another, provide an excellent approach to problem solving through the means of PATTERN RECOGNITION.

The production of dot-type maps pose fewer technical problems, as I have said. Unfortunately, most disease dot-type maps are of low resolution (large groups of cases represented by a single dot), and give considerable misinformation because of distortions that reflect improper groupings of data. Despite their limitations, however, dot-type maps can be very helpful in the special situation where every case or small group of cases of a particular disease is depicted by a dot on the map. This requires that the problem be a suitable, one, also, of course, that the cartographic techniques be appropriate. As a matter of fact, the only absolute way of presenting geographic distribution of disease data is by "high resolution" dot-type maps that indicate individual cases, since this is the only way to show precisely where the person was when he had his disease.*

*There is fuzziness even with this kind of presentation, however. The dot does not necessarily indicate where the patient contracted his disease, or even where he was when the disease became evident, since "registration" of the case--related to specific diagnosis or definitive treatment--may have occurred in a medical center far removed both in place and time from the real point of exposure/development.

Disease data mapped in this manner may be appropriate for CLUSTER ANALYSIS, which can be a precise and highly valuable analytical tool. I wish to illustrate such effective use of dot-type maps by presenting some of the material that has been produced by Carl Marienfeld's Health Surveillance group at the University of Missouri.

The basic objective of Dr. Marienfeld's group was-- and still is--to determine whether or not environmental factors are associated with birth defects and, if so, whether or not the association is casual. The many critically important parts of the experimental design that concern selecting appropriate times and places for sampling, actually getting and validating the data, then subjecting them to statistical scrutiny, etc., are not pertinent to our major area of interest and I shall not consider them here. Our interest is more with how the information can be displayed in a problem-oriented contest and, in this particular instance, a form suitable for cluster analysis.

The several maps I shall present are but a small part of the total information, and I am using them to illustrate two points: First, that dot-type maps can be effectively used together with contour-or shading-type maps (which present supplementary information in context). Second, and more important, that dot-type maps can provide a means of displaying data in a form suitable for cluster analysis, toward the goal of determining cause-effect relationships in diseases.

This kind of approach, which I have illustrated, is the one that we plan to use in our geographic pathology study to determine causal relationships between geochemical environment and a wide variety of diseases.

We ordinarily think of two ways to detect something that no one has seen before: one, to aim at the finest detail, to get as close to the object as possible, to use the best analytical instruments; the other, to look at it from a new angle, where it shows hitherto unexposed facets. If we accept the view of Laplace that "to discover is to bring together two ideas which were separate," there is a third way of detecting something that no one has seen before. And this third way closely approaches the primary objectives of our Conference as I see it: to develop better methods for the manipulation and display of data to yield new information.

REFERENCES

Cannon, H. L. and Hopps, H. C., Environmental geochemistry: health and disease. Science 162:815 (1968).

Cannon, Helen L. and Hopps, Howard C., Minor metals of the geochemical environment, health and disease. Science 170:1232 (1971).

Hopps, H. C., Cuffey, R. J., Morenoff, J., Richmond, W. L., and Sidley, J. D. H., Computerized mapping of disease and environmental data, The Government Printing Office, Washington, D. C., 1969. 419 pages.

Hopps, Howard C., Data versus information (an editorial) International Pathology 8:39 (1967).

Hopps, Howard C., Computers and pathologists (an editorial). International Pathology 10:55 (1969).

Hopps, Howard C., Environmental geochemistry and geographic pathology (an editorial). International Pathology 9:64 (1968).

Khalili, A., Marienfeld, C. J., Wright, H. T., Weiss, E. S., An approach to the estimation of the true numbers of congenital malformations. Pediatrics 46:712 (1970)

Wright, H. T., Marienfeld, C. J., Silberg, S. L., The definition of 'place' in environmental epidemiology, a rectangular coordinate method. Public Health Report 83:427-434 (1968).

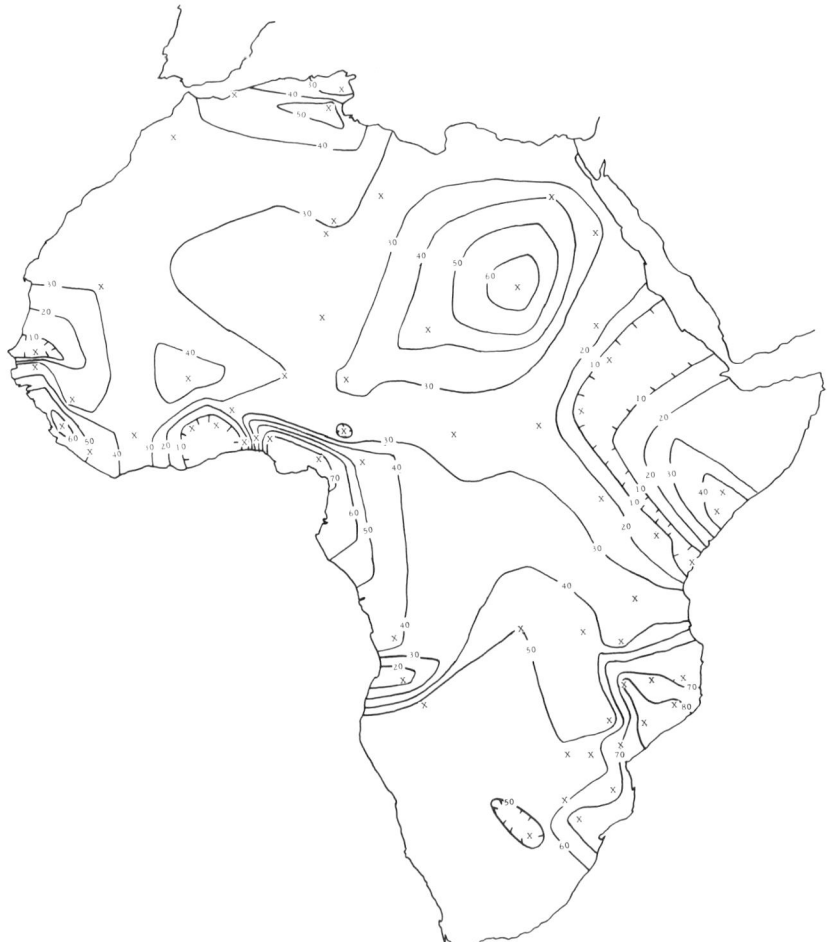

Figure 1. This contour-type map shows infection rates of schistosomiasis in Africa (based on data no longer current). Computer interpolation techniques were used to develop the contour lines (isopleths).

DOCUMENTATION OF LABORATORY DATA

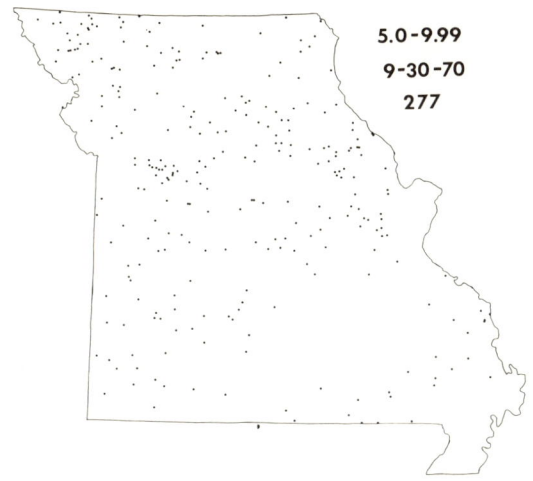

Figure 2

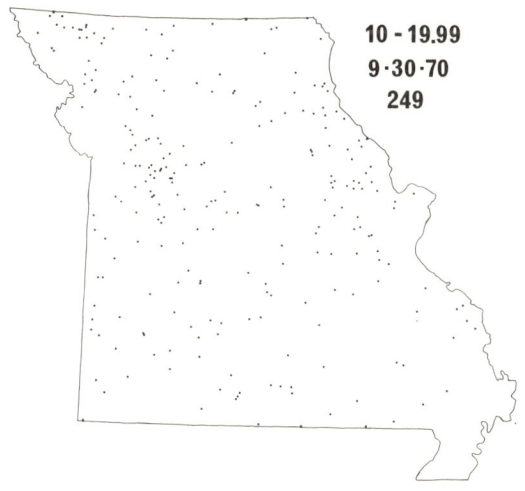

Figure 3

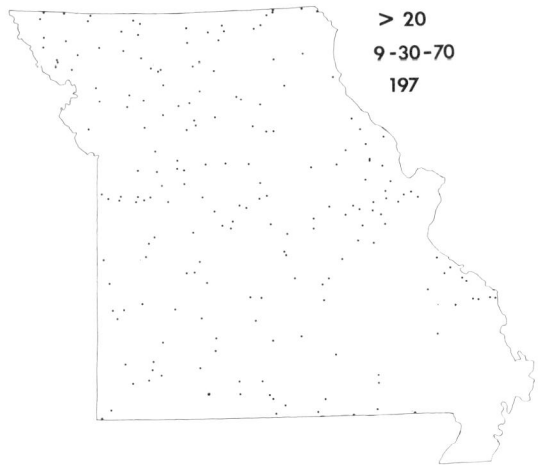

Figure 2
3 and 4. This series of three computer-produced maps shows the location of individual farms in Missouri on which swine were raised, where the incidence rate of congenital anomalies (during a particular six month period) was as indicated: 5.0 - 9.99 or 10.0 - 19.99 or greater than 20 per thousand births. (The lowermost of the three figures on each map is the number of farms, i.e., dots, represented). The original maps were produced on transparent stock so that by overlaying the maps, one on another, the different incidence groups can be combined, preserving the information that relates to precise geographic location. Obviously, data displayed in this form are highly suitable for cluster analysis. Moreover, such maps as these can be overlayed on base maps (of the same projection and scale) that show the geographic distribution of soil types, geologic substratum, specific sources of surface water, etc., allowing comparison of patterns with respect to possible causal factors.

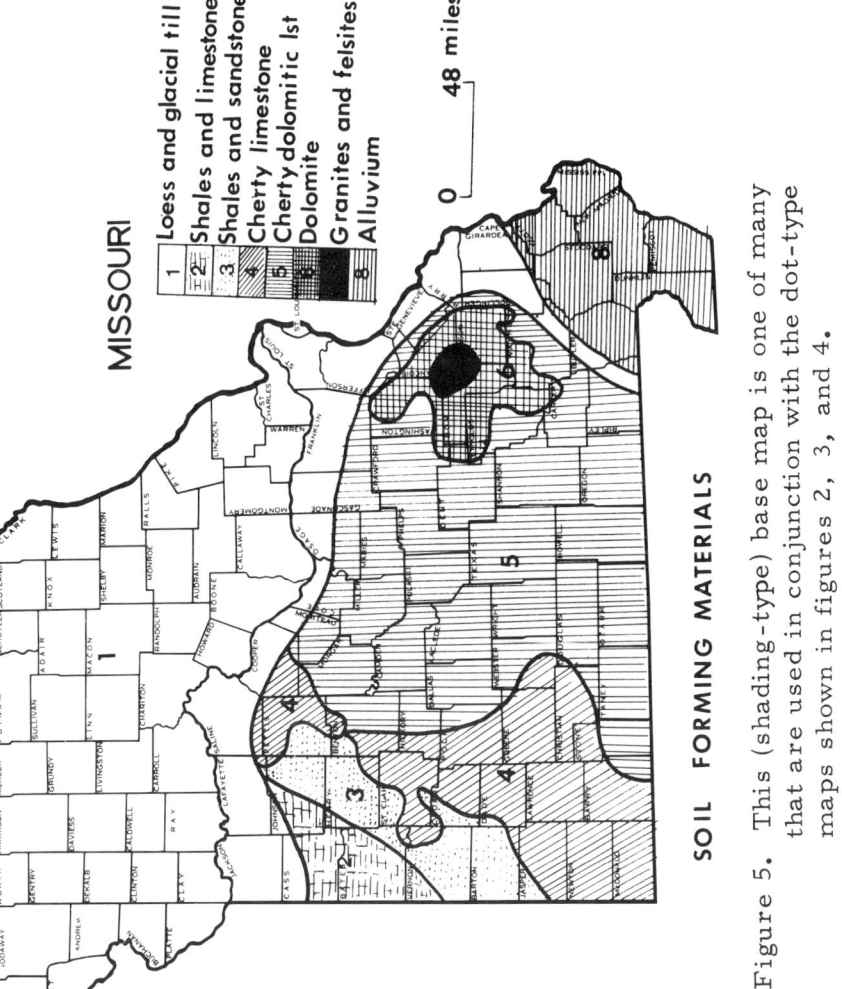

Figure 5. This (shading-type) base map is one of many that are used in conjunction with the dot-type maps shown in figures 2, 3, and 4.

NORMAL RANGES OF VALUES DERIVED FROM LARGE SCALE MULTITEST SURVEYS

David C. Hohnadel, Ph. D.

Introduction

Recent publications in the medical literature have indicated the increasingly complex role that laboratory medicine is fulfilling in patient care (1, 9, 10). The complexity has developed from major changes that have occurred in the way laboratory scientists carry out biochemical tests and evaluate the data produced. The clinical laboratory has become highly sophisticated in the technical aspects of testing and the variety of procedures that can be accomplished. In addition, the data obtained contains more inherent information if evaluated properly by the practitioners of clinical medicine. At the same time, the fruits of extensive research in cell biology have vastly expanded the amount of information available for clinicians and has increased the understanding of disease processes on a molecular level.

Unfortunately this increasing specialization of both the producers and users of clinical laboratory data may lead to a profound decrease in the information content of the data passing between these two groups. The laboratory scientist in trying to present the data in the most informative manner has become involved in describing a "normal population" and defining a "normal range" from such a population. Because it is very difficult to do this the laboratory scientist has to estimate the "normal range" in the best way possible, using statistical terminology such as parametric and non-parametric statistics, frequency distributions, estimates, and confidence intervals. The laboratory scientist may aid the users of the results by providing an accurate measure of the uncertainty in the data. The uncertainty of the estimate of the "normal range" is associated with the reproducibility of individual results and accuracy with which the results can be placed within the population of data. In most cases the reproducibility of individual results is a small factor in the population uncertainty (26). Since every estimate has at least a little uncertainty associated with it, then the presentation of the laboratory results with the uncertainty explicitly expressed may make the users of the results less sure rather than more sure of the data. Thus, although the data may be more informative, the growing body of knowledge associated with clinical medicine and the increasing sophistication of laboratory data may make the proper evaluation of laboratory results a very difficult task.

It has been known for some time that many factors including age, sex, race, diet, geographic location, occupation, physiological state and biological rhythms influence the normal ranges obtained. However, only recently has enough data been compiled to begin to separate and quantitate the relative effects of each of these factors (2, 11, 20).

The advent of automation to laboratory testing methods has been the single advance that has made most of the large scale studies of normal values possible. The most significant change effected by automation has been to greatly reduce the time required for an analysis, Conversely, many analyses can now be completed in a relatively brief time. In many cases, rapid availability of test results has definite benefits for patient care, but this advantage, in some cases, may be reduced by the proliferation of test results that are now generated automatically, concealing those results that may be the most important. Large amounts of data are being produced as automated analysis equipment has become readily

confidence intervals. The laboratory scientist may aid the users of the results by providing an accurate measure of the uncertainty in the data. The uncertainty of the estimate of the "normal range" is associated with the reproducibility of individual results and accuracy with which the results can be placed within the population of data. In most cases the reproducibility of individual results is a small factor in the population uncertainty (26). Since every estimate has at least a little uncertainty associated with it, then the presentation of the laboratory results with the uncertainty explicitly may make the users of the results less sure rather than more sure of the data. Thus, although the data may be more informative, the growing body of knowledge associated with clinical medicine and the increasing sophistication of laboratory data may make the proper evaluation of laboratory results a very difficult task.

It has been known for some time that many factors including age, sex, race, diet, geographic location, occupation, physiological state and biological rhythms influence the normal ranges obtained. However, only recently has enough data been compiled to begin to separate and quantitate the relative effects of each of these factors (2, 11, 20).

The advent of automation to laboratory testing methods has been the single advance that has made most of the large scale studies of normal values possible. The most significant change effected by automation has been to greatly reduce the time required for an analysis. Conversely, many analyses can now be completed in a relatively brief time. In many cases, rapid availability of test results has definite benefits for patient care, but this advantage, in some cases, may be reduced by the proliferation of test results that are now generated automatically, concealing those results that may be the most important. Large amounts of data are being produced as automated analysis equipment has become readily available and widely distributed.

Discussion

A representative sample of multitest surveys that have been published recently has been compiled in Table I. The table summarizes the population studied, age distribution, number of individuals, location and number of constituents tested. The first study is that of the Kaiser-Permanente group and involved large numbers of healthy outpatients ranging in age from 20 to 79 years. In this case, eight constitutents were routinely tested and healthy individuals were judged to be those with "no significant abnormality". The second study of Keating and co-workers demonstrated an age and sex distribution of values for seven constitutents in healthy subjects at the Mayo Clinic. The study by Werner et al. was conducted on ambulatory individuals at the San Francisco Health Fair and the influence of age and sex on results was determined. The study of Cunnich and co-workers was that of the Metropolitan Life Insurance Company on their own employees. In this case distributions of many of the twelve constitutents were shown to be different for men and women. The data of O'Halloran and co-workers compares the values obtained in South Australia for twelve constituents between inpatients, outpatients, and healthy members of the hospital staff but does not break down the values by age or sex. The study by Roberts has indicated the types of distributions that were obtained for seventeen components of serum from blood donors in Great Britain.

Kannel and co-workers have examined portions of the general population of Framingham, Massachusetts, in a long term study looking for correlations between levels of cholesterol, lipoproteins and heart disease. The last study shown was an examination of IBM Company employees between 41 and 65 years for six serum constituents. In all the studies cited groups of both men and women were included but they were not always separated. Some of the authors have carried out limited comparisons to demonstrate differences between subgroups in the population, but even with the large amount of data available, it is sometimes difficult or impossible to compare the data between these various authors.

Some of the fundamental conceptual problems which are associated with the interpretation of multitest screening results have been illustrated using data that was taken from the last survey. These concepts are: first, the distribution of results for a particular constituent, and second, the normal ranges of values. They are interdependent, and are profoundly influenced by technical, clinical and economic factors as well as the physiological and environmental ones previously mentioned.

It is most important to emphasize the term multitest screening in contrast to the testing of hospitalized individuals. Certain fundamental concepts of a statistical nature are common to both situations and must be understood to obtain the maximum amount of information from the data. The clinical interpretation of results of a multitest screening program on normal individuals should not be the same as the clinical interpretation of laboratory results on hospital patients since the relative incidence of disease is very different. The probability that a positive test is a true positive is very different in each population (23). Recommendations have been made regarding the utilization of results of multitest surveys which incorporate these statistical concepts.

A large scale multiphasic screening program is being carried out by the IBM Company for its employees (6, 7). A preliminary report of the data has been presented (13). The total population which was selected for consideration included IBM employees in the U.S. and Canada between the ages of 41 and 65 who were examined in the first year of this screening program from September, 1968 through August, 1969. The population consists of 22,100 men and 3,000 women. The IBM examination included the following diagnostic procedures: a computerized medical history, morphometry, audiometry, chest X-ray, electrocardiogram, hematocrit, hemoglobin and urinalysis. These procedures were performed at thirty-six locations throughout the United States and Canada. Serum samples were obtained and sent to the IBM Medical Data Center in White Plains, New York, where the chemical and enzymatic analyses were performed, including fasting glucose, urea-nitrogen, uric acid, cholesterol, SGOT and LDH. The analyses were performed by means of single and dual channel AutoAnalyzers to maintain flexibility in the testing program. Standardization was carried out using National Bureau of Standards material for all chemical procedures.

For the delineation of normal ranges, a healthy subgroup of the total population has been selected on the basis of the computerized medical history questionnaire. The questions used as a criteria of health were designed to eliminate individuals with a personal or family history of systemic disease; those with an excessive intake of coffee, or alcohol; and those taking drugs, medication or vitamins. All individuals considered their health to be good or excellent. The healthy subjects in this cohort are truly representative of the population to be tested, in regard to age, sex, race and geographic distribution as well as occupations. Large variation in biological rhythms were minimized by drawing all blood specimens between 8:30 and 10:00 A.M.

Figure 1 shows several superimposed probit plots of glucose measurements for subgroups of the population. In the probit graphical presentation, the ordinate axis is expressed as the cumulative percentage of the population and has a logarithmically spaced scale such that a Gaussian distribution is described by a straight line.

A superimposition has been made of the values obtained in an apparently healthy subgroup (curve C) with the values obtained from those who considered their health to be good or excellent (curve B), and with the values obtained from all men (curve A). The three populations appear to be indistinguishable from the 5th to 90th percentiles with the same mean and standard deviation. It is noteworthy that the group of individuals who considered their health to be good or excellent did not contain a substantially lower number of subjects with elevated glucose values. The differences between curves A and B are 5 - 15 mg/dl at various percentiles and are not very large. Results closer to a Gaussian distribution were obtained by using a more complete questioning procedure as indicated by the lessening of the deviation of the tail of the distribution in curve C, but the results still do not conform to a Gaussian distribution indicated by the dots at the tails of the three distributions. The observed difference between curve C and the other distributions is 30 - 70 mg/dl at various percentiles and is not negligible.

An intensive evaluation of the statistical methods used for the delineation of normal ranges has been evident in recent publications (2, 8, 11, 17, 20, 21). The percentiles method of Herrera (12) and the critical values method of Murphy and Abbey (18) are generally regarded as the most reliable techniques for delineation of normal ranges. However, these techniques need refinement in order to provide an adequate solution to the problems of multitest screening.

The power of the percentiles and the critical values methods are derived from the non-parametric nature of the criteria used to set "normal ranges". The parametric statistical methods which were commonly used in the past for computation of normal ranges were based on the assumption that test results in healthy subjects adhere to the Gaussian frequency distribution. In practice, such measurements as seen in Figure 1 seldom conform precisely to the Gaussian distribution curve, even after logarithmic transformation. Therefore, recent investigators have emphasized that parametric statistical indices (that is, mean $\pm$ 2 or 3 S.D.) are unreliable for demarcation of normal ranges of values, and that it is preferable to employ non-parametric techniques, for example, the percentiles method, which are independent of the shape of the frequency distribution curve. The effect that the frequency distribution has upon the selection of normal ranges has been illustrated by consideration of two examples in detail, one taken from a distribution of results that is approximately Gaussian, and one taken from a distribution of results that is approximately log-Gaussian. In addition, comparisons of analytical results for the total group and the healthy subgroup have been considered.

The frequency histogram of measurements of fasting glucose concentrations in the healthy cohort was close to the Gaussian distribution. Figure 2 is a computer-generated frequency distribution curve for concentrations of serum glucose collected from healthy, fasting men between the ages of 41 and 45 years. The histogram appears to be approximately Gaussian, since the vertical dashed lines giving the mean $\pm$ 2 standard deviations are close to the 2.5th and 97.5th percentiles represented by the lower triangles, and the curve appears to be bell-shaped.

The magnitude of the deviation of this sample of apparently healthy individuals from a true Gaussian distribution is illustrated by the probit plot given in Figure 3. A superimposition has been made of the values obtained from the healthy individuals (curve B) and the values obtained from all the men in this age range (curve A). Theoretical adherence to a Gaussian distribution is illustrated by a series of dots at the tails of the other distributions. The frequency distribution of glucose concentration in the healthy subjects is approximately linear from the 5th to the 97.5th percentiles which corresponds to an upper limit of 120 mg/dl. There is little difference in the two distributions at low glucose concentrations but there is a significant difference between the two curves at high glucose concentrations. The data appears to follow a Gaussian distribution for about 92 percent of the values.

The concentrations in mg/dl of serum glucose at specific percentiles in the healthy subgroup have been compared with the corresponding values for the entire male population in Table II. The median and the 95th percentile values are only slightly different in the two categories for all ages. On the other hand, the 97.5th and 99.5th percentile values in the two categories are much more widely disparate. For example: in the 99.5 percentile column a difference of 24 mg/dl is seen in the 41-45 age group which increases to a difference of 122 mg/dl in the 61-65 age group. Such differences would, of course, be expected due to the presence of men with undiagnosed diabetes mellitus in the total group. Progressive increases in median values were observed in advancing quintiles for both males and females.

The frequency histogram of measurements of SGOT activity was close to a "log-Gaussian" distribution. Figure 4 is a computer-generated histogram of SGOT activities in serums from healthy male subjects between the ages 41 and 45 years. SGOT activities are definitely skewed to the higher side of the histogram, and the mean $\pm$ 2 S.D. lines no longer correspond to the central 95 percentile limits indicated by the lower triangles. Obviously, the normal ranges cannot be derived by the standard deviation technique. This is true of all non-symmetric distributions since skewing will cause the ranges derived from the mean $\pm$ 2 or 3 standard deviations to no longer coincide with the central 95 or 99 percentiles. In addition, symmetric distribution curves with significant kurtosis will cause the normal range to

in the healthy subjects is approximately linear from the 5th to the 97.5th percentiles which corresponds to an upper limit of 120 mg/dl. There is little difference in the two distributions at low glucose concentrations but there is a significant difference between the two curves at high glucose concentrations. The data appears to follow a Gaussian distribution for about 92 percent of the values.

The concentrations in mg/dl of serum glucose at specific percentiles in the healthy subgroup have been compared with the corresponding values for the entire male population in Table II. The median and the 95th percentile values are only slightly different in the two categories for all ages. On the other hand, the 97.5th and 99.5th percentile values in the two categories are much more widely disparate. For example: in the 99.5% column a difference of 24 mg/dl is seen in the 41-45 age group which increases to a difference of 122 mg/dl in the 61-65 age group. Such differences would, of course, be expected due to the presence of men with undiagnosed diabetes mellitus in the total group. Progressive increases in median values were observed in advancing quintiles for both males and females.

The frequency histogram of measurements of SGOT activity was close to a "log-Gaussian" distribution. Figure 4 is a computer-generated histogram of SGOT activities in serums from healthy male subjects between the ages 41 and 45 years. SGOT activities are definitely skewed to the higher side of the histogram, and the mean $\pm$ 2 S.D. lines no longer correspond to the central 95 percentile limits indicated by the lower triangles. Obviously, the normal ranges cannot be derived by the standard deviation technique. This is true of all non-symmetric distributions since skewing will cause the ranges derived from the mean $\pm$ 2 or 3 standard deviations to no longer coincide with the central 95 or 99 percentiles. In addition, symmetric distribution curves with significant kurtosis will cause the normal range to be underestimated using the standard deviation technique if the distribution is leptokurtic and overestimated using the standard deviation technique if the distribution is platykurtic.

The deviation of this sample of apparently healthy subjects from a log-Gaussian distribution is illustrated in Figure 5 by a probit plot of the same measurements. Again, a superimposition has been made of the values in the healthy cohort (curve B) and the values obtained from all men in this age range (curve A). Both curves are seen to deviate from log-Gaussian distributions beyond the 90th percentile and below the 5th percentile with much greater deviation shown in the category of total men. Eighty-five percent of the population corresponds to a log-Gaussian distribution. The difference in the elevated range would be expected since the total population includes men with known hepatic disease, as well as men suffering from alcoholism.

In Table III, the SGOT activities in Karmen units of the healthy cohort were compared at various percentiles with the activities in corresponding segments of the entire male population. The medians are the same for both populations for all age groups examined. A greater and greater difference between the populations is seen by moving to more extreme percentiles. No age trend was observed for SGOT activities in men. Women, however, exhibited a slight age trend which increased to comparable values with men in the 61-65 age group.

The results for uric acid concentrations of men in the 41 to 45 age group are given in probit graphical format in Figure 6. The values for the apparently healthy subgroup (curve B) are superimposed on the values for all men in this age group (curve A). The deviation of curve A from a log-Gaussian distribution is seen above the 90th percentile and below the 10th percentile which indicates only an 80 percent correspondence with a log-

Gaussian distribution. Although corresponding tabular data has been omitted, the medians are the same for both populations in all age groups examined except for the 61 to 65 grouping. No trend with age was seen in this data for men; however, an age trend was observed in corresponding data for healthy women.

The cholesterol results obtained from the 41 to 45 year old men in the apparently healthy subgroup is given by curve B in Figure 7 with the values for all men in this age group given by curve A. The difference between the two populations was observed to be small. Both appear to be similar to log-Gaussian distributions from the 5th to the 95th percentiles, but more divergent outside these limits. There was approximately a 90 percent correspondance to a log-Gaussian distribution. The medians were similar for both populations for all age groups. An age trend was observed for men which was found to increase to age 60 and to decrease in the 61 to 65 age range.

The distribution of urea nitrogen concentrations is given in Figure 8 which compares the values obtained from apparently healthy men (curve B) with the values of all men in the 41 to 45 age range (curve A). Very few differences were observed between the two distributions at any percentile level. Both curves are seen to deviate from log-Gaussian distributions below the 10th percentile and above the 99th percentile, indicating an 89 percent correspondence to a log-Gaussian distribution.

The distribution of lactic dehydrogenase activities for the healthy subgroup (curve B) and the corresponding segment of the male population (curve A) is given in Figure 9. It is readily apparent that no difference existed between these groups. There is a slight but significant increase in the medians with age in healthy men up to age 55.

DOCUMENTATION OF LABORATORY DATA

Data has been presented in Figures 6 through 8 to show that uric acid, cholesterol and urea nitrogen all resembled SGOT in seeming to be closer to log-Gaussian than arithmetic Gaussian distributions. Conversely, the distributions of results for glucose and lactic dehydrogenase seemed to be closer to arithmetic Gaussian rather than log-Gaussian distributions. Similar results for these analyses have been found by some previous investigators (22, 25), but there is some disagreement as to the nature of the distributions for these parameters in healthy groups. It seems likely that the different types of distributions observed by various investigators may be due to variations in sampling of genetic, dietary, geographic and occupational factors or perhaps to variations in biological rhythms or methodology that are as yet unknown.

It is most important to emphasize that the data presented here demonstrate that the actual distributions obtained are not completely consistent with either the Gaussian or log-Gaussian distributions. It has been observed that the frequency distributions of results are similar to the Gaussian and log-Gaussian distributions for only an 80 to 90 percent portion of the distribution. Two problems that are immediately evident are first, the similar portion to the theoretical distribution varies from constitutent to constituent preventing broad generalizations, and second, a 5 to 15 percent error results in the normal ranges that are based on the assumption of a 95 percent correspondence to the theoretical distribution (mean $\pm$ 2 standard deviations). These problems persist even with extremely large sample populations. This distribution disparaity has been noted by others in recent publications (8, 17, 21).

The observations which have been made regarding the frequency distributions of test results must be considered in order to decide on normal ranges for multi-test surveys. As has been indicated earlier, the most practical solution which avoids the problems related to the type of distribution is to utilize the percentiles of the actual distribution in a healthy cohort. Once the criteria has been set for evaluating the health of the subgroup, it is necessary to obtain relatively large groups of individuals to make comparisons. In most multiphasic surveys large groups of individuals are usually screened.

An example of a subdivision that must be made in order to obtain normal values is given in Figure 10. Data for the glucose distributions are compared for the total groups of apparently healthy women (curve A) and apparently healthy men (curve B). Differences were obtained between these subgroups in the population. Since curve B contains the data on more individuals it has been extended to more extreme percentages. The medians of these two populations differ by 5 mg/dl and the standard deviations which are related to the slopes of the lines differ by about 3 mg/dl. By conventional calculations of mean $\pm$ 2 standard deviations, the normal ranges would be about 12 mg wider for men than women and would be displaced 5 mg toward higher concentrations. Calculations based on the actual percentages show the 95 percent range for men to be about 6 mg/dl wider and shifted about 4 mg to higher concentrations than the range for women. A comparison of the central 95 percent between these groups and the composite total population indicates that a narrower range can be obtained by using the separated populations. Such a finding is highly significant and cannot be ignored if the maximum information is to be obtained from the laboratory data.

An illustration of the method involving percentiles is given in Table IV. The 2.5th and 97.5th percentile limits have been picked to further demonstrate the differences obtained between the subgroups of healthy men and women in the 41 to 45 age group. The differences shown in the table for the 50th percentiles and the other percentile limits were significant at the 0.001 probability level for glucose, urea nitrogen, uric acid and SGOT. Cholesterol and LDH were not significantly different in healthy men and women in this age group. Two types of non-parametric tests have been used to establish the significance of the differences seen in this table. The median test (5) has been used to evaluate whether the 50th percentiles were significantly different and the Kolmogorov-Smirnov "two sample" test (16) was used to indicate whether the cumulative percentage distributions were the same. It appears to be fortuitous that the same level of significance was found for both types of test; such is not always the case.

The significance of the increasing median values for the chemical parameters with advancing age were evaluated using the Von Neumann ration (24) and are given for all the determinations for both healthy men and women in Table V. Men show progressions with age for all six determinations at the 1 percent or 5 percent probability level. On the other hand, healthy men showed no increase in either uric acid or SGOT activity in the age ranges from 41 to 65, and show a slight decrease in cholesterol in the 61 to 65 age group. These data further demonstrate the necessity for defining the normal ranges in multitest surveys by categorization of results by age and sex.

One of the goals of multiphasic screening programs is to estimate the relative "health" of the individual. In order to approach this goal and to aid in the interpretation of the results of multitest surveys, the author proposes that the simplistic concept of a single "normal range" for a given population be discarded just as the single "normal value" was discarded in favor of a "normal range". A graded series of signals can then be provided to the clinician to indicate the degree of aberrance of test values in individuals who have no clinical evidence of disease. This is not to indicate that such individuals are necessarily ill, but only that they be evaluated further. Urea nitrogen concentrations in the serums of "healthy men" from age 41 to 45 may be taken as an example: those results which fall outside the 5th to 95th percentile range (11-22mg/dl) may be designated with one asterisk: those results which fall outside the 2.5th to 97.5th percentile range (10-24 mg/dl) may be designated with two asterisks: and those beyond the 0.5 to 99.5th percentile range (8-27 mg/dl) may be designated with three asterisks. The complete data for healthy men and women are given in Tables VI and VII.

Alternatively, the exact percentile rank of each test result relevant to the healthy population can be indicated in parentheses after the concentration. It is the author's considered opinion that these alternatives constitute the most practical solutions to the problem of delineating normal values for interpretation of multitest surveys.

Summary

The shape of the frequency distribution curve or analytical results obtained in a healthy population profoundly affects the "normal range" for the analyses when parametric statistical methods are used to delineate this range. The frequency distributions of results of the six biochemical tests which were considered in this study were found to deviate from the Gaussian or log-Gaussian curves and hence it was concluded that parametric methods could not be used reliably to define the "normal ranges" for these tests. To avoid this source of error, non-parametric statistical methods were employed to set normal percentile limits and to test for differences between various subsets of the population. In the author's opinion, the most practical method of reporting and interpreting the results of multitest surveys is to abandon the concept of a single "normal range" for a given test, and instead to consider test results according to their location on the percentile distributions of values in relevant healthy populations.

REFERENCES:

1. Barnett, R. N., Civin, W. H., and Schaen, I., Multiphasic screening by laboratory tests - an overview of the problem. Amer. J. Clin. Path. 54:483-492 (1970).

2. Cotlove, E., Harris, E. K., and Williams, G. Z., Biological and analytic components of variation in long-term studies of serum constituents in normal subjects III. Physiological and medical implications. Clin. Chem. 16:1028-1032 (1970).

3. Cunnick, W. R., Cromie, J. B., Beach, E. F. Seltzer, F., Tobin, J., and Culberson, S., Biochemical profiles in a healthy employee-population: Distribution of Values classified by age and sex, in Advances in Automated Analysis, Volume III, pp. 85 - 88 Mediad, White Plains, New York, (1969).

4. Cutler, J. L., Collen, M. F., Siegelaub, A. B., and Feldman, R., Normal values for multiphasic screening blood chemistry tests in Advances in Automated Analysis, Volum III, pp. 67-73, Mediad, White Plains, New York, (1969).

5. Dixon, W. J. and Massey, F. J., Jr., Introduction to Statistical Analysis 3rd Ed., p. 351-352, McGraw-Hill, New York, (1969).

6. Duffy, J. C., Health screening on an international basis, J. Kentucky Med. Assoc., 68:154-158 (1970).

7. Duffy, J. C., and Moonan, K. F., Applying the computer to an international health screening program. Industrial Med. 39:35-38 (1970).

8. Elveback, L.R., Guillier, C.L., and Keating, F.R., Jr., Health, normality, and the ghost of Gauss. J. Amer Med. Assoc. 211:69-75 (1970).

9. Feinleib, M., and Zelen, M., Some pitfalls in the evaluation of screening programs. Arch. Environ. Health, 19:412-415 (1969).

10. Gabrieli, E.R., Enhancing the meaning of clinical laboratory data. Critical Reviews in Clinical Lab. Science, 1:65-85 (1970).

11. Harris, E.K., Konofsky, P., Shakarji, G., and Cotlove, E., Biological and analytical components of variation in long-term studies of serum constituents in normal subjects II. Estimating biological components of variation. Clin. Chem. 16:1022-1027 (1970).

12. Herrera, L., The precision of percentiles in establishing normal limits in medicine. J. Lab. Clin. Med. 52:34-42 (1958).

13. Hohnadel, D.C., Duffy, J.C., Godbold, E.O., Hillman, G., Pomper, I.H., Reid, F.H., and Sunderman, F.W., Jr. Frequency Distributions of Results of Chemical Analyses in Multitest Profiles of Adults Categorized According to Age and Sex, in Technicon International Congress, 1970, Halos Associates, Miami, Florida, in press.

14. Kannel, W.B., Castelli, W.P., Gordon, T., and McNamara, P.M. Serum cholesterol, lipoproteins, and the risk of coronary heart disease. Annals of Inter. Med. 74:1-12, (1971).

15. Keating, F. R. Jr., Jones, J. D., Elveback, L. R., and Randall, R. V., The relation of age and sex to distribution of values in healthy adults of serum calcium, inorganic phosphorous, magnesium, alkaline phosphatase, total proteins, albumin, and blood urea J. Lab. Clin. Med. 73:825-834 (1969).

16. Kraft, C. H., and Van Eeden, C., A nonparametric introduction to statistics, p. 172, Macmillan Co., New York, (1968).

17. Mainland, D., Remarks on Clinical "Norms", Clin. Chem., 17:267-274 (1971).

18. Murphy, E. A., and Abbey, H., The normal range - a common misuse. J. Chronic Dis. 20:79-88 (1967).

19. O'Halloran, M. W., Studley-Rux on, J., and Wellby, M. L., A comparison of conventionally derived normal ranges with those obtained from patients' results Clin. Chim. Acta. 27:35-46 (1970).

20. O'Kell, R. T. and Elliott, J. R., Development of normal values for use in multitest biochemical screening of sera, Clin. Chem. 16:161-165 (1970).

21. Reed, A. H., Henry R. J., and Mason, W. B. Influence of statistical method used on the resulting estimate of normal range. Clin. Chem. 17:275-284 (1971).

22. Roberts, L. B. The normal ranges, with statistical analysis for seventeen blood constituents, Clin. Chim. Acta. 16:69-78 (1967).

23. Sunderman, F. W., Jr. and van Soestbergen, A. A. Laboratory Suggestions: Probability computations for clinical interpretations of screening tests. Amer. J. Clin. Path., 55:105-111 (1971).

24. Von Neumann, J., Kent, H., Bellinson, H., and Hart, B. F., Mean square successive difference, Anal. Math. Stat., 12:153 (1941).

25. Werner, M., Tolls, R. E., Hultin, J. V. and Mellecker, J., Influence of sex and age on the normal range of eleven serum constituents, Z. Klin. Chem. u. Klin. Biochem. 8:105-115 (1970).

26. Williams, G. Z., Young, D. S., Stein, M. R. and Cotlove, E., Biological and analytic components of variation in long-term studies of serum constituents in normal subjects I. Objectives, subject selection, laboratory procedures, and estimation of analytic deviation. Clin. Chem. 16:1016-1021 (1970).

DOCUMENTATION OF LABORATORY DATA

Table I

Selected Large Scale Multitest Surveys of Men and Women

Author	Population	Age Distribution	Number	Location	No. of Constituents	Reference
Cutler, et.al.	Outpatients	20-79	33,900	U.S. (Calif.)	8	4
Keating, et.al.	Ambulatory Individuals	20-80	576	U.S. (Minn.)	7	15
Werner, et.al.	Ambulatory Individuals	0-79	3,000	U.S. (Calif.)	11	25
O'Halloran, et.al.	Patients, Hospital Staff	Averages (22-51)	1,300	South Australia	12	19
Roberts, et.al.	Blood Donors	Adults	3,211	Great Britain	17	22
Kannel, et.al.	Framingham	30-62	5,100	U.S. (Mass.)	2	14
Cunnick, et.al.	White Collar Workers	18-65	2,300	U.S. (New York)	12	3
Hohnadel, et.al.	Industrial workers	41-65	25,100	U.S. and Canada	6	13

Table II

Fasting Glucose Concentrations in Serums from "Healthy" Men Versus All Men in Tested Population

Age (Years)	No. of Subjects	Percentiles*			
		50.0	95.0	97.5	99.5
41-45	2247/9449	100/101	116/118	120/123	133/157
46-50	1356/6293	102/102	120/122	126/132	148/200
51-55	695/3531	102/103	121/126	125/138	145/232
56-60	367/1973	104/104	126/131	134/146	152/249
61-65	142/853	104/104	122/133	127/148	136/258

* Units = mg/dl. Data for "healthy" men are in regular type; data for all men in population are in expanded type.

Table III

SGOT Activities in Serums from "Healthy" Men
Versus All Men in Tested Population

Age (Years)	No. of Subjects	Percentiles* 50.0	95.0	97.5	99.5
41-45	1901/7959	19/19	29/32	33/37	42/56
46-50	1140/5313	19/19	31/32	35/37	48/62
51-55	596/2982	19/19	29/32	34/37	44/55
56-60	305/1624	19/19	30/33	35/38	47/60
61-65	119/685	19/19	30/31	31/35	38/59

* Values are in Karmen units. Data for "healthy" men are in regular type; data for all men in population are in expanded type.

Table IV

Comparisons of Normal Values for Serum Constituents
in "Healthy" Men and Women, Age 41 to 45

Constituent	Percentiles* 2.5	50.0	97.5	Units	P**
Glucose (Fasting)	79/77	100/96	120/114	mg/dl	<0.001
SGOT	11/8	19/16	33/29	Karmen units	<0.001
LDH	68/63	99/98	139/143	Wacker units	N.S.
Cholesterol	148/150	205/211	283/284	mg/dl	N.S.
Uric Acid	4.2/2.4	6.1/4.4	8.7/6 5	mg/dl	<0.001
Urea Nitrogen	10/8	16/13	24/21	mg/dl	<0.001

*Data for men in regular type; data for women are in enlarged type.
**P = Probability of significance based on the median test, and Kolmogorov-Smirnov "two sample" test. N.S. = Not Significant.

Table V

THE SIGNIFICANCE OF THE INCREASING MEDIAN VALUES WITH ADVANCING AGE*

Constituent	Healthy Men	Healthy Women
Glucose (Fasting)	.01	.05
Urea Nitrogen	.01	.01
Uric Acid	NS	.01
Cholesterol	.05**	.01
LDH	.05	.01
SGOT	NS	.05

* Computed by the Von Neumann Ratio
** Omits 60 to 65 age group where trend is reversed.

Table VI

Normal Values for Healthy Men

Constituent	Age (Years)	Percentiles			
		5.0	95.0 *	97.5 **	99.5 ***
Glucose (Fasting) (mg/dl)	41-45	83	116	120	133
	46-55	85	120	126	147
	56-65	87	124	131	144
Urea Nitrogen (mg/dl)	41-45	11	22	24	27
	46-55	11	23	25	29
	56-65	11	24	26	31
LDH (Wacker units)	41-45	73	131	139	168
	46-55	74	135	145	169
	56-65	74	138	146	164
Cholesterol (mg/dl)	41-45	157	268	283	314
	46-55	162	269	282	326
	56-65	164	278	296	326
Uric Acid (mg/dl)	41-45	4.5	8.2	8.7	9.5
	46-55	4.5	8.2	8.7	9.5
	56-65	4.5	8.2	8.7	9.5
SGOT (karmen units)	41-45	12	30	33	42
	46-55	12	30	33	42
	56-65	12	30	33	42

*Values greater than the 95th percentile are denoted with one asterisk, greater than the 97.5th percentile are denoted with two asterisks and greater than the 99.5th percentile are denoted with three asterisks.

Table VII

Normal Values for Healthy Women

Constituent	Age (Years)	Percentile			
		5.0	* 95.0	** 97.5	*** 99.5
Glucose	41-45	81	112	115	123
(Fasting	46-55	82	113	118	124
(mg/dl)	56-65	86	116	120	127
Urea Nitrogen	41-45	9	21	24	28
(mg/dl)	46-55	11	23	26	30
	56-65	13	25	28	32
LDH	41-45	73	142	149	170
(Wacker units)	46-55	79	148	155	176
	56-65	85	154	161	182
Cholesterol	41-45	163	284	303	313
(mg/dl)	46-55	165	286	305	315
	56-65	167	289	307	318
Uric Acid	41-45	3.0	6.5	7.1	8.3
(mg/dl)	46-55	3.3	6.8	7.4	8.6
	56-65	3.6	7.1	7.7	8.9
SGOT	41-45	10	28	31	38
(Karmen units)	46-55	11	29	31	29
	56-65	13	30	33	40

*Values greater than the 95th percentile are denoted with one asterisk, greater than the 97.5th percentile are denoted with two asterisks and greater than the 99.5th percentile are denoted with three asterisks.

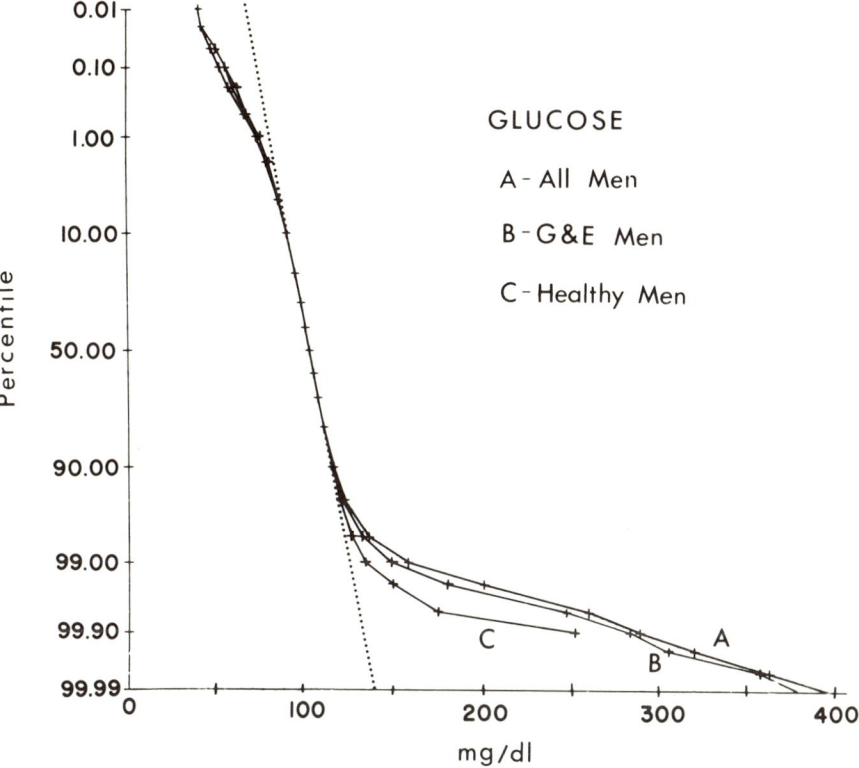

Figure 1 - Cumulative Percent Distribution of Glucose Concentrations for All Men.

The concentrations of serum glucose for subgroups of the population have been plotted as a cumulative percent distribution on a probability scale. The values given in curve A are for the entire population of men; curve B contains the values of those men who considered their health to be good or excellent; and curve C presents the values of those men judged to be apparently healthy.

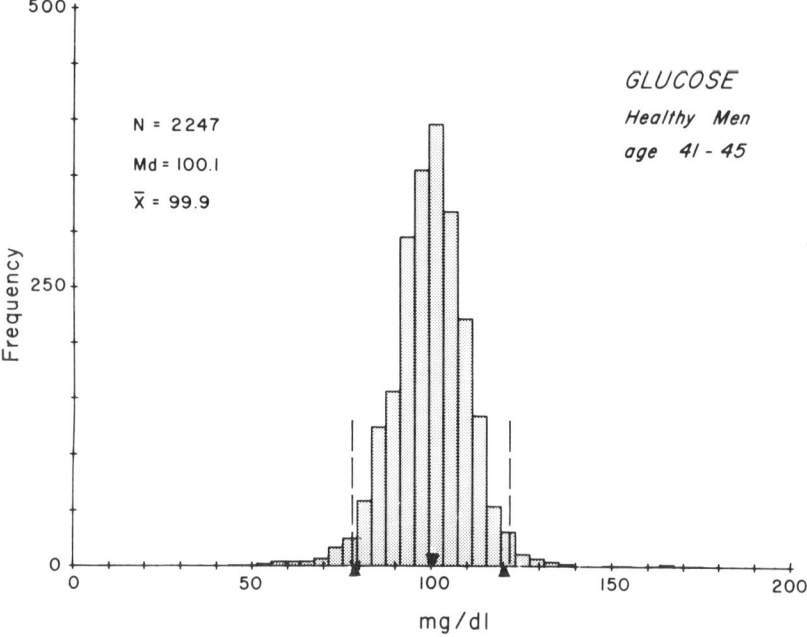

Figure 2 - Histogram of Serum Glucose Concentrations from Apparently Healthy Men.

The values of serum glucose concentration are presented for 2,247 healthy, fasting men, age 41 to 45 years. The median (Md) and mean (X̄) glucose concentrations for this age range were 100.1 and 99.9 mg/dl respectively. The vertical dashed lines designate the mean ± 2 S. D. and the lower triangles represent the 2.5th and 97.5th percentiles. The 50th percentile is indicated by the upper triangle. This figure is reprinted by permission, from Hohnadel et. al. (13).

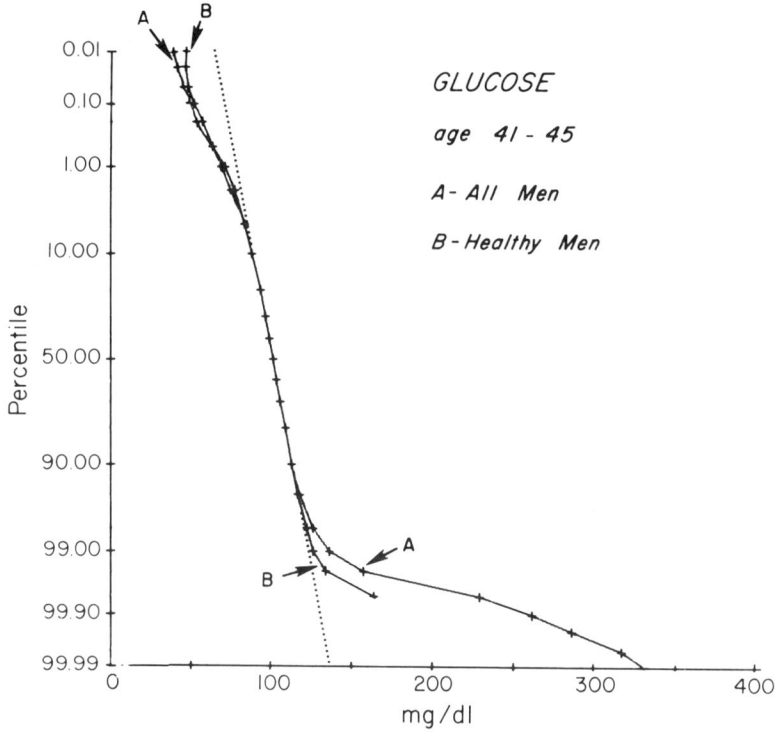

Figure 3 - Cumulative Percent Distribution of Glucose Concentrations for Men.

The values of serum glucose concentration are presented in curve A for 9,449 fasting men, age 41 to 45 years. The values obtained for the 2,247 healthy, fasting men in this age range are given in curve B. The results of an arithmetic Gaussian distribution are presented as a series of dots at the tails of the other distributions. This figure is reprinted, by permission,

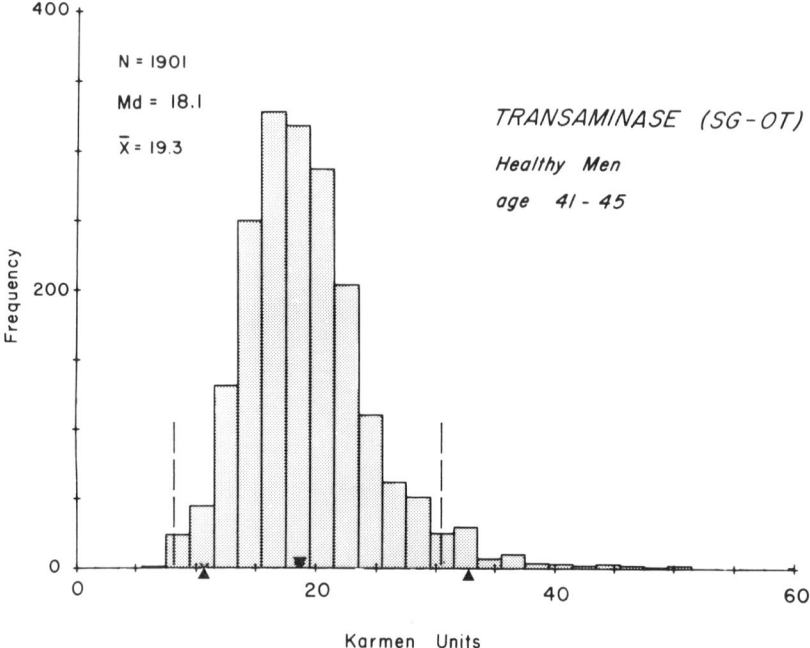

Figure 4 - Histogram of Serum SGOT Activity from Apparently Healthy Men,

The values of serum SGOT activity are presented for 1,901 healthy men, age 41 to 45. The median (Md) and mean ($\bar{X}$) SGOT activities for this age range were 18.1 and 19.3 Karmen units, respectively. The vertical dashed lines designate the mean $\pm$ 2 S. D. and the lower trangles represent the 2.5th and 97.5th percentiles. The 50th percentile is indicated by the upper triangle. This figure is reprinted, by permission, from Hohnadel, et. al. (13).

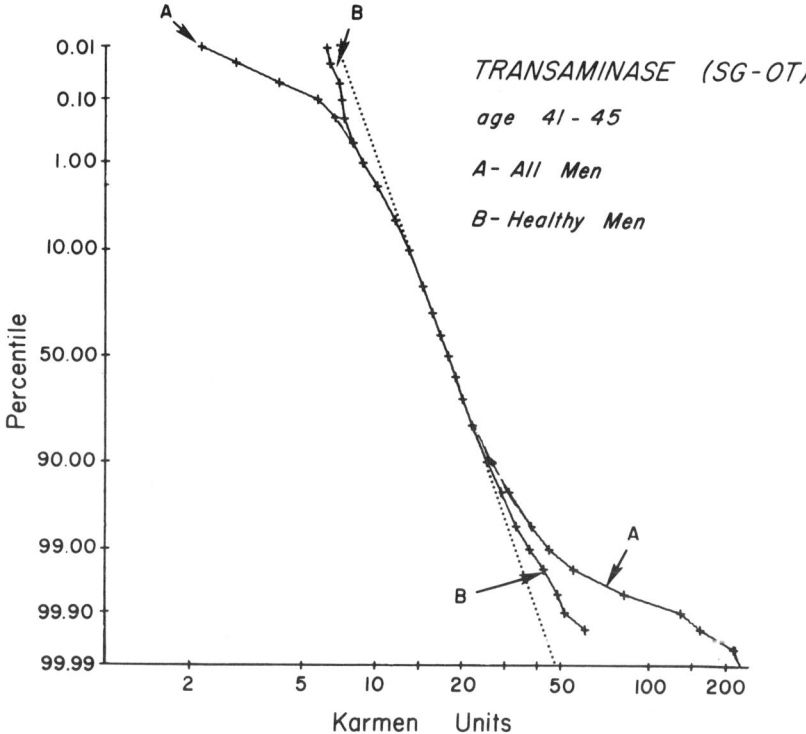

Figure 5 - Cumulative Percent Distribution of SGOT Activities for Men.

The values of serum SGOT activity are presented in curve A for 7,959 men, age 41 to 45 years. The values obtained for 1,901 healthy men in this age range are given in curve B. The abscissa is a logarithmic scale expressed in Karmen units. The results of a logarithmic Gaussian distribution are presented as a series of dots at the tails of the other distributions. This figure is reprinted, by permission, from Hohnadel, et. al. (13).

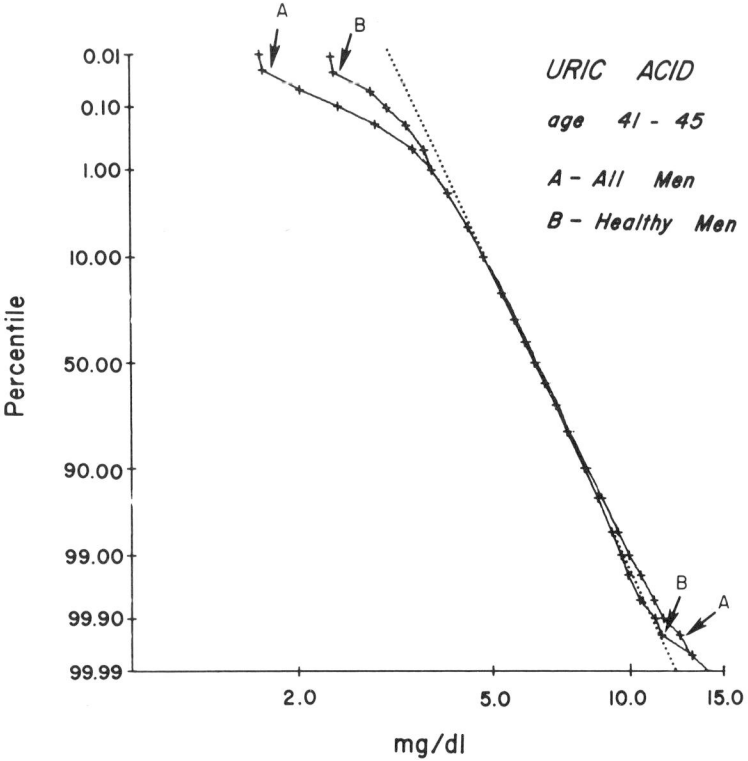

Figure 6 - Cumulative Percent Distribution of Uric Acid Concentrations for Men.

The values of serum uric acid concentrations are presented in curve A for 9,462 men, age 41 to 45 years. The values obtained for 2,247 healthy men in this age range are given in curve B. The abscissa is a logarithmic scale expressed in mg/dl. The results of a logarithmic Gaussian distribution are presented as a series of dots at the tails of the other distributions. This figure is reprinted, by permission, from Hohnadel, et.al. (13).

DOCUMENTATION OF LABORATORY DATA

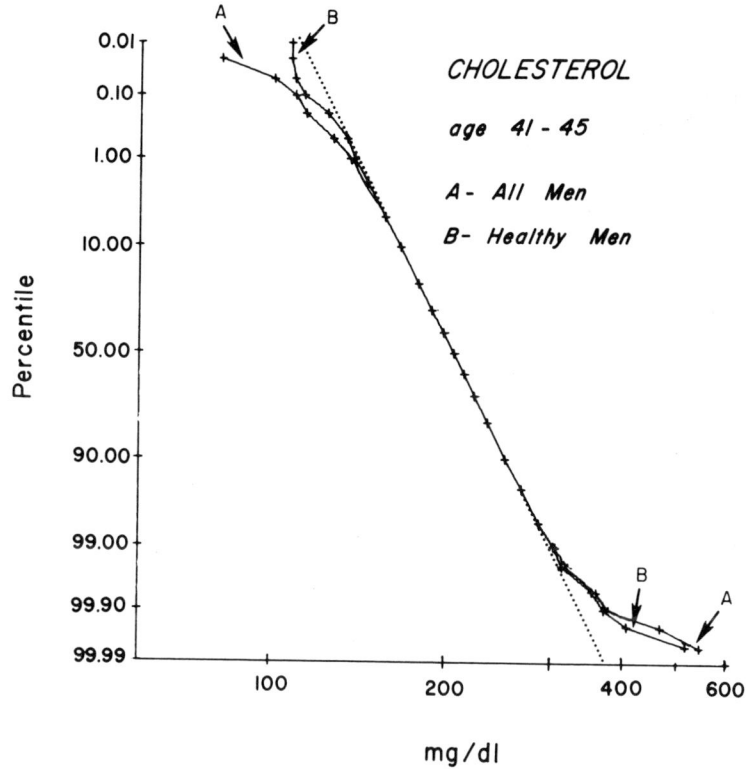

Figure 7 - Cumulative Percent Distribution of Cholesterol Concentrations for Men.

The values of serum cholesterol concentrations are presented in curve A for 9,289 men, age 41 to 45 years. The values obtained for 2,215 healthy men in this age range are given in curve B. The abscissa is expressed as a logarithmic scale in mg/dl. The results of a logarithmic Gaussian distribution are presented as a series of dots at the tails of the other distributions. This figure is reprinted, by permission, from Hohnadel et. al. (13).

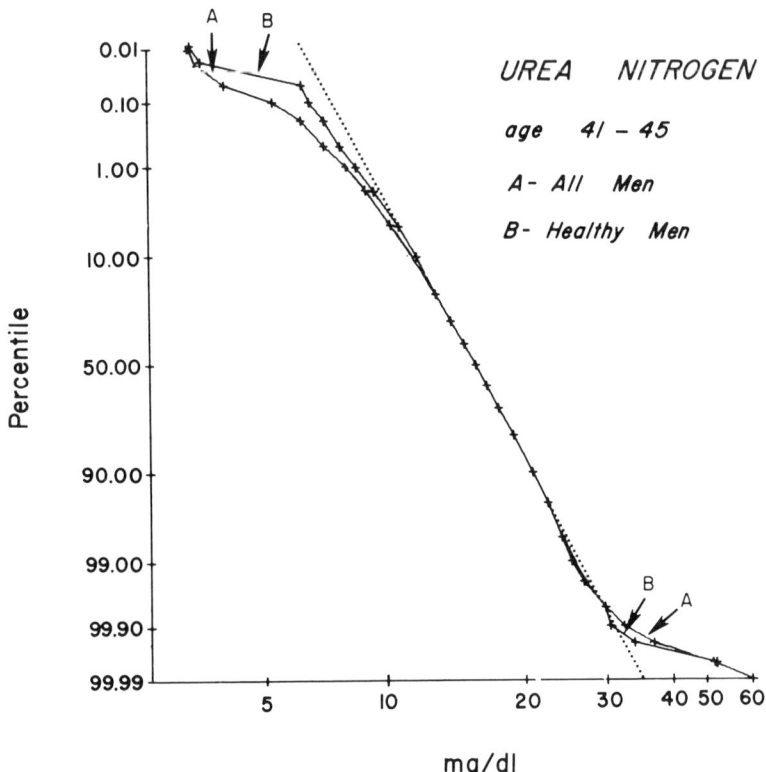

Figure 8 - Cumulative Percent Distribution of Urea Nitrogen Concentrations for Men.

The values of serum urea nitrogen concentrations are presented in curve A for 9,462 men, age 41 to 45 years. The values obtained for 2,247 healthy men in this age range are given in curve B. The abscissa is expressed as a logarithmic scale. The results of a logarithmic Gaussian distribution are presented as a series of dots at the tails of the other distributions. This figure is reprinted, by permission, from Hohnadel, et.al. (13).

DOCUMENTATION OF LABORATORY DATA

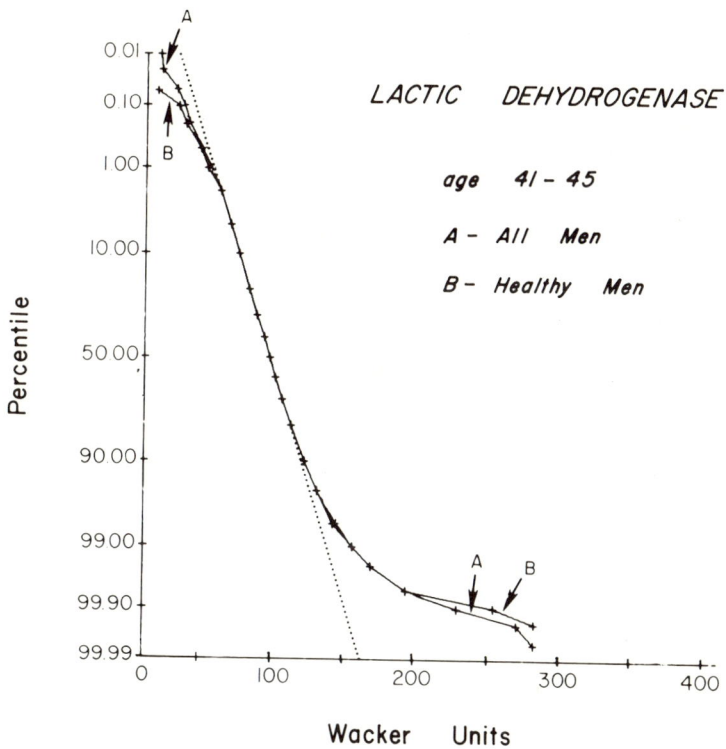

Figure 9 - Cumulative Percent Distribution of Lactic Dehydrogenase Activity for Men.

The values of serum lactic dehydrogenase activity are presented in curve A for 7,953 men, age 41 to 45 years. The values obtained for 1,905 healthy men in this age range are given in curve B. The results of an arithmetic Gaussian distribution are presented as a series of dots at the tails of the other distributions. This figure is reprinted by permission, from Hohnadel, et. al. (13).

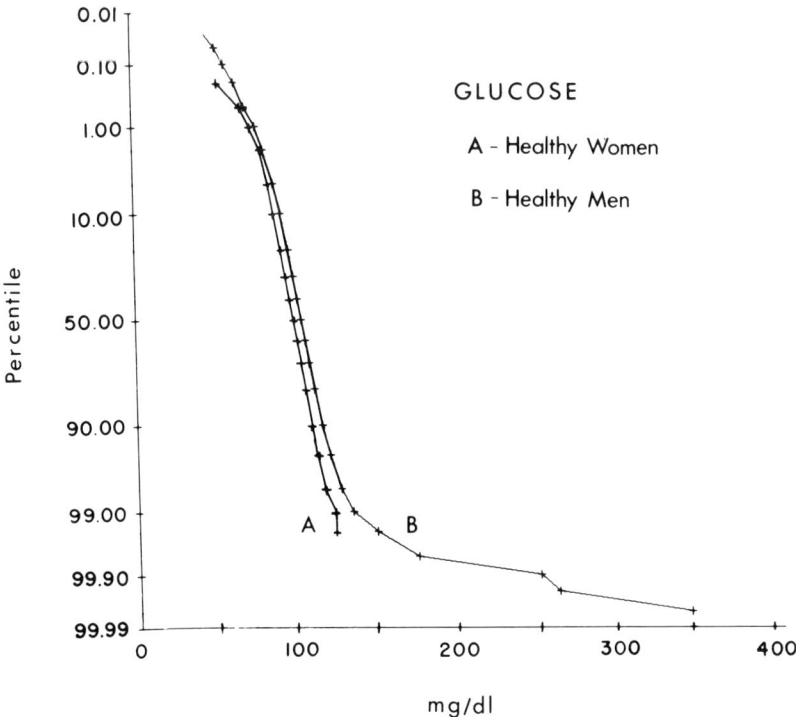

Figure 10 - Cumulative Percent Distributions of Glucose Concentrations for Healthy Men and Women.

The values of serum glucose given in curve A are for the entire population of healthy women. The values given in curve B are for the entire population of healthy men.

A DISCUSSION OF SOME ESTIMATION PROBLEMS ENCOUNTERED IN ESTABLISHING "NORMAL VALUES"

Lila Elveback, Ph. D.

The general subject of statistical methods for laboratory data would be appropriate for a three-day symposium of this sort. My assigned topic is necessarily limited to a few rather specific problems.

As a result I shall omit further reference to laboratory error, both short and long term, true physiologic variation within the individual both in terms of diurnal and circadian rhythm, and long-term changes associated with season, diet, or other factors. Further I shall omit consideration of geographic variation and proceed under the tacit assumption that we all agree that "norms" should be local.

Most of the discussion will center about variability between persons, although at the close I have a few words to say about intralaboratory differences.

I shall begin with the simplest of the problems and leave the importance of age and sex differences for later consideration.

Problem I

Given a list of numbers which result from running a lab test on n healthy persons, what shall we do in response to a request for so-called "normal values"? Dr. Gabrieli has asked us for practical solutions rather than academic theorizing. I will attempt to comply. However, it is impossible to know what to do without considering what it is we wish to accomplish. Obviously the basic purpose is to give the clinician information which will assist him in interpreting the results of the lab test in question. What information shall we give him? The fact that "normal values" have been requested suggests that this information should consist of some estimates of the 2.5 percent point and the 97.5 percent point of the distribution of values in healthy persons. I agree that the information needed concerns the distribution of values in healthy persons, but why the 2.5 and 97.5 percentiles? There are arguments pro and con.

The chief argument in favor of giving the 2.5 and 97.5 percentile points goes something like this: "Why not? Another and equally arbitrary selection of percentile points, such as 5, and 95% have no obvious advantages. Besides, clinicians are accustomed to the 2.5 and 97.5 points, are used to working with them, and are expecting them. If you give them some other points they will probably treat them as bracketing the central 95% of healthy persons no matter what you say."

The chief argument against giving the 2.5 and 97.5 percent points is that this is far too little information. I will come back to this point since I regard it as critical. For the moment, however, let us direct our attention to the problem of estimating the 2.5 and 97.5 points of the distribution in healthy persons. There are three methods of procedure which deserve attention.

The first, which is appropriate when n is small, is to recognize that the information at hand is inadequate for estimation of the required percentiles. Until such a time as an adequate number of healthy persons have contributed test values, any questions about the distribution in healthy persons must receive an answer such as "Well I don't really know, I only have 47 values, and so that I can hardly guess about the shape of the distribution, let alone any percentiles out in the tails. In the meantime, here are my 47 values." I not only propose this procedure quite seriously and use it frequently, but hold that there is no admissable alternative if estimates of the 2.5 and 97.5 percentiles are really what is wanted.

The next question, of course, is how big an n do you need before it is all right to start estimating? In the April, 1971 issue of <u>Clinical Chemistry</u>, Reed, Henry, and Mason[1] of Bioscience Labs propose n = 120 as a minimum. I don't have any other numbers to propose because I believe that the question of how large the sample must be cannot be divorced from the question of what accuracy is needed in the estimates. Since the accuracy needed in the estimates depends crucially on what test we are talking about, I reject the concept that any such adequate sample size exists. Another way of saying it is "All generalizations are false - including this one". The education, wisdom, and experience of a well-trained statistician as part of a collaborative effort with medical colleagues must be directed to one specific problem at a time. On the whole, I regard 120 as rather small.

The other two procedures to be considered are methods of estimation of the required percentile points by

(a) $\bar{x} \pm 2s_x$, a procedure which is far too widely used, since it usually gives the wrong answer,

(b) by the corresponding sample percentiles, a non-parametric method which has the advantage that, on the average, it gives the correct answer.

Let us consider the first procedure, that is the use of the estimate $\bar{x} \pm 2s_x$ which involves the assumption that the distribution is Gaussian (or normal). Dr. Mainland, in his guest editorial in the April, 1971 issue of <u>Clinical Chemistry</u> [2] says, "In the world of real (nongaussian) distributions, the obviously preferable tool is the percentile tool, and it strikes me as odd that, 13 years after the publication of Herrera's article, (3) this problem of choice between the percentile tool and the Gaussian tool should persist." It is almost a century since it was realized that, while the gaussian error curve is appropriate, as Gauss proposed, as a description of the random errors asssociated with repeated measurements made on the same physical object, it is not adequate for the description of physiologic measurements made on different people. Nor did Gauss ever propose that it was. However, the myth persists in the medical sciences along with another equally mistaken idea concerning the standard deviation. The statement that "the mean $\pm$ 1.96 σ's contains the central 95% of the frequency" is a statement about a property of the Gaussian error curve, not about the standard deviation. For example, if we consider magnesium in adult males, the 2.5 and 97.5 percentiles are approximately 1.7 o's below and 2.3 o's above the mean. If we pool the male and female distributions they lie at approximately 2 o's below and 2.7 o's above the mean. It is a sad fact that the estimate $\bar{x} \pm 2s_x$ is, in general, not a good estimate. If we cannot assume that the distribution is the Gaussian normal distribution, then we have no clue as to what percentages will be cut off in the two tails by $\bar{x} - 2s_x$. It takes a great deal of evidence (a very large n) to demonstrate that the distribution is well enough approximated by the normal curve (including the tails of the distribution) to justify the use of the $\bar{x} \pm 2s_x$ estimate. It is, on the other hand, precisely when n is small, say 47, that the $\bar{x} \pm 2s_x$ is inviting, possibly on the grounds that a bad estimate is better than none. It should be remembered that while getting good estimates is very difficult, getting rid of bad ones may be even more difficult.

Figure 1 shows six distributions that have exactly the same mean and standard deviations. In only one of these (the top one) can $\bar{x} \pm 2s_x$ estimate be expected to cut off 2.5 percent in each tail.

Figure 2 illustrates the point that, in the presence of non-normality, skewness or kurtosis, the Gaussian estimates do not, on the average, give the right answer since they are biased.

Consider the problem of estimating P_{95} in sampling from the X_9^2 distribution. The 95th percentile is 16.9. In 100 samples of size 100 the average value of the appropriate Gaussian estimate, $\bar{x} + 1.645\ s_x$ was 15.9, which is the 93rd percentile.

The standard error this estimate (which is a measure of how far away from its own average value the estimate is apt to be) is 0.13. If on the other hand we use the mean square error, (which is a measure of how far away from the right answer the estimate is apt to be) we get a corrected SE, appropriate when the estimate is biased as in this case, of 1.01, almost eight times as large.

Alkaline phosphatase is highly skewed to the right. The skewness can be seen in the next figure. However, if we sample repeatedly from this distribution with n = 50, only 40% of our samples will show skewness detectable by the test at the 5% level. If n = 100, the probability of failing to detect skewness is still 20%. The fact that non-normality is not detectable in your data (by any standard test) is not at all reassuring for n's of the order of 100 or less.

Question: Will the logarithm transform cure the ills? probably not. It may make matters worse and you can't tell without very large n's.

Conclusion: First, we have become accustomed to sample size requirements for the estimation of means. We must recognize and remember that the sample sizes required for estimation of percentiles in the tails are many times greater. Second, the sample percentiles are the safest and most logical estimates of the population percentiles.

Part 2 - Age and Sex

Problem 2

In a study of Dr. Raymond Keating [5], seven biochemical variables were considered. In all except one there were differences between males and females. Of the 14 regressions on age, only three were not significant. In 11 of the 14 problems, it was necessary to consider the scatter of the points about the regression line for males and females separately.

Figure 4 shows the distribution of serum calcium in healthy males. Here the sample size is N = 298. While the distribution of calcium values in males is skewed the distribution of the residuals (the vertical distances of the points to the regression line) is not detectable non-normally. In this case for the estimates of the age specific 97.5 percentile we used a line, parallel to the regression line and two residual standard deviations above it, that is $y + 2s_{y.x}$. And here is the Gaussian assumption to which I have been so valuably opposed. In this case, (n = 298) there is some justification for using it. More on this subject in a moment. While this slide is on, I would like to comment on the confidence interval shown for the line given by $y + 2s_{y.x}$. This has been constructed [3] by allowing for sampling variability in both y, the regression line and in $s_{y.x}$ the standard deviation of the residuals. Note that no allowance is made for the contribution of whatever undetected non-normality exists in the distribution of the residual.

Since the article by Reed [1] et. al. in the April, 1971 issue of Clinical Chemistry discusses the use of tolerance intervals as estimates of the percentiles, I would like to point out that the tolerance interval estimates are equivalent to the outer dotted lines and represent an attempt to assure ourselves that at least 95% of the frequency is included between them, or that not more than 5% is excluded. This represents an attempt to protect ourselves against false positives. Since a false positive on a single lab result is unlikely to result in any action more decisive than ordering further tests, I believe this is exactly the wrong approach. If I had to choose, I would elect the inner dotted lines and thus protect myself against the false negative or failure to detect some incipient disease state. Luckily we don't have to choose. We can have the hopefully unbiased estimate and its confidence interval. I am happy to say that Reed and co-authors also reject the tolerance interval approach in the case of normal values.

Now to look at the question of why I don't stick to my guns and insist on using percentile estimates in that regression on age problem. Figure 5 shows the regression of serum urea on age in the same 298 healthy males. In this example it is the 95th percentile we are estimating. To use the sample percentile method, we must divide the 298 into age subclasses and our answers, of course, will depend on which divisions we use. I have chosen decades 20-29, 30-39, etc. for which the n values drop to 67, 77, 61, 54, and 39 over age 60. Again the distribution of the residuals shows no significant non-normality. However, this does not really justify the use of the Gaussian estimate given by the upper solid line. Despite this fact, I have adopted it because I believe that the 95th percentile must be some smooth function of age and that it is only logical to estimate it as some smooth function. It may not be linear, it is true, but I don't have enough data to justify some other smooth function. The nonparametric estimates are erratic, and I find the jagged function they give just too illogical to accept. You may have reservations about accepting the straight line Gaussian estimate, and I do too. On the basis of an n of 298,

this is the best I know how to do, and I recognize that
my estimate may have error larger than that given by
the dotted lines and that this will be true if (1) the residuals are non-normal or (2) the true function is nonlinear.

Problem 3

So far we have discussed methods of estimating the
2.5 and 97.5 percentiles. I would like now to come to
the question of whether or not this is the information
which should be given to the physician.

I hold that we can do a lot better. As a medical statistician I cannot believe that life is so simple, patients so
much alike, the meaning of different laboratory tests
so similar, the cost of failure to diagnose different diseases so much the same, and different physicians so
much alike, that one single percentile, whatever it will
be, will suffice. Is it true that a serum iron below the
2 1/2% point in a 25 year old woman, a serum calcium
above the 97.5% point in a 70 year old man, a sweat
sodium just at the 97.5 in a 9 year old child all represent the same indication for further testing, watching,
and checking? Besides, how much below, how much
above? With our present method of communication with
the physician, he can't tell unless he has made a special
study on the test in question.

In a sense, in giving him only the 2 1/2 and 97 1/2%
points, we are limiting his privilege to use a 90% critical point on one patient on one test and a 99% point on
another patient on another test.

For example, our "norms" on serum calcium in adults
are 8.9 to 10.1. How can we interpret a serum calcium
of 9.9? It is 2 mg./100ml. below 10.1. But how unusual
is this in "healthy adults"? All we know from the
"norms" is that more than 2 1/2% of healthy adults have
calciums this high or higher. How much more than

DOCUMENTATION OF LABORATORY DATA

2 1/2%? It turns out that, in males, the answer depends on the age of the patient. For age 20, 18% of healthy males have calciums of 9.9 or above, while at age 70 only 2% have calcium values of 9.9 or above. In adult women, the answer need not be age specific, the corresponding percent this high is 8%. In the opinion of the large majority of my colleagues this type of information would be of great value to the clinician. The problem is one of communication between the laboratory and the clinician. A solution must be one which makes this type of information readily available to him without added demands either on his memory or his time.

First, let us look at the fairly obvious solution. In all laboratories, a report goes to the physician. It might say, for example, John Doe:
PO_4 = 4.0 mg./100ml. or Mrs. F. Smith:
PO_4 = 4.0 mg./100ml.

If, instead of this the report says:

    Mr. John Doe   Male   Age: 60
    Serum inorganic phosphorus <u>4.0 mg./100ml</u>
    Percentile for this patient <u>97</u>

and

    Mrs. F. Smith   Female   Age: 70
    Serum inorganic phosphorus <u>4.0mg./100ml</u>
    Percentile for this patient <u>69</u>

the physician is presented with the information relevant to each patient at the time he needs it. This information can be univariate or multivariate and can include information on the discriminant function when a single alternative is involved.

Dr. J. D. Jones of the Mayo Clinic has prepared the following figure which shows sweat sodium values for healthy persons, for those with cystic fibrosis, and six patients whose values fall into the "grey zone" between the healthy and the cystic fibrosis. A report to the physician which represents his patient by a red x superimposed on this graph would, I believe, constitute an excellent report. The graph not only gives the relative position of the patient with respect to the two populations, but also shows the number of persons in each of the two groups on whom we have data, so that the physician would know that in the case of sweat sodium a careful study based on a large number of healthy persons has been carried out.

This method gives the physician a great deal more information than the current norms. It does so without asking him for any additional memory work, in fact it relieves him of remembering, or looking up, a lot of so-called norms. It not only leaves him free to use his clinical judgement for each patient, for each test, to choose the appropriate critical percentage, but it gives him the quantitative information he must have to do so optimally.

The examples here have been univariate, but the same method can be used on the discriminant function to give, for any patient, his position relative to the healthy.

This proposal is simple to grasp both for the physician and the laboratory. Its implementation demands the background of the measurements on a large number of carefully checked healthy persons that was discussed earlier.

Problem 4

Who are the so-called healthy and how can we get information about them?

I realize that any definition of health must contain arbitrary elements and fall far short of perfection. I am not unduly impressed by this argument. I believe that for any specific study a protocol can be written defining eligibility which, as properly documented, can give useful results. I have never, for example, heard any criticism of the protocol used by Dr. Keating [4]. The problem of how the protocol should be written is a medical one. I will confine myself to saying that it should be well documented.

I have also been assigned the task of discussing the question of how information on the distribution of values for healthy individuals can be obtained. I have already expressed myself somewhat vigorously on the subject [5]. I consider it to be self evident that to obtain information on the healthy we must identify some large number n of healthy persons and study them. The fact that this is difficult, time consuming, and expensive is beside the point. This is the price tag on the information we want and all the wishful thinking in the world will not change it.

I will summarize briefly my conclusions [5] concerning the Hoffman method of attempting to extract from routine laboratory records information concerning the unidentified healthy persons included. This method is based on certain assumptions which Hoffman himself has characterized as untested. The assumptions are:

(1) the distribution in healthy persons is Gaussian (or a normal curve)

(2) the distribution in the ill is Gaussian

(3) the mean for the healthy is given by the mode of the entire lab load distribution

(4) the standard deviation for the healthy can be estimated from the total distribution.

First: Not one of these assumptions has any support whatsoever from logic, mathematics, or biological fact.

Second: Since Hoffman's statement about the unknown truth of the assumptions they have been adequately tested by several investigators, (5, 6, 7, 8) and each in turn has been shown to be contrary to fact.

Third: It has also been adequately demonstrated that the method doesn't work and that it can lead to serious errors.

I have already devoted enough time to the assumption concerning the Gaussian distribution in the healthy. Let me point out that the assumption is even more disasterous when applied to the highly nonhomogeneous collection of ill persons.

The assumption which states that the mean of the distribution for the healthy is given by the mode of the laboratory distribution is profoundly disturbing from a logical point of view. It is obvious that the relationship between the distribution in the healthy and the total laboratory distribution depends in large part on what proportion of the laboratory load is made up of healthy persons. And yet we are asked to accept this assumption for screening tests such as hemoglobin and white counts on the one hand and for serum iron, copper, and zinc on the other. It is not surprising that these assumptions do not perform well in practice.

Problem 5

Statisticians cause and create problems too - partly because of their training, and partly because they are constantly asked to evaluate precision and discover which of two methods are more precise. As a result, they frequently find the lack of precision in certain laboratory methods distrubing. They may, for example, give undue importance to the fact that a differential white count based on counting 200 cells does not have a very great precision.

Recently our laboratory set out to determine what the results of a rule based on differentials based on a 100 cell count would be if the following safeguards were built in: Count 200 cells if the WBC is abnormal or the result of the first 100 is abnormal. With these safeguards the only error of concern was that the first 100 cells would fail to detect an abnormality apparent in 200. In two weeks, using the entire lab load, we had 1,775 tests in which the WBC was normal. In 370 of these, the 200 count was abnormal by a very strict application of our current norms. Among these, we found 80 cases in which the 100 cell count would have been reported as normal. We proceeded to print out the 100 counts, the 200 count, and the WBC for these 80 cases.

The majority of cases in which the 100 and 200 cell counts disagreed as to classification as normal or abnormal represented trivial differences, such as 79% and 81% neutrophils. We submitted the entire list to a panel of clinicians who unanimously characterized all of the differences as trivial. The study continues. It appears that the question is not one of numerical evaluation of the precision of the proposed rule, but whether or not the precision is such as to fulfill the needs defined by current clinical know-how in interpretation of moderate departures from stipulated "norms" for differential white counts. It is of real interest to ask, however, whether the limitations of clinical know-how have, at least in some part, been imposed by the limitations of the precision of the data the laboratory has been giving them. Is it possible, for example, that when we have a Technicon which does differentials based on 10,000 cells that clinical meaning of at least some of these moderate departures from "normal" will become apparent? It remains to be seen.

Problem 7

I have also been asked to discuss the question of what can be done to help the small laboratory that cannot afford to identify and study a large number of healthy persons.

Is it possible that a small laboratory can attach itself to a reference laboratory in a nearby large city, and by some calibration procedure, earn the right to use their "norms"? This idea received some attention at the May 1970 Washington, D.C. meeting sponsored by the National Research Council. I was interested and I set out to get some data. I have very little such data, but what I have is not encouraging. First we did a very small study with Dr. Benson at the University of Minnesota on serum calcium. The results, shown in Figure 7 were encouraging. But the problem is not one for two large reference laboratories both using the atomic absorption method. The laboratory of our local community hospital which uses the flurometric method was kind enough to send us their samples for duplicate measurement. The results shown in Figure 8 are very discouraging. At present, a large part of their calcium test load is being checked by our laboratory. The small laboratory often has a number of factors working against it which may include less than optimum equipment and training of technicians. In addition, the basic problem of the small laboratory is present - small volume, resulting in sporadic experience, which in turn results in problems of keeping the procedure in control.

The amount of information I have on the small laboratory is extremely limited. What I have has led me to the conclusion that the small laboratory problem is, at least in some instances, one in which statistical methods

DOCUMENTATION OF LABORATORY DATA

can contribute very little until more basic problems are solved.

In conclusion, while I have discussed methods of estimation of specific percentiles which are to serve as "norms", I am basically opposed to use of norms, basically opposed to the suggested dichotomy of "normal" and "abnormal". I believe that little defense can be made for presenting the clinician with such oversimplified, predigested, and censored information. In presenting to the clinician, along with each laboratory report, the patient's percentile rank among the healthy (and if we know it his percentile rank among patients with a specific allerative disease) we can help him use his clinical judgement optimally with respect to a particular patient rather than forcing him to be content with the small glimpse at reality provided by the so-called norms.

Bibliography

1. Reed, A. H., Henry, R. J., and Mason W. B.: Influence of statistical method used on the resulting estimate of normal range. Clin. Chem. 17(4):275-284, April, 1971.

2. Mainland, D.: Remarks on clinical "norms". Clin. Chem., 17(4): 267-274, April, 1971.

3. Herrera, L.: The precision of percentiles in establishing normal limits in medicine. J. Lab. Clin. Med., 52:34-42, 1958.

4. Elveback, L. R. and Taylor, W. F.: Statistical methods of estimating percentiles. Annals of the N. Y. Acad. of Sciences, 161:538-548, September 30, 1969.

5. Keating, F. R., Jr., Jones, J. D., Elveback, L. R., and Randall, R. V.: The relation of age and sex to distribution of values in healthy adults of serum calcium, inorganic phosphorus, magnesium, alkaline phosphatase, total proteins, albumin, and blood urea. J. Lab. Clin. Med., 73(5):825-834, May, 1969.

6. Elveback, L. R., Guillier, C. L., and Keating, F. R., Jr.: Health, normality, and the ghost of Gauss. J. Am. Med. Assoc., 211:69-75, January 5, 1970.

7. O'Halloran, M. W., Studley-Ruxton, J., and Wellby, M. L.: A comparison of conventionally derived normal ranges with those obtained from patients' results. Clinica Chimica Acta, 27:35-46, 1970.

8. Van Pennen, H. J., and Lindberg, D. A. B.: The limitations of laboratory quality control with reference to the "number plus" method. Am. J. Clin. Path., 44(3):322-330, September, 1965.

9. Amador, E. and Hsu, B. P.: Indirect methods for estimating the normal range. Am. J. Clin. Path. 52:538-546, November, 1969.

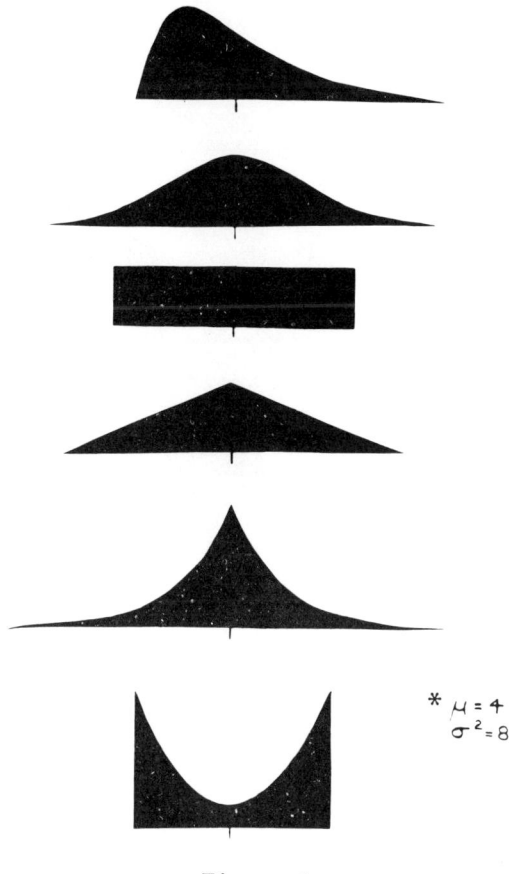

* $\mu = 4$
$\sigma^2 = 8$

Figure 1

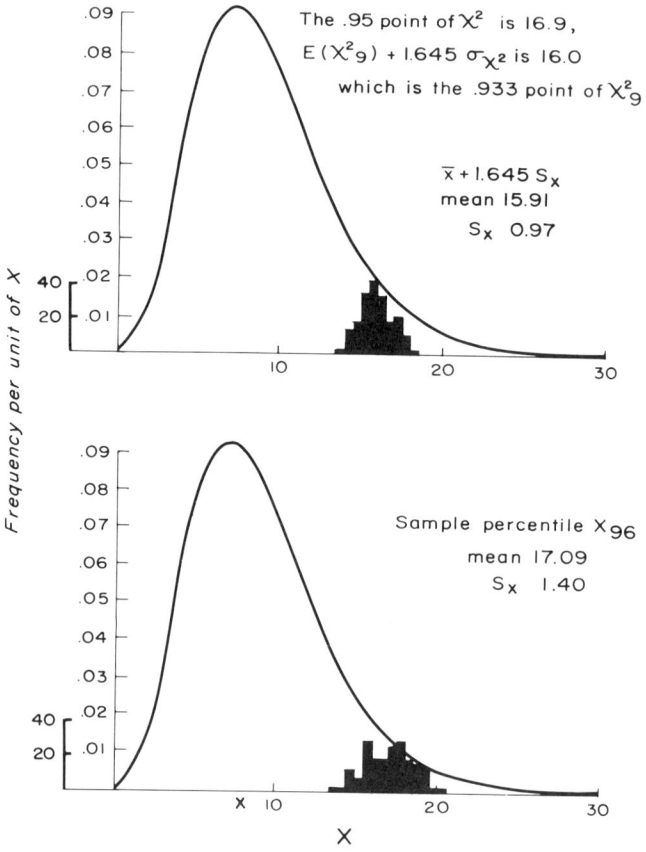

Figure 2

DOCUMENTATION OF LABORATORY DATA

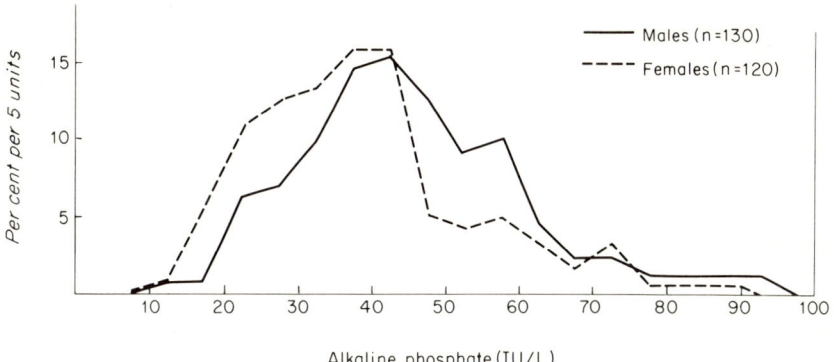

Figure 3

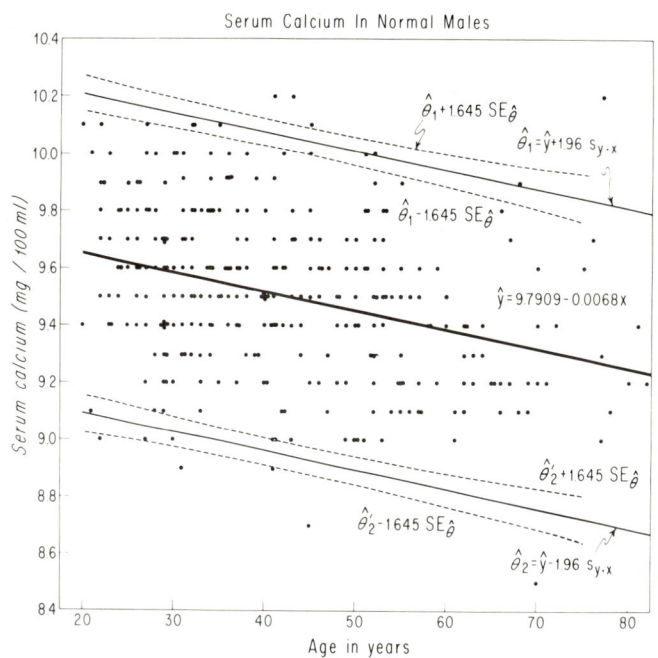

Figure 4

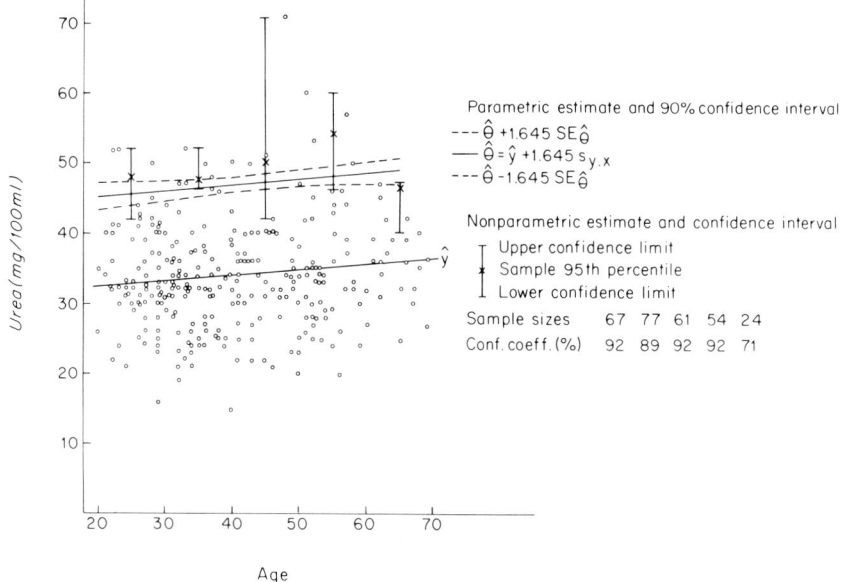

Figure 5

DOCUMENTATION OF LABORATORY DATA

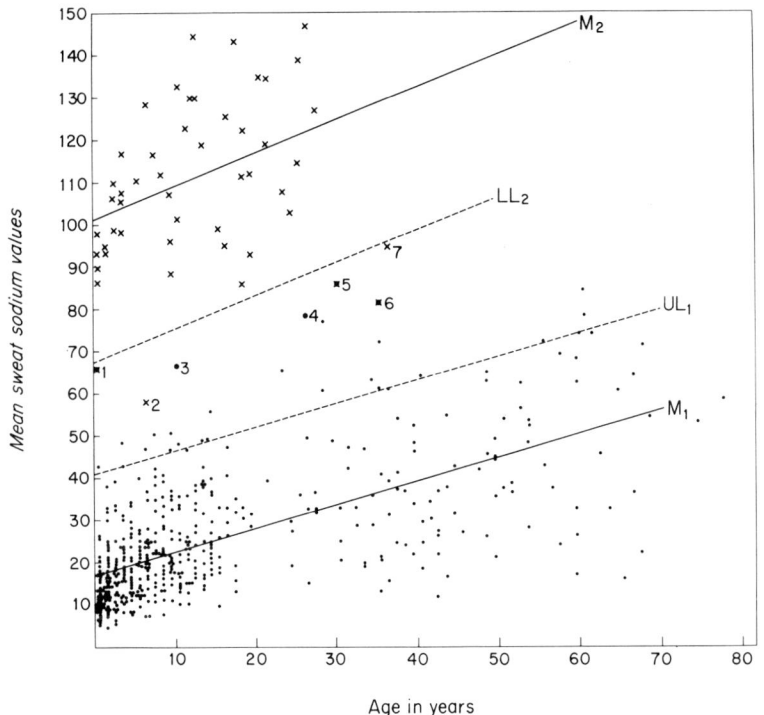

Figure 6

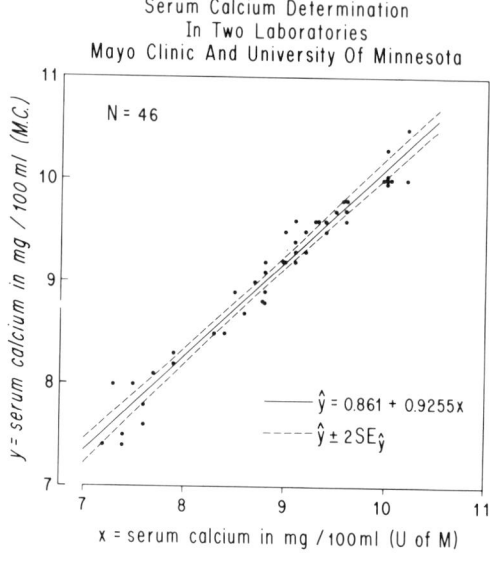

Figure 7

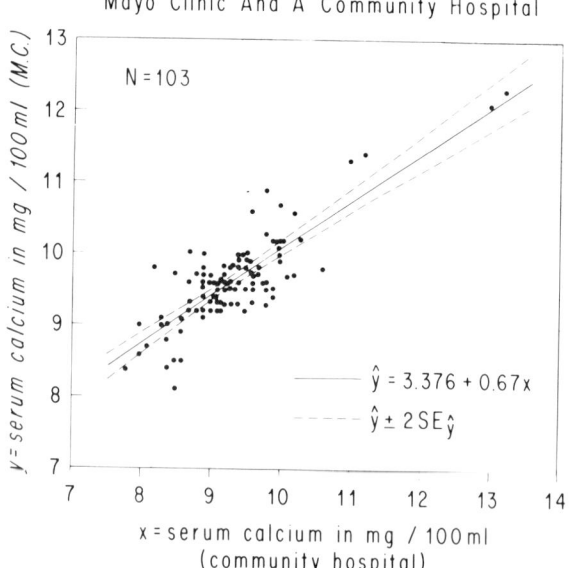

Figure 8

EVALUATION OF CLINICAL LABORATORY COMPUTERS

Chairman: Marion J. Ball
Panel: Paul R. Finley, The Fairview Hospitals
Sidney A. Goldblatt, Conemaugh Valley
Memorial Hospital
L. E. Loveless, Clinical Laboratories of
St. Louis
William W. McLendon, The Moses Cone
Memorial Hospital
David Seligson, Yale University School of
Medicine
Wellington B. Stewart, University of Missouri
School of Medicine
Thomas O. Swallen, North Memorial Hospital

*I would like to gratefully acknowledge the assistance of Barbara A. Heisler in the preparation and editing of the material contained in this section.

MARION J. BALL

Introduction

The introduction of computing techniques has opened up a vast array of new possibilities for the expansion and improvement of the services which the pathologist can render. It also has deepened his insight in many problems. Scope and nature of this influence of computer science should, I feel, be assessed within the framework of the history of pathology in the United States. This history covers less than a century; its beginning is linked with the life's work of William Henry Welch (1850-1934), "the Dean of American Medicine," as Simon and James Thomas Flexner have called him. At the age of twenty-seven, Welch sailed for a study trip to German, "a voyage of exploration that was in its results perhaps the most important event taken by an American doctor." This is how the story was put in 1937 by Henry Sigerist, Welch's successor as Professor of the History of Medicine at John Hopkins University Medical School.

On his arrival in Europe in April, 1877, Welch decided to go to Breslau to work under Professor Julius Cohnheim who accepted and came to like the young American. The liking was mutual as the following passage indicates. It is part of a letter written by Welch to his father shortly after his first meeting with Cohnheim:

"It is not enough for Cohnheim to know that congestion of the kidney follows heart disease or that hypertrophy of the heart follows contraction of the kidney, or that atheroma occurs in old age, he is constantly inquiring why does it occur under these circumstances. The result is that Cohnheim has taken for his special studies such common subjects as inflammation, dropsy, embolism, and through his investigations these have become perhaps the only subjects in pathology in which our knowledge approaches in exactness what is known concerning physical or chemical process."

It was at Cohnheim's recommendation that Welch received his appointment at Johns Hopkins where he is remembered as one of the "Four Doctors", together with Osler, Kelly, and Halsted.

In 1897 when his reputation as a pathologist was firmly established, Welch delivered his great paper on "Adaptation in Pathological Processes," before the Congress of American Physicians and Surgeons in Philadelphia. In this paper he reviewed Cohnheim's teachings which have ever since remained alive in the United States.

During Welch's long life, the science of pathology expanded by leaps and bounds. Biochemistry, biophysics, and biomathematics became satellite branches of pathology. In turn, biostatistics developed as a quasi-independent branch of biomathematics.

A common denominator of the advancement of pathology thus engendered was that more and more observed phenomena became amenable to measurement. The axiom first pronounced in 1888 by the great British mathematician, James Cleark Maxwell, that "one of the main functions of science is the measurement of quantities" was applied at an increasing scale to pathology, a trend whose importance young Welch had anticipated, to judge from the concluding sentence of the letter which I have just read. The two first American pathologists who were awarded Nobel Prizes in medicine, Karl Landsteiner, Austrian born, and Thomas Hunt Morgan of Lexington, Kentucky, were recognized not only for their original discoveries but also because they had presented their findings as measured quantities. It is interesting in this context to point out that both Landsteiner and Morgan handled the facts from which they developed their concepts, "in their heads."

Things are different today. The number of entities with which pathologists are nowadays expected to deal is so great that it is quite impossible to evaluate them all "in the head." This is where the science of computing comes into the picture. The computer can manipulate facts and figures better and more rapidly than "one head" can do. Nevertheless, the computer is and will always remain the servant of the scientist. It is the scientist who programs the computer in the image of his thinking. The computer is a tool of man.

Sir Charles Sherrington, the "philosopher of the nervous system," made the distinction between the nervous system as the "tenement" of the mind which, he said, is the "tenant." I like to apply Sherrington's simile to the theme of today's meeting. The computer is the tenement. The pathologists are the tenants. It is the pathologist's lot to establish a profitable relationship between "tenant" and "tenement" in his attempt to alleviate the increasing workload in the laboratory.

Because hospital services continue to expand to accomodate the increasing demand for medical care, the expediency with which laboratory work is handled has become correspondingly important. The problem of effective data acquisition and reporting in the clinical laboratory inevitably leads to the consideration of implementing a computer system in the clinical laboratory. Many discussions concerning how to computerize a clinical laboratory have been held. One must, of course, first realize that there is no single solution: problems seldom repeat themselves specifically, and each laboratory has an equal task in implementing a smoothly operating system according to the unique organization of that laboratory.

DOCUMENTATION OF LABORATORY DATA

The following presentations are offered as examples of how a diverse group of pathologists have effectively applied the concept of computer technology in the clinical laboratory. Their opinions and advice are invaluable testimonials concerning management, organization, and the quality of available computerized laboratory systems. It is anticipated that their experiences in university hospitals, community hospitals, and private laboratories will present alternative approaches to computerization in the laboratory for their colleagues' consideration.

OFF-LINE BATCH PROCESSING

Paul R. Finley, M.D.

Introduction

Automation has greatly increased the capacity of the laboratory for undertaking repetitive work, but problems relating to specimen collection and identification, to the preliminary handling of the specimens and request forms in the laboratory before analytical work can begin, to the collection and processing of raw data generated by the automatic machines, to the storage of laboratory records and to the best methods of presenting laboratory results following completion of analytical work-all of these problems have been magnified. Mr. Robert Townsend, in his book "Up the Organization" has written entertainingly and trenchantly about "computers and their priests". He has written, "first get it through your head that computers are big, expensive, fast, dumb adding machine-typewriters. Then realize that most of the computer technicians that you are likely to meet or hire are complicators, not simplifiers. They are trying to make it look tough. Not easy. They are building a mystique, a priesthood, their own mumbo-jumbo ritual to keep you from knowing what they, and you--are doing. At this state of the art, keep decisions on computers at the highest level. Make sure the climate is ruthlessly hard-nosed about the practicality of every system, every program, and every report. Otherwise the programmers will be writing their doctoral papers on your machines, and your managers will be drowning in ho-hum reports they've been conned into asking for and are ashamed to admit are of no value. Make sure your present report system is reasonably clean and effective before you automate. Otherwise your new computer will just speed up the mess. No matter what the experts say, never, never automate a manual function without a long period of dual operation. When in doubt discontinue the automation. And don't stop the manual system until non-experts in your organization think that automation is working. I've never known a company seriously injured by automating too slowly but there are some classic cases of companies bankrupted by computerizing prematurely."

THE INQUIRY

When a laboratory is considering the installation of a computer or the sharing of a computer with another facility or with other departments in their own hospital, they should draw up a list of pertinent questions which should be answered before any undertaking regarding the computer is carried out. There should be a series of questions which would encompass all of the aspects of the laboratory function and these questions might involve the following:

1. Is a computer-prepared master log required?

A master log is a listing of the work requested of the laboratory. Further, the sequence of the individual entries in the master log should be specified as to whether they should be chronological by patient number, by patient name, or some other sequence. In addition, the entries should be specified as to their grouping for printing. That is, should the entries be printed as one unit, should they be subdivided by laboratory, or should they be subdivided by tests?

2. Is a computer-prepared collection schedule required?

A specimen pick-up list is particularly applicable where the requisition arrives in the laboratory without the associated specimen. It is generally assumed that entries on the collection schedule are to be in a ward-room-bed sequence. If some other sequence is desired it should be stated. Also, the assigning of the accession number should be done either by the computer or by the laboratory personnel.

3. Are computer work lists needed?
A work list itemizes, in sequence, the work to be performed by a given laboratory work station. There may be work lists required for manual test procedures as well as automated test procedures.

4. Are laboratory instruments to be attached directly to the computer, for the automatic acquisition and analysis of data? Additionally, are these instruments to be monitered for error conditions as the run progresses?

5. Are test result reports to be prepared by the computer? Is the patient summary type of reporting desired? That is to say, a summary of the results grouped by test over a specified period of time for inclusion in the patient's chart may be desirable.
The format of these reports is particularly important and this aspect of the electronic data processing system should be scrutinized very carefully. In addition, the aspect of ward reports should be considered. A ward report is a summary of all the test results requested on all patients in a given ward.

6. Are individual test reports required?
This would suggest a report of a result or a group of results for a single patient. The computer may also be required to produce reports of unfinished tests at specified periods of time during the day. The whole problem of the actual introduction of data is a major one. There are a variety of ways for the data to be introduced into the computer for reporting and the type of input best suited to the individual laboratory should be obviously used. One should, in the reporting of the data, be able to produce narrative reports of any type. This gives the

system a flexibility that is necessary for unusual reporting.

7. Is a computer-prepared quality control listing required?
Each laboratory can take advantage of the great capability of the computer to store data and to produce a variety of statistical measurements which may be of great use to the laboratory before the results are released as well as sometime after the results are released.

8. Are inquiries to be processed by the computer?
Should the inquires be made from the laboratory as well as from various stations throughout the hospital? Consideration should be given to placing inquiry terminals in certain emergency wards and in critical care units, particularly. A decision concerning the maximum acceptable response time and the mode of input must be made.

Certain considerations should be given to a variety of more general questions regarding the computer operation. A general knowledge of the environment in which the system will operate is mandatory. If the hospital already has a large general purpose digital computer the laboratory should consider time sharing as a means of introducing computerization into the laboratioy. If the laboratory desires its own computer it encounters a host of special problems that would not occur if time sharing were a possibility. It is useful to know if the hospital itself has long range plans regarding data processing and if there are capable data processing people in the institution. There is no question that the management aspects of the laboratory are greatly aided if the hospital already has a computer which has the capability of producing many of the financial and management reports of the hospital to the laboratory. If other hospitals are involved in the computerization, the concept of teleprocessing can be entertained with the assurance that this technique of time sharing via telephone wires has been successfully employed in a variety of institutions.

DOCUMENTATION OF LABORATORY DATA

THE SYSTEM

The clinician should expect laboratory data to be presented to him in a logical, sequential and readily decipherable form at the same time the laboratory experiences a significant reduction in clerical functions. Since July of 1965 the laboratories at Fariveiw Hospital and its satellite Fairview-Southdale Hospital have been solely dependent on on electronic data processing of all in-patient and out-patient clinical laboratory data except bacteriology, which was incorporated into the system in 1966. Situated 14 miles apart, the twohospitals with a combined bed capacity of 700, provide both long-term and acute care, and have a combined annual laboratory test load of 400,000 tests, The primary concept of satellite hospitals is to increase efficiency and reduce costs by sharing central services such as laboratory, purchasing and data processing. The first computer installed at the data center in Fairview Hospital was an IBM 1440 which was later replaced by an IBM 360/40. In January of 1970 the IBM system was replaced with a Univac 9400 system. The computer is located in the main hospital and linked by high speed teleprocessing to terminals at the satellite hospital. The Univac 9400 general purpose digital computer provides the mechanism for processing information from either laboratory and directing such information to the appropriate patient hospital record. The current equipment consists of the computer with 124 K core storage, two magnetic tape drives, six disc storage drives providing random access capabilities, and 0711 card reader and 0604 card punch, a line printer capable of printing 1600 lines per minute, two DCT 2000 line printer terminals which are located at Fairview-Southdale and a DC2 1000 line printer terminal located at a recently acquired hospital 120 miles to the south of the main hospital, eight keypunches, five of which are located at the main hospital two of which are located at Fairview-Southdale and one which is located at the satellite hospital 120 miles away. All of the punches are interpreting as well as verifying punches. Recently a number of cathode ray tubes were purchased. These will function as inquiry terminals in various areas in the hospital as well as in the laboratory.

Requests for laboratory tests identified by addressograph originate at the nursing stations and either accompany specimens to the laboratory or act as requests for specimen collection. These requests are in two-part forms. The top sheet is the request and worksheet for the technologists' use and the second sheet, in the case of hematology, urinalysis and other miscellaneous tests exclusive of chemistry, is the input form used by the key punch operator to enter the laboratory data as well as the automatic charge into the file. Only one number is punched for both of these functions. Once the test results are recorded by the technologist, the form is separated providing the top copy for the laboratory and the second copy for the data center.

In chemistry, the second sheet of the request, after having been given an accession number, is detached and sent to the data center to initiate the production of protocol sheets, log sheets, a master work chart, a log chart for the SMA 12/60 and labels for the blood tubes. This same procedure is followed for prothrombin times in hematology. The first sheet functions as the blood drawing request.

The laboratory data is entered on the protocol sheet by the technologist and the first sheet is sent to the data center for key-punching and the second is kept in the laboratory. The second copy then serves as a source document and a permanent log record.

This system of combined work sheets and report forms, all on the original source document generated by the com-

DOCUMENTATION OF LABORATORY DATA

puter virtually eliminates transcription errors. Approximately 90% of all test results are reported on the original request from the station or on the portocol sheets generated by the data center. For the remaining results not handled in this manner protocol sheets without the patient names but with all the proper coding may be used as well as standard key punch cards designed in the exact format of the reporting system. All of these sheets and cards are available in each department. The sheets and cards are identified by patients' case numbers and include the date, the technologists code and test results.

Currently 14 applications are in operation on the Univac 9400, although the laboratory program is one of the lesser operations (computer time estimated at one hour daily for both hospitals). Priority based on the immediacy of laboratory needs is guaranteed at scheduled times of the day. The data center provides 24 hours of coverage 7 days a week. Cumulative ward reports in room number sequence containing all current tests not yet incorporated in the patient's record are processed at 11 p.m., 7 a.m., 1:30 p.m., and 4:30 p.m.

The daily update of patient records is done at 2 a.m. This affords all work done during the previous day up until midnight to be on the chart in the morning when the doctor makes his rounds. These records are cumulative, sorted into categories, in chronological and alphabetical order and are generated each day the patient has new test results. The previous chart record is discarded and replaced by the current print-out.

The keypunch time for all laboratory functions is estimated at six hours daily. Once a patient's vitat statistics are incorporated into the laboratory file all subsequent test results are linked to the patient's file by case number alone. The use of self check digits and a verifier has virtually eliminated the possibility of identification errors in the data center. The record of a discharged patient is held in storage for 48 hours to accomodate late results, after which a three part final document is generated. This document provides one copy for the laboratory, one for the physician's office and one for the patient's record in those instances where new information has been added to the record since the previous printing. The computer flags those copies that are to be directed to the record room for incorporation into the patient's record.

Bacteriology data processing presented some organizational problems which were solved by using separate color coded chart records and by independent storage of the cumulative records. Because the physician wants the hospital laboratory record available for the first post-hospitalization office visit, holding discharged patient records on disc for late bacteriology reports was unacceptable to the staff. Cumulative in nature, bacteriology reports are updated each day that new information is available, and a copy is sent to the physician as soon as the cultures on a given patient are completed.

Because an initial attempt at straight narrative key punching resulted in numerous errors and was time consuming, a system of coding was devised which was far simpler for both the technologist and the operator. All input is done with three forms: a form for direct smear results, a form for culture results, and a form for sensitivity results. Narrative reports are done by numerically linking phrases, modifiers, nouns or adjectives. Since the same code can be used repeatedly, only one form is necessary for any given report.

Every month the computer generates two quality control reports; one which calculates the standard deviation and coefficient of variation based on the computed mean and the other which repeats the operation based on the established mean of the pool. A more sophisticated program using student "T" scores and "F" scores to

DOCUMENTATION OF LABORATORY DATA

test the statistical significance of the variance of means and standard deviations is in preparation. An additional program now in operation produces frequency distribution curves in the form of histograms with the following information: size of sample, numerical distribution, size of interval, percentiles and cumulative percentiles.

A number of refinements have been added to the original program to insure the quality of the reports and to make them more meaningful to the clinician. These include: an extensive edit routine; reasonableness limits by which the computer judges the validity of a report; flagging of chemistry results exceeding the 95% confidence limits adjusted to age and sex where these factors pertain; calculations from raw data for such things as protein electrophoresis calculations, cell indices calculations, checks for percentage totals, creatinine clearance calculation and other simple mathematical calculations. In addition to program checks for validity and verifications, two administrative technologists independently scan the records each morning, an exercise in quality control found to be indispensable to the operation. Of particular value is the opportunity to observe within-day and between-day variations in patient test results, especially in an organizational framework where the same test may be done in either laboratory, or an SMA 12/60, single autoanalyzer or by manual methods.

Computer-generated management reports of great merit to laboratory administration include: the monthly revenue report cumulative for the fiscal year with each test item categorized by branch of hospital service; bi-monthly departmental payroll reports including budget control; cumulative employee payroll records logging hours worked in the fiscal year, sick leave, vacation and holidays used and available; monthly cost accounting of all supplies issued from both general stores and outside vendors, and a cumulative budget report including current operating costs, the estimated budget and the year to

date budget. In addition, the data center together with
one of the staff physicians has devised a history questionnaire which can be given to a patient prior to entry into
the hospital. The patient fills out the questionnaire and
mails it back to the data center, where the information
is entered by key-punching. The computerized history is
then available on the chart for the doctor when he is investigating the patient. Approximately 60 histories are
processed in this way each day.

CONCLUSION

Because of a comparatively low laboratory test volume,
divided laboratory service, and a non-tax basis of support, time sharing offers some distinct advantages in
our type of institution.

First and probably the most generally appealing is
the low cost of the operation. The cost per patient day
is approximately $0.07, including amortization of programming costs over a 5 year period. Although cost
accounting was done to establish this figure count, in
actual practice no direct computer costs are allocated
to the laboratory budget. The rental of the computer is
justified solely for business and accounting needs, and
the laboratory, by utilizing computer time otherwise
idle, becomes a beneficiary.

Second-Sharing of data center personnel affords coverage equal to four shifts daily or four full time equivalents with only a fraction of the time actually devoted to
laboratory functions.

Third-The large computer provides versatility, flexibility, high speed and virtually unlimited storage and
random access retrieval. The resources for future
expansion of laboratory programs are unrestricted by
computer size and storage capacity.

DOCUMENTATION OF LABORATORY DATA

Fourth-Staffed by professional data processing personnel, the data center offers access to a high level of programming talent.

Fifth-The data center assumes responsibility for data collection, processing and distribution of reports. Once the test results are recorded on the appropriate form, the laboratory personnel are relieved of all clerical functions associated with charting.

The disadvantage encountered in our operation can be listed as follows:

First-On a digital computer no direct analog input is possible without first interphasing with an analog to digital converter.

Second-The success of the operation is dependent on a continually close inter-departmental relationship. Mutual patience and understanding are critical necessities.

Third-Sharing programming time and talent, without top priority on such services, often results in delays not only in instituting new programs but also in correcting existing programs.

At present all data acquisition is manual. Under consideration for off-line data acquisition is some type of data reduction system which would be attached to the SMA 12/60. However, the cost of installation and monthly rental fee is difficult to justify at our present level of operation. The pattern of daily staff visits to patients except for the critically ill or emergencies makes the cost of on line acquisition with the accompanying necessity for extensive backup an unnecessary luxury for this type of hospital practice.

In conclusion, this systems approach is an example of a simple and economical utilization of centralized computer facilities. The cost is extremely small. This type of program can be organized step by step in a logical fashion. It is completely flexible and requires a minimal period of orientation for new employees in all areas affected by the operation. The contribution of the computer services to the laboratory and medical staff is of great value in both management and services directly related to patient care.

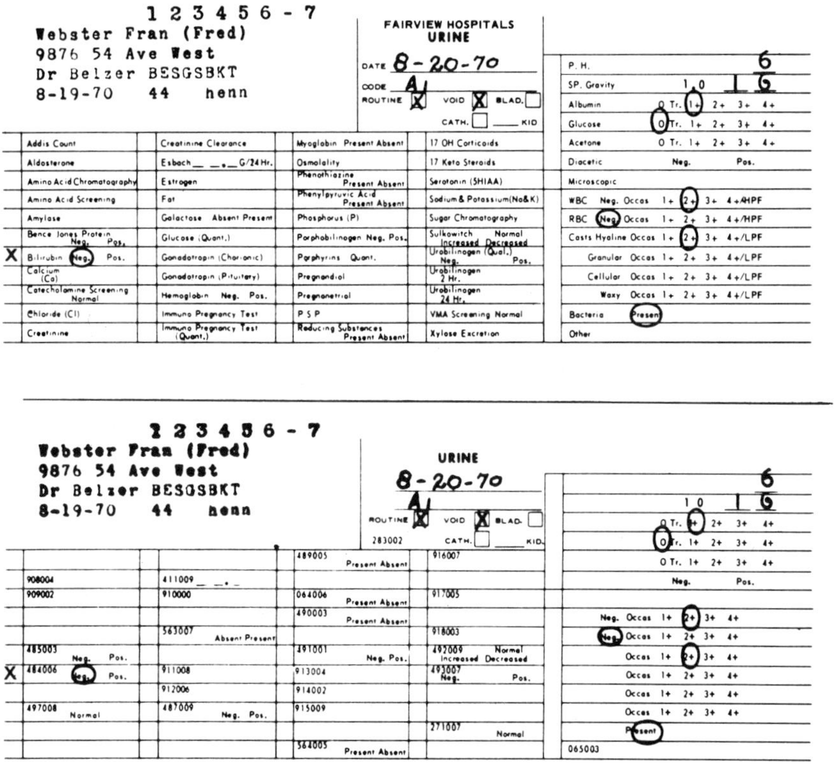

DOCUMENTATION OF LABORATORY DATA

FIGURE 1. Combination request and report form (two-part) for Urinalysis

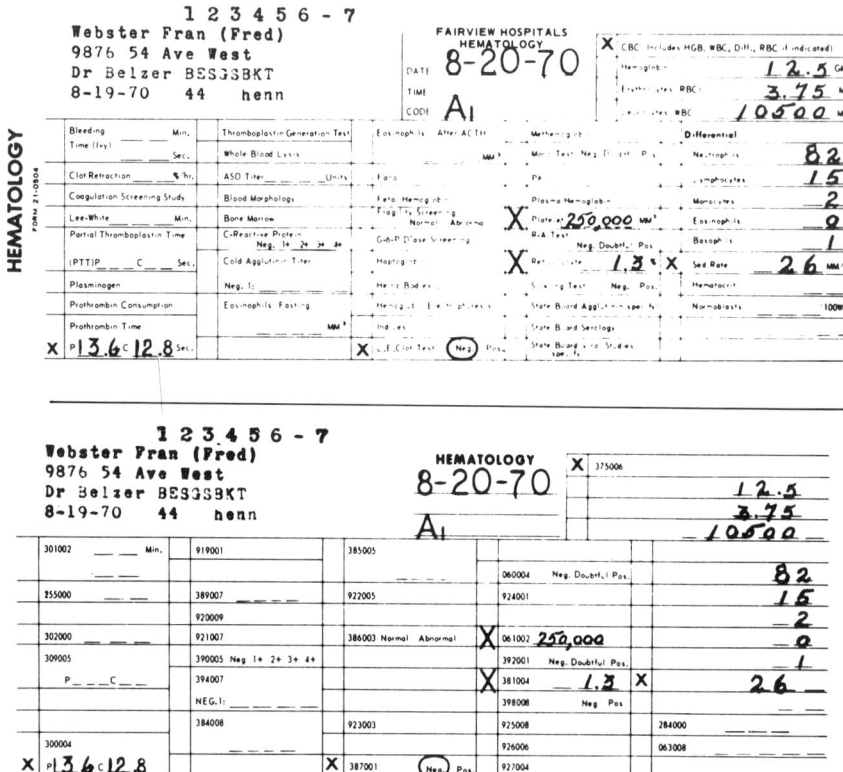

FIGURE 2. Combination request and report form (two part) for Hematology.

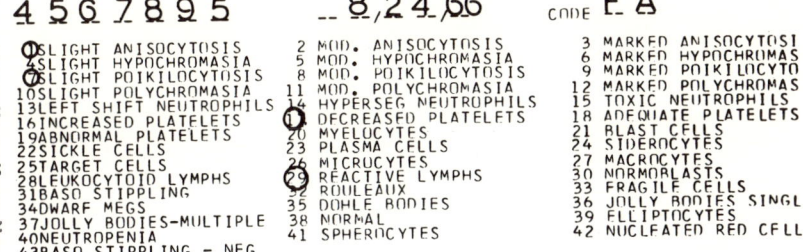

```
4 5 6 7 8 9 5            _ 8,24,66         CODE  E A
 5LIGHT ANISOCYTOSIS       2  MOD. ANISOCYTOSIS        3  MARKED ANISOCYTOSI
 4SLIGHT HYPOCHROMASIA     5  MOD. HYPOCHROMASIA       6  MARKED HYPOCHROMAS
 6SLIGHT POIKILOCYTOSIS    8  MOD. POIKILOCYTOSIS      9  MARKED POIKILOCYTO
10SLIGHT POLYCHROMASIA    11  MOD. POLYCHROMASIA      12  MARKED POLYCHROMAS
13LEFT SHIFT NEUTROPHILS  14  HYPERSEG NEUTROPHILS    15  TOXIC NEUTROPHILS
16INCREASED PLATELETS     17  DECREASED PLATELETS     18  ADEQUATE PLATELETS
19ABNORMAL PLATELETS      20  MYELOCYTES              21  BLAST CELLS
22SICKLE CELLS            23  PLASMA CELLS            24  SIDEROCYTES
25TARGET CELLS            26  MICROCYTES              27  MACROCYTES
28LEUKOCYTOID LYMPHS      29  REACTIVE LYMPHS         30  NORMOBLASTS
31BASO STIPPLING          32  ROULEAUX                33  FRAGILE CELLS
34DWARF MEGS              35  DOHLE BODIES            36  JOLLY BODIES SINGL
37JOLLY BODIES-MULTIPLE   38  NORMAL                  39  ELLIPTOCYTES
40NEUTROPENIA             41  SPHEROCYTES             42  NUCLEATED RED CELL
43BASO STIPPLING - NEG
```

FIGURE 3. Blood smear morphology report card. Technologist merely circles the appropriate entries and sends card to data center for keypunching.

```
    GLUCOSE                         FAIRVIEW HOSPITALS
    TECH ----               PROTOCOL SHEET         06/11/69
    STANDARD     S1-----    S2-----    S3-----    S4-----    S5-----
    CONTROL
    ---------------         -- -- -- --MGX    - - - - - 331009
    PATIENTS                         RESULT           HOUR     CODE

17  SWANSON, ELENA  6319990          -- -- -- --MGX    - - - - - 331009
    AGE 63    F

20  WESTERGAARD, NE 6355317          -- -- -- --MGX    - - - - - 331009
    AGE 59    M

22  ANDERSON, SADIE 6357818          -- -- -- --MGX    - - - - - 331009
    AGE 83    F

23  ALBRECHT, ESTHE 6317341          -- -- -- --MGX    - - - - - 331009
    AGE 63    F

24  VASATKA, FLOREN 6334643          -- -- -- --MGX    - - - - - 331009
    AGE 71    F

26  NELSON, RUTH N  6354922          -- -- -- --MGX    - - - - - 331009
    AGE 63    F

27  STEWART, RUTH   6358311          -- -- -- --MGX    - - - - - 331009
    AGE 46    F

28  THERREIN, WILFR 6329163          -- -- -- --MGX    - - - - - 331009
    AGE 64    M

32  FILIPEK, ALBERT 6359285          -- -- -- --MGX    - - - - - 331009
    AGE 74    M

33  COLE, LUCY      6347611          -- -- -- --MGX    - - - - - 331009
    AGE 52    F

35  PETERSON, NEAL  6358568          -- -- -- --MGX    - - - - - 331009
    AGE 51    M

    ---------------         -- -- -- --MGX    - - - - - 331009

    ---------------         -- -- -- --MGX    - - - - - 331009
```

FIGURE 4. Computer-produced protocol sheet for reporting chemistry data. The form is in two parts; the first sheet is sent to data processing and the second is retained in the laboratory as the permanent record of the log system.

CHEMISTRY WORK SHEET 09/08/66

NO.	NAME	ROOM	Glucose	BUN	Uric Acid	CO2	Chloride	Na	K	pH	Bili	Thymol	Ceph	Phos	BSP	Ca	P	Mg	T. Prot.	ELP	Chol	Fe	SGOT	LDH	SGPT	CPK	NBD	Amylase	Creat	Catechol	VMA	PBI
1	GNAGY, MAYME	465								1	1	1	1						1												
2	SHEEHY, LISA	686			2	2	2	2	2																						
3	O BLENESS, STEPHE	329		3															3												
4	LINDEEN, WILBUR	270	4	4						4		4																			
5	HALKIS, JAMES	1		5	5																		5								
6	HOHLER, CHARLES	229								6		6													6						
7	FREDELL, ELLEN	257	7	7													7		7												
8	DREYER, ANNA	340			8	8	8	8				8																			
9	VAUGHAN, MOSES	354																					9	9							
10	DONNELY, ELIZABET	374			10	10	10	10	10																						
11	JORGENSON, KATHLEE	374	11											11														11			
12	KENNEDY, THOMAS	389																					12		12						
13	HALL, KATHERINE	393	13						13		13	13											13								
14	HUEMOLLER, MARGAR	429	14	14	14																											
15	DANELZ, ED	434	15		15	15																										
16	JOHNSON, ELIZABET	456	16																													
17	STIEHM, EVE	2104			17	17	17	17										17													
18	CLARK, JOHN	397																					18								
19	WINEBRENNER, HARR	524																			19										
20	SAVAT, JOE	439		20																			20								
21	JOHNSON, ELIZABET	456	21	21																			21								
22	CLEVEN, HAROLD	386								22	22	22	22	22																	
23	AHRENS, MARY	328								23	23	23	23													23					
24	HARMS, HARRIET	232	24			24																										
25	HOHLER, CHARLES	229				25							25																			
26	DALY, JOSEPH	298	26	26																												

FIGURE 5. Computer-produced work sheet for use in the chemistry laboratory. The accession number of the patient is used in each request box that is relevant.

DOCUMENTATION OF LABORATORY DATA

```
50            4:30PM           WARD REPORT        04/03/70      PAGE 1

    PATIENT              ROOM    NO         RESULT


TCHELISNIG,MARY  J       524  663012   R F RISCH
    08 03            P1         SOURCE                    VOID
    08 03            P1         P. H.                     5
    08 03            P1         SP. GRAVITY               1.012
    08 03            P1         ALBUMIN                   0
    08 03            P1         GLUCOSE                   0
    08 03            P1         WBC                       OCCASIONAL
    08 03            P1         RBC                       NEG
    08 03            P1         HEMOGLOBIN                13.6 GM%
    08 03            P1         LEUCOCYTES                7000    /MM3
    08 03            P1         NEUTROPHILS               69 %
    08 03            P1         LYMPHOCYTES               28 %
    08 03            P1         MONOCYTES                 3 %
    08 03            P1         EOSINOPHILS               0 %
    08 03            P1         BASOPHILS                 0 %
    08 03            S1         ALBUMIN                   4.8 GM%
    08 03            S1         ALK. PTASE                46 MU/ML
    08 03            S1         BILIRUBIN TOTAL           0.7 MG%
    08 03            S1         CALCIUM                   9.6 MG%
    08 03            S1     a   CHOLESTEROL               340 MG%
    08 03            S1         GLUCOSE                   91 MG%
    08 03            S1         L D H                     80 UNITS
    08 03            S1     a   PHOSPHORUS                4.9 MG%
    08 03            S1         SGOT                      17 UNITS
    08 03            S1         TOTAL PROTEIN             7.1 GM%
    08 03            S1         UREA NITROGEN             16 MG%
    08 03            S1         URIC ACID                 6.8 MG%


CUNDY, MARY              524  663039   S  SOLHAUG JR
    08 02            12         HEMOGLOBIN                12.2 GM%
    08 02            12         LEUCOCYTES                14700   /MM3
    08 02            12         NEUTROPHILS               83 %
    08 02            12         LYMPHOCYTES               15 %
    08 02            12         MONOCYTES                 2 %
    08 02            12         EOSINOPHILS               0 %
    08 02            12         BASOPHILS                 0 %
    08 02            F2         BLOOD GROUPING
    08 02            F2             ABO GROUP             A
    08 02            F2             RH GROUP              POS


MC LAUGHLIN, CAROL A     528  662879   P  KOONTZ
    08 03            C1         HEMOGLOBIN                10.1 GM%
```

FIGURE 6. A typical ward report. The data are listed in room number sequence.

PAUL R. FINLEY

FAIRVIEW HOSPITALS
LABORATORY RECORD
FINAL   07/23/70

SCHONSTEDT,OLAF   #662120   DR M   DANYLUK   ROOM DIS1   AGE 95

URINALYSIS

	DATE	HOUR	SOURCE	PH	SP.GR	ALB	GLUC	ACET	DIAC	WBC	RBC	CASTS
?1	6/16		VOID	7	1.010	0	0			NEG	NEG	
W1	6/23		VOID	6	1.022	TR	0			OCCAS	NEG	*
G1	7/01		VOID	5	1.023	1+	0			2+	3+	
W1	7/08		VOID	5	1.026	1+	0			2+	1+	
W1	7/11		CATH	6	1.026	1+	0			3+	2+	
W1	7/16		VOID	6	1.016	1+	0			OCCAS	1+	

MISC. URINALYSIS

W1	6/23	MICR. CASTS HYALINE	
W1	7/16	URINE OTHER	YEAST

HEMATOLOGY

	DATE	HOUR	HGB	RBC	WBC	N	L	M	E	B	ESR	HCT
G1	6/16		16.9		10600	69	13	8	5	0		
T1	6/24		15.7		9200	77	19	0	3	1		
W1	6/28				23500	91	2	6	1	0		
I1	7/01				23500	88	7	1	4	0		
E1	7/08				46400	79	19	2	0	0		
W1	7/11				19300	79	14	1	6	0		
P1	7/16				11700	82	10	3	5	0		

CHEMISTRY

S1	6/16	a ALBUMIN	3.4 GM%
S1	6/16	ALK. PTASE	51 MU/ML
S1	6/16	BILIRUBIN TOTAL	1.2 MG%
S1	6/16	CALCIUM	9.2 MG%
S1	6/16	CHOLESTEROL	235 MG%
S1	6/16	GLUCOSE	80 MG%
S1	6/16	L D H	95 UNITS
S1	6/16	PHOSPHORUS	3.0 MG%
H1	6/16	POTASSIUM	3.9 MEQ/L
S1	6/16	SGOT	25 UNITS
H1	6/16	SODIUM	135 MEQ/L

FORM 21-084 SCHONSTEDT,OLAF   662120   07/23/70
                                 CLINICAL LAB REPORT   PAGE 18

FIGURE 7. A patient summary report. The technologist code and shift are the first data to the left of the date.

DOCUMENTATION OF LABORATORY DATA

		3A		SUMMARY					11/14/69		
SCHULTZ, EARL			#631288	DR D C OLSON			ROOM	398	AGE 55		
URINALYSIS											
	DATE	HOUR	SOURCE	PH	SP.GR	ALB	GLUC	ACET	DIAC	WBC	RBC	CASTS
FI	3/27		VOID	5	1.025	0	0			NEG	NEG	
PW	8/29		VOID	8	1.017	0	0			NEG	NEG	
LD	9/01		VOID	6	1.024	0	0			OCCAS	OCCAS	*
LB	9/03		VOID	8	1.012	0	0			NEG	NEG	

MISC. URINALYSIS

LD	9/01		MICR. CASTS HYALINE		OCCAS

HEMATOLOGY

	DATE	HOUR	HGB	RBC	WBC	N	L	M	E	B	ESR	HCT
SS	3/27		14.4		6100	69	22	6	3	0		
SS	4/16				6400							
KS	4/22		13.7		6100						62	
KS	4/23				5000							
JH	5/05				6100							
SO	5/08		14.2		5700							
KD	5/18	0400PM	13.3									
SO	6/04				8100							
NA	6/05				8500							
LB	6/06				9100							
JG	6/07				7100							
PV	6/08				7500							
JG	6/09	AM			5900							
SO	6/10				5000	81	17	2	0	0		
JG	6/11				5400							
JB	6/12		13.3		4900							
KS	6/13				4700							
FH	6/14				4500							
FH	6/15				3800							
KS	6/16				3200							
KS	6/17				3400							
JG	6/18				2400							
JG	6/19				2300							
LB	6/20				1900							
JG	6/21				2200							
CU	6/22				2100							
JG	6/23				1300							
KS	6/24				1300							
KS	6/25				2000							
JG	6/26				2600							
JG	6/27				3800							
JG	6/28				4700							
KD	6/29				6200							
SS	6/30		12.4									
JG	6/30				7400							

E SCHULTZ, EARL   631288   11/14/69

FIGURE 8. A patient summary report showing the utility of this type of format. Recorded on one sheet are fully three months of intermittent white counts. The asterisk under the heading "CASTS" refers the reader to the next category. "MISC. URINALYSIS", where the actual report of the casts appears.

```
                    28              SUMMARY                      01/07/70

        TERHO, EARL              #647942   DR J C GIERE    ROOM  252       AGE 57
        URINALYSIS

              DATE    HOUR   SOURCE   PH   SP.GR  ALB  GLUC  ACET  DIAC  WBC  RBC  CASTS
        PW    12/08          VOID     7    1.020   0    0                NEG  NEG

        HEMATOLOGY

              DATE    HOUR   HGB    RBC    WBC    N    L    M    E    B    ESR   HCT
        MD    12/08          15.2          9900   63   33   2    0    2
        SS    12/10   AM                  12900                            4
        NA    12/12                        9100                             68
        NA    1/06           15.8          6000   65   28   0    7    0     22

        COAGULATION

        MD    12/08          PROTHROMBIN TIME             15.7  C12.8  SEC
        PW    12/09          PROTHROMBIN TIME             14.0  C13.7  SEC
        PW    12/10          PROTHROMBIN TIME             20.6  C12.3  SEC
        PW    12/11          PROTHROMBIN TIME             20.4  C12.7  SEC
        PW    12/12          PROTHROMBIN TIME             18.3  C12.5  SEC
        MD    12/13          PROTHROMBIN TIME             21.1  C12.4  SEC
        SS    12/14          PROTHROMBIN TIME             23.1  C13.7  SEC
        PW    12/15          PROTHROMBIN TIME             22.8  C13.2  SEC
        PW    12/16          PROTHROMBIN TIME             23.3  C13.5  SEC
        MJ    12/17          PROTHROMBIN TIME             25.4  C13.9  SEC
        PW    12/18          PROTHROMBIN TIME             22.3  C12.5  SEC
        PW    12/19          PROTHROMBIN TIME             22.0  C13.1  SEC
        JG    12/20          PROTHROMBIN TIME             22.4  C13.7  SEC
        FI    12/21          PROTHROMBIN TIME             20.5  C11.8  SEC
        PW    12/22          PROTHROMBIN TIME             21.4  C13.2  SEC
        PW    12/23          PROTHROMBIN TIME             22.6  C12.8  SEC
        PW    12/24          PROTHROMBIN TIME             22.9  C13.8  SEC
        PW    12/25          PROTHROMBIN TIME             12.9  C11.8  SEC
        LB    12/26          PROTHROMBIN TIME             22.8  C12.1  SEC
        KM    12/27          PROTHROMBIN TIME             22.7  C12.5  SEC
        FI    12/28          PROTHROMBIN TIME             23.9  C12.0  SEC
        PW    12/29          PROTHROMBIN TIME             22.4  C13.2  SEC
        PW    12/30          PROTHROMBIN TIME             20.8  C13.8  SEC
        PW    12/31          PROTHROMBIN TIME             20.8  C13.6  SEC
        FI    1/02           PROTHROMBIN TIME             23.0  C12.9  SEC
        PW    1/03           PROTHROMBIN TIME             21.9  C12.9  SEC
        PW    1/04           PROTHROMBIN TIME             21.3  C12.2  SEC
        PW    1/05           PROTHROMBIN TIME             21.1  C11.8  SEC
        FI    1/06           PROTHROMBIN TIME             20.3  C13.3  SEC
        KB    1/07           PROTHROMBIN TIME             20.3  C12.3  SEC

        CHEMISTRY

        JB    12/08          B GLUCOSE                    136 MG%


               TERHO, EARL              647942              01/07/70
```

FIGURE 9. A patient summary report showing daily prothrombin times over a period of one month. This is a useful kind of sequential presentation of data.

DOCUMENTATION OF LABORATORY DATA

JS	11/22	∂ BILIRUBIN	1 MIN	1.6	MG%
JS	11/22	∂ BILIRUBIN	TOTAL	4.3	MG%
LG	11/24	∂ BILIRUBIN	TOTAL	5.4	MG%
KB	11/26	∂ BILIRUBIN	1 MIN	1.5	MG%
KB	11/26	∂ BILIRUBIN	TOTAL	4.3	MG%
CC	12/04	∂ BILIRUBIN	1 MIN	0.9	MG%
CC	12/04	∂ BILIRUBIN	TOTAL	1.8	MG%

FIGURE 10. Example of original presentation of bilirubin data. The text is awkard and difficult to follow sequentially.

O1	4/26	BILIRUBIN	1 MIN	11.8 MG%-TOTAL 17.8 MG%	0006
Y1	4/27	BILIRUBIN	1 MIN	11.0 MG%-TOTAL 17.8 MG%	0009
G1	4/30	BILIRUBIN	1 MIN	10.2 MG%-TOTAL 17.0 MG%	0013
B1	4/24	CALCIUM		9.4 MG%	0004
B1	4/24	CHOLESTEROL		238 MG%	0004
B1	4/24	GLUCOSE		75 MG%	0004
B1	4/24	∂ L D H		179 UNITS	0004
H1	4/30	∂ L D H		171 UNITS	0011
B1	4/24	PHOSPHORUS		3.7 MG%	0004
L1	4/24	∂ SGOT		185 UNITS	0007
H1	4/30	∂ SGOT		348 UNITS	0012
B1	4/24	TOTAL PROTEIN		6.5 GM%	0004
B1	4/24	UREA NITROGEN		10 MG%	0004

HUBERTY, STEVEN   680847   04/30/71

FIGURE 11. The new format for presentation of bilirubin data is seen at the top of the report. The data are more logically displayed and are easier to follow sequentially. The ability to change format simply and quickly is a distinct advantage of the system.

CHEMISTRY

FA	11/26	BLOOD PH	7.420
KD	11/26	CHLORIDE	96 MEQ/L
PV	11/26	a CO2 CONTENT	33 MEQ/L
FA	11/26	a OXYGEN SATURATION	88.0 %
FA	11/26	PCO2 ARTERIAL	36 MM/HG
FA	11/26	PO2	55 MM/HG
JB	11/26	POTASSIUM	5.0 MEQ/L
JB	11/26	SODIUM	137 MEQ/L

FIGURE 12. Example of original presentation of electrolyte data. The data are only in alphabetical arrangement with no logical sequential formulation.

ELECTROLYTES

	DATE	HOUR	NA	K	CO2	CL	PH	PCO2	SOURCE
O1	2/02		144	4.9	a35	102			
I1	2/18		139	a5.9	a21	105			
Z2	2/18	0400PM	138	a6.0					
Z3	2/18	1200PM	138	5.5					
L1	2/19	0700AM	a133	5.4	25	101	a7.140		
C1	2/20		137	5.3	a20	100			
C1	2/22		143	4.4	24	105			
F1	2/24		a151	4.0	29	a108	7.374	a43	ARTERIAL
O1	2/24					a110			
I1	2/25		a151	4.2	30				
H1	2/28		a146	4.2	29	a107			
B1	3/26		134	5.4	24	98			
B1	3/29		a133	5.0	25	100			
L1	3/30		136	a6.0	29	104			
E2	3/30	0500PM	a130						
F1	3/31		137	a5.6	27	a94			
G1	4/01						7.400	a42	ARTERIAL
L1	4/05						7.436	40	ARTERIAL

BRYANT, HOLLIS   672908   04/14/71

FIGURE 13. A recent example of the newer format for presentation of electrolyte data. The display is more logical and more useful to the clinician. It should be noted that the report covers a period of two months.

DOCUMENTATION OF LABORATORY DATA

BACTERIOLOGY DIRECT SMEAR RESULTS

PATIENT NO. 325679-4   ACQ. NO. 184   TECH M.G.

A

---10108 NO
(3,4)---10207 FEW
---10306 MODERATE NUMBER OF
(1,2)---10405 LARGE NUMBER OF
---10603 NO INCREASE IN
---10702 MODERATE INCREASE IN
---10801 MARKED INCREASE
---10900 DECREASE IN
---11007 PREDOMINANCE OF
---11106 NO PREDOMINATING ORGANISM
---11205 QNS
---11304 SMALL AMOUNT MATERIAL
---11403 SPECIMEN UNSATISFACTORY

B

---12510 INTRACELLULAR
---12609 EXTRACELLULAR
(4)---12708 SMALL
---12807 LARGE
---12906 SLENDER
---13003 ELONGATED
---13102 LANCET SHAPED
---13201 COCCOID
---13310 ENCAPSULATED
---13409 BRANCHING
---13508 BUDDING
---13607 PLEOMORPHIC
---13706 DISINTERGRATING
---13805 FILIFORM

C

---15305 GRAM POS COCCI PAIRS CHAINS
(3)---15404 GRAM POS COCCI PAIRS CLUSTERS
---15503 GRAM POS BACILLI
---15602 GRAM VARIABLE BACILLI
---15701 MIXED BACTERIAL FLORA
---15800 BACTERIA
---15909 YEAST
---16006 MYCELIA
---16105 ACID FAST BACILLI
---16204 SPIROCHETES
---16303 FUSIFORM BACILLI
(1)---16402 PMNS
---16501 EOSINOPHILS
---16600 TRICHOMONAS

C

---15008 GRAM NEG COCCI
---15107 GRAM NEG DIPLOCOCCI
(2,4)---15206 GRAM NEG BACILLI
---10504 GRAM POS COCCI PAIRS

D

---17509 PROBABLE HEMOPHILUS
---17608 PROBABLE PNEUMOCOCCUS
---17707 PROBABLE NEISSERIA MENINGITIDES
---17806 PROBABLE COLIFORM
---17905 PROBABLE STAPH
---61101 FINAL

---10009--
---10009--

FIGURE 14. The report form used by the bacteriologist to report the results of direct smears. The key-puncher in the data center merely follows the numbers from left to right by columns. The report is then printed in narrative form because of the linking of phrases.

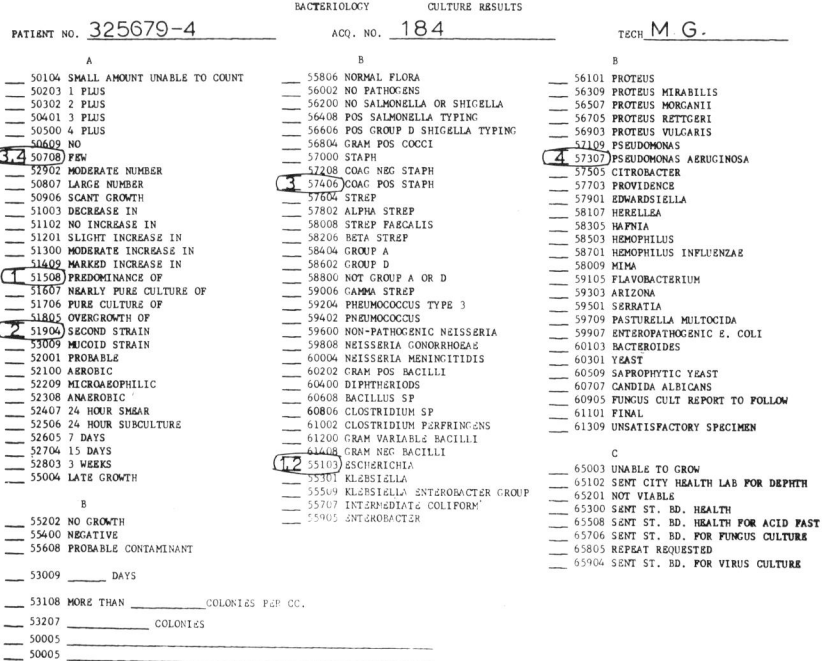

FIGURE 15. The culture report form used by the bacteriologist. The number given to the organism is the number used in the sensitivity reporting. The numbers are read from left to right by the keypuncher. The resultant report will be in narrative form because of the linking of phrases.

DOCUMENTATION OF LABORATORY DATA

BACTERIOLOGY   SENSITIVITY RESULTS

CASE NO. 325679-4   ACQ. NO 184 _ _

--77776 INSUFFICIENT GROWTH FOR SENS TESTS

70102	①	②	③	④	⑤	61101 FINAL
AMPICILLIN	S	R	R	R		—
CARBENICILLIN	S	R	R	R		—
CEPHALOTHIN	S	R	S	R		—
CHLORAMPHENICOL	S	S	S	R		—
COLYMYCIN	S	R	R	S		—
ERYTHROMYCIN	R	R	S	R		—
GANTRISIN	R	R	R	R		—
GENTAMICIN	R	S	S	R		—
KANTREX	S	S	S	R		—
LINCOCIN	—	—	S	—		—
MACRODANTIN	S	S	S	R		—
NALIDIXIC ACID	—	—	—	—		—
NEOMYCIN	L	S	R	L		—
OXACILLIN	S	R	R	S		—
PENICILLIN	R	R	R	R		—
STREPTOMYCIN	S	R	L	R		—
TETRACYCLINE	R	R	S	R		—

70003 --

70003 --

FIGURE 16. The sensitivity report form used by the bacteriologist. The form can be filled out rapidly and key-punched rapidly. The code at the bottom of the form (70003) is used for narrative entries which the key-puncher may type into the key-punch card.

```
07/14/70    OP                  FAIRVIEW HOSPITALS
                                LABORATORY RECORD

SJOBERG, MARION      #659524   DR R M SILAS      ROOM OP         AGE 51

06/11   SOURCE URINE VOID CLEAN                  CULTURE # 749


LB CULTURE RESULTS

    1     MORE THAN 100,000 COLONIES PER CC
          GRAM NEG BACILLI
          ESCHERICHIA

    2     MORE THAN 100,000 COLONIES PER CC
          GRAM NEG BACILLI
          SECOND STRAIN ESCHERICHIA

    3     SMALL AMOUNT PROTEUS
          PROTEUS MIRABILIS
          UNABLE TO COUNT

ORGANISM  1  RESISTANT                SENSITIVE

             CHLORAMPHENICOL          AMPICILLIN
                                      CEPHALOTHIN
                                      GENTAMICIN
                                      KANTREX
                                      NALIDIXIC ACID
                                      NEOMYCIN
                                      STREPTOMYCIN
                                      TETRACYCLINE
                                      GANTRISIN           SLIGHTLY
                                      MACRODANTIN         SLIGHTLY

ORGANISM  2  RESISTANT                SENSITIVE

             AMPICILLIN               CHLORAMPHENICOL
             CEPHALOTHIN              GENTAMICIN
             GANTRISIN                MACRODANTIN
             TETRACYCLINE             NALIDIXIC ACID
                                      KANTREX             SLIGHTLY
                                      NEOMYCIN            SLIGHTLY
                                      STREPTOMYCIN        SLIGHTLY

ORGANISM  3  RESISTANT                SENSITIVE

             AMPICILLIN               CEPHALOTHIN
             CHLORAMPHENICOL          GENTAMICIN
             GANTRISIN                KANTREX
             MACRODANTIN              NEOMYCIN
             NALIDIXIC ACID           STREPTOMYCIN
             TETRACYCLINE




SJOBERG, MARION         CULTURE 749        FINAL        07/14/70

                         BACTERIOLOGY REPORT
```

FIGURE 17. A final bacteriology report. The actual color of the report is magenta, and is printed separately from the other data from the laboratory, all of which appears on white sheets. The bacteriology data are constantly updated every time new information is reported.

DOCUMENTATION OF LABORATORY DATA

FAIRVIEW HOSPITAL

STATISTICAL ANALYSIS OF CONTROL POOL 03/31/71

SGOT HAU WITH ESTABLISHED MEAN

TECH	DATE	TEST RESULT		MEAN		DIFF.	SQUARE
S1	03/01	71.00	MINUS	68.00	EQUALS	3.00	9.0000
S1	03/02	70.00	MINUS	68.00	EQUALS	2.00	4.0000
S1	03/02	66.00	MINUS	68.00	EQUALS	2.00	4.0000
S1	03/04	60.00	MINUS	68.00	EQUALS	8.00	64.0000
S1	03/05	62.00	MINUS	68.00	EQUALS	6.00	36.0000
C1	03/06	70.00	MINUS	68.00	EQUALS	2.00	4.0000
S1	03/08	75.00	MINUS	68.00	EQUALS	7.00	49.0000
S1	03/09	70.00	MINUS	68.00	EQUALS	2.00	4.0000
L1	03/11	70.00	MINUS	68.00	EQUALS	2.00	4.0000
F1	03/12	70.00	MINUS	68.00	EQUALS	2.00	4.0000
S1	03/13	68.00	MINUS	68.00	EQUALS	0.00	0.0000
S1	03/16	63.00	MINUS	68.00	EQUALS	5.00	25.0000
C1	03/17	61.00	MINUS	68.00	EQUALS	7.00	49.0000
F1	03/18	67.00	MINUS	68.00	EQUALS	1.00	1.0000
O1	03/19	72.00	MINUS	68.00	EQUALS	4.00	16.0000
O1	03/20	72.00	MINUS	68.00	EQUALS	4.00	16.0000
H1	03/22	65.00	MINUS	68.00	EQUALS	3.00	9.0000
S1	03/23	65.00	MINUS	68.00	EQUALS	3.00	9.0000
L1	03/24	63.00	MINUS	68.00	EQUALS	5.00	25.0000
C1	03/25	62.00	MINUS	68.00	EQUALS	6.00	36.0000
C1	03/26	61.00	MINUS	68.00	EQUALS	7.00	49.0000
Y1	03/27	69.00	MINUS	68.00	EQUALS	1.00	1.0000
S1	03/29	73.00	MINUS	68.00	EQUALS	5.00	25.0000
F1	03/30	65.00	MINUS	68.00	EQUALS	3.00	9.0000
JB	03/31	67.00	MINUS	68.00	EQUALS	1.00	1.0000
LB	03/03	66.00	MINUS	68.00	EQUALS	2.00	4.0000
LB	03/10	65.00	MINUS	68.00	EQUALS	3.00	9.0000
S1	03/15	75.00	MINUS	68.00	EQUALS	7.00	49.0000

SUM OF SQUARES 515.0000

SUM OF SQUARES DIVIDED BY N-1 19.07407

28 RESULTS IN THIS CONTROL POOL 1 S.D. 4.36739

COEFFICIENT OF VARIATION 6.422630

FIGURE 18. Computer printout of standard deviation and coefficient of variation calculated from the analyses of a lyophilized serum pool. The serum in this case is Hyland Unassayed Abnormal serum. (HAU). The standard deviation is calculated from the previously established mean.

FAIRVIEW HOSPITAL

STATISTICAL ANALYSIS OF CONTROL POOL   03/31/71

SGOT HAU   WITH CALCULATED MEAN

TECH	DATE	TEST RESULT		MEAN		DIFF.	SQUARE
S1	03/01	71.00	MINUS	67.25	EQUALS	3.75	14.0625
S1	03/02	70.00	MINUS	67.25	EQUALS	2.75	7.5625
S1	03/02	66.00	MINUS	67.25	EQUALS	1.25	1.5625
S1	03/04	60.00	MINUS	67.25	EQUALS	7.25	52.5625
S1	03/05	62.00	MINUS	67.25	EQUALS	5.25	27.5625
C1	03/06	70.00	MINUS	67.25	EQUALS	2.75	7.5625
S1	03/08	75.00	MINUS	67.25	EQUALS	7.75	60.0625
S1	03/09	70.00	MINUS	67.25	EQUALS	2.75	7.5625
L1	03/11	70.00	MINUS	67.25	EQUALS	2.75	7.5625
F1	03/12	70.00	MINUS	67.25	EQUALS	2.75	7.5625
S1	03/13	68.00	MINUS	67.25	EQUALS	0.75	0.5625
S1	03/16	63.00	MINUS	67.25	EQUALS	4.25	18.0625
C1	03/17	61.00	MINUS	67.25	EQUALS	6.25	39.0625
F1	03/18	67.00	MINUS	67.25	EQUALS	0.25	0.0625
O1	03/19	72.00	MINUS	67.25	EQUALS	4.75	22.5625
O1	03/20	72.00	MINUS	67.25	EQUALS	4.75	22.5625
H1	03/22	65.00	MINUS	67.25	EQUALS	2.25	5.0625
S1	03/23	65.00	MINUS	67.25	EQUALS	2.25	5.0625
L1	03/24	63.00	MINUS	67.25	EQUALS	4.25	18.0625
C1	03/25	62.00	MINUS	67.25	EQUALS	5.25	27.5625
C1	03/26	61.00	MINUS	67.25	EQUALS	6.25	39.0625
Y1	03/27	69.00	MINUS	67.25	EQUALS	1.75	3.0625
S1	03/29	73.00	MINUS	67.25	EQUALS	5.75	33.0625
F1	03/30	65.00	MINUS	67.25	EQUALS	2.25	5.0625
JB	03/31	67.00	MINUS	67.25	EQUALS	0.25	0.0625
LB	03/03	66.00	MINUS	67.25	EQUALS	1.25	1.5625
LB	03/10	65.00	MINUS	67.25	EQUALS	2.25	5.0625
S1	03/15	75.00	MINUS	67.25	EQUALS	7.75	60.0625

SUM OF SQUARES   499.2500

SUM OF SQUARES DIVIDED BY N-1   18.49074

28 RESULTS IN THIS CONTROL POOL   1 S.D.   4.30009

COEFFICIENT OF VARIATION   6.39418O

FIGURE 19. Computer printout of standard deviation and coefficient of variation calculated from the analyses of a lyophilized serum pool. The serum in this case is Hyland Unassayed Abnormal serum. (HAU). The standard deviation is calculated from the actual calculated mean of the values. This technique affords a comparison to the standard deviation calculated from the previously established mean, and gives information about the significance of the changing of the mean.

DOCUMENTATION OF LABORATORY DATA

```
STATISTICAL ANALYSIS OF CONTROL POOL              04/13/71

FAIRVIEW * SPINAL PROTEIN FROZEN POOL    CALCULATED MEANS      63.94
                              SUM OF SQUARES                  134.9448
                  SUM OF SQUARES DIVIDED BY N-1                 8.17322
   18 RESULTS IN THIS CONTROL POOL         1 S.D.              2.43460
   COEFFICIENT OF VARIATION                                    3.815930

FAIRVIEW * SPINAL PROTEIN FROZEN POOL    ESTABLISHED MEANS     63.00
                              SUM OF SQUARES                  121.0000
                  SUM OF SQUARES DIVIDED BY N-1                 7.11765
   18 RESULTS IN THIS CONTROL POOL         1 S.D.              2.66749
   COEFFICIENT OF VARIATION                                    4.234740

FAIRVIEW * SGOT HAU                      CALCULATED MEANS      67.68
                              SUM OF SQUARES                  446.7728
                  SUM OF SQUARES DIVIDED BY N-1                21.27490
   22 RESULTS IN THIS CONTROL POOL         1 S.D.              4.61247
   COEFFICIENT OF VARIATION                                    6.815110

FAIRVIEW * SGOT HAU                      ESTABLISHED MEANS     68.00
                              SUM OF SQUARES                  449.0000
                  SUM OF SQUARES DIVIDED BY N-1                21.38095
   22 RESULTS IN THIS CONTROL POOL         1 S.D.              4.62395
   COEFFICIENT OF VARIATION                                    6.799920

FAIRVIEW * LDH HAU                       CALCULATED MEANS     175.93
                              SUM OF SQUARES                  608.9286
                  SUM OF SQUARES DIVIDED BY N-1                46.84065
   14 RESULTS IN THIS CONTROL POOL         1 S.D.              6.84402
   COEFFICIENT OF VARIATION                                    3.890190

FAIRVIEW * LDH HAU                       ESTABLISHED MEANS    170.00
                              SUM OF SQUARES                 1101.0000
                  SUM OF SQUARES DIVIDED BY N-1                84.69231
   14 RESULTS IN THIS CONTROL POOL         1 S.D.              9.20284
   COEFFICIENT OF VARIATION                                    5.413430

FAIRVIEW * CHLORIDE HNU                  CALCULATED MEANS     108.19
                              SUM OF SQUARES                   36.0386
                  SUM OF SQUARES DIVIDED BY N-1                 1.44154
   26 RESULTS IN THIS CONTROL POOL         1 S.D.              1.20064
   COEFFICIENT OF VARIATION                                    1.109750

FAIRVIEW * CHLORIDE HNU                  ESTABLISHED MEANS    109.00
                              SUM OF SQUARES                   53.0000
                  SUM OF SQUARES DIVIDED BY N-1                 2.12000
   26 RESULTS IN THIS CONTROL POOL         1 S.D.              1.45602
   COEFFICIENT OF VARIATION                                    1.335790

FAIRVIEW * BUN HNU                       CALCULATED MEANS      11.91
                              SUM OF SQUARES                    9.0386
                  SUM OF SQUARES DIVIDED BY N-1                 0.32154
   26 RESULTS IN THIS CONTROL POOL         1 S.D.              0.56704
   COEFFICIENT OF VARIATION                                    4.801350

FAIRVIEW * BUN HNU                       ESTABLISHED MEANS     12.00
                              SUM OF SQUARES                    9.0000
                  SUM OF SQUARES DIVIDED BY N-1                 0.36000
   26 RESULTS IN THIS CONTROL POOL         1 S.D.              0.60000
   COEFFICIENT OF VARIATION                                    5.000000
```

FIGURE 20. A statistical report which summarizes all the more detailed computer analyses, which are used primarily to check for obvious keypunch error enteries. The entire body of data from both hospitals can be printed on several sheets such as the one pictured.

THE CLINICAL LAB-12 LABORATORY COMPUTER SYSTEM- ITS EVOLUTION AND ITS OPERATION

Sidney A. Goldblatt, M. D.

In 1965 our laboratory began to explore methods for organizing patient reports. Our aim was to present data in summary format so that we could easily check for discrepancies and errors.

In a first attempt, we employed scribes to copy the data in organized form. But we soon found that the scribes themselves made errors. Next we tried machine copying of test slips and documents. But with the half million tests per year, this method quickly became expensive as well as cumbersome. After a careful cost accounting, we discovered that the problem was even more acute. Excluding technicians time, we were spending over $30,000 per year to simply record and report laboratory information. Since this inadequate single sheet report system was surprisingly expensive, it seemed time to investigate a hardware solution - to look for equipment that could help organize the laboratory portion of the hospital chart.

We began our quest for cumulative summary reporting by developing our own IBM tab system. Since this system required a card for each of our 1500 to 2000 tests per day, the volume of cards soon became unmanageable.

Next we sought help from computer manufacturers in developing the kind of system useful to the laboratory. It was then that we established our relationship with Digital Equipment Corporation of Maynard, Mass., and Dr. Hicks of the University of Wisconsin in developing the Clinical Lab-12 System.

Our experiences were educational, occasionally humorous, and in the end very rewarding.

We learned that hard work and motivation are the keys to success of any laboratory computer system. And motivation means that the entire hospital staff must be motivated - doctors, nurses, administration - if the system is to work well and be totally accepted.

On the humorous side, the computer made a considerable change in laboratory life. Not only was the lab run by a pathologist turned computernik, but it became a feature attraction with an imposing schedule of visitors requesting guided tours. We are always happy to share our knowledge and experiences, but it never seemed to fail that the visitors would arrive during a frozen section or when an irate clinician was complaining about a serum iron. A few visiting pathologists showed their gratitude by making job offers to my better looking technologists.

In the end, we achieved our goal of organizing the patient record and providing the reports necessary for better laboratory operation. At the same time, we relieved the clerical burden on our technologists. As a bonus, we were able to interface the system directly to our AutoAnalyzer^R and achieve better consistency and improved quality control.

Professionally, I believe a computer system helps the pathologist become a more integral part of the clinical team. It provides better use of the laboratory information in his consultations with the physician at the bed-side.

^{R} AutoAnalyzer is a registered trademark of Technicon Corporation

The Clinical Lab-12 System in Operation

The Clinical Lab-12 System shown in Figure 1 requires no operator per se; the person with me in the photograph is a laboratory technician. Amazingly enough, a laboratory person at CLA level can be trained as a system operator in only three days. Programmer training, of course, takes longer.

A partial list of system programs is shown in Figure 2. For simplicity, the list uses names that are familiar to the technician such as requisition entry, accession number entry, etc.

Most os these programs can produce reports in a variety of forms. For example, Fig. 3 shows some of the reports from the Patient Summary Printout (SU): Cumulative Summaries, Incomplete and Complete Tests for the Day, Master Worksheets, Ward Reports, and Billing Reports. These reports can be requested for specific patients or for all patients, listed in alphabetical order, by patient name, or by ward. Early every morning, one of our technicians arrives and enters approximately 2000 test requests for some 350 of our 500 patients and administration data for 50-60 new admissions per day.

Using the Administrative Update program, he types in the names of new patients via his keyboard terminal, entering as shown in Figure 4; name, patient number, etc. If the technician makes an error in format, the program automatically prints an error message. Next, he enters test requisitions. Both the updates and requisitions are completed in an hour to an hour and 15 minutes.

A sample of Requisition Entry is shown in Figure 5. The technician can assign an accession number, have the computer assign, it, or give the computer a starting

number for a particular day or time and let the computer
assign sequential numbers. The technician also enters
the time that the specimen was collected. The first patient on this list, for example, requires a glucose test and
the computer has assigned an accession number of 325.

As the computer receives this information, it
searches the patient file on disk storage and returns with
the patient name to verify that the entry was made for
the proper patient.

The work sheet shown in Figure 6 is simple, since
it is only for glucose. Work sheets for a particular
work area can contain up to 12 tests on the same report.
The work sheet for electrolytes in Figure 7 contains
four tests.

The AutoAnalyzer^R and Coulter Counter^R Model
"S" operate "on-line", being directly connected to the
computer system. The AutoAnalyzer^R interface is a
simple 0 to 2 volt potentiometer which is connected to
the pen of the recorder. As the pen moves, a potential
proportional to the reading is created which is converted
to digital form for acceptance by the computer system.

The technologist finds that it takes very little time
to perform set-up analysis for the analyzer. Again it's
a simple keyboard entry which indicates which analyzer
is to be used. As the work sheet indicates, the chemistry
technologist can organize the cups and choose any cup
sequence for a particular patient grouping.

After results are entered, there is an automatic
printout from the Print Test Results Program, Figure 8.
This printout not only records the results, but it also

---

^{R} Coulter Counter is a registered trademark of
Coulter Electronics, Inc.

indicates whether or not the result is within acceptable limits. The system also includes an automatic correction for drift which is quite useful for some types of analysis.

Quality control calculations, Figure 9, may be performed on-line while the auto-analyzers are collecting data. The system will print out the mean, and standard deviations of new quality control pools in familiar graphical form, a task which is commonly done manually.

After results are verified, they are accepted by the operator of the instrument who enters the accession number. As the accession and patient numbers are given, the system positively confirms patient identity by responding with the correct patient name.

If a test is not requested, the result will not be entered. If, for example, only a glucose test was ordered and the specimen run on the Technicon SMA 12/60, only glucose will be filed.

Manual tests are entered using the Update Test Results program as shown in Figure 10. At the work station, the technician types in the accession and patient numbers and the system responds with patient name for verification.

The Clinical Lab-12 System may include a card reader for system input to simplify such complex entries as hematology and urinalysis data. Because our present teletype entry method works so well, we don't plan to use cards for requisition entry.

In the early part of the day, as results are completed, cumulative patient summaries, Figure 11, are issued. Note the various groupings possible and that the information is classified by day and time. These reports are prepared for each patient, each day.

Since a patient's work may not be completed by the

end of the day, we produce a Ward Report, Figure 12, in the morning, particularly for those critical values such as blood sugar or prothrombin times. This report is printed each day- at noon- for delivery to the nurses stations. One of the most important steps in training the staff and nurses was to get them to examine these reports. It took many months before the staff fully realized the benefits of this procedure.

The various business routines are carried out in the early morning. When requisition entry is completed, billing report may be produced. Because our hospital billing system does not have its own computer, we greatly value the Clinical Lab-12 Billing Report shown in Figure 13.

The technician that operates the system produces the daily test census, Figure 14, which lists the total tests of each kind for the day as a tally for the monthly report. We are also using this census information as the basis for developing a reagent inventory system.

The patient list, Figure 15, which is printed each day is also sent to the administration. We have created much good will by providing them with this daily inpatient list.

Preventing System Downtime

No computer dexription would be complete without a discussion of downtime. In the very early days of our pilot installation, downtime was a way of life. However, after installation was complete, system outages were much less frequent, occurring several months apart. Over the last six months, we have had no prolonged downtime.

What causes downtime? Elecrical storms with their "brown" or "black-outs" invariable cause system

DOCUMENTATION OF LABORATORY DATA

failures. Static electricty from nylon dresses and uniforms can also cause problems. However, failure from this source can be controlled by regulating computer room humidity.

Several features of the Clinical Lab-12 allow the laboratory to recover from these failures without loss of patient information, Figure 16.

For example, we use the Clinical Lab-12 magnetic tape system to duplicate patient information stored on disk. As a routine precaution, we copy patient files in the morning, after requisitions are entered, and again at the end of the day. Interim tapes are run should the lab receive advanced warnings of storms or possible power difficulties. If results are documented in card form, we have additional information backup.

To make sure that information on the disk has not become garbled, we use the Clinical Lab-12's Filesafe^R feature. This feature checks the integrity of the pointer words which link related information on disk storage. It takes only a few seconds each day to totally check patient files and assure that data is intact. I regard Filesafe^R and the system's on-line editing capability as two of the most important features of the Clinical Lab-12 System.

A laboratory should also practice manual backup. If a system is down for less than 12 hours, only stat and critical results need be manually recorded. If longer downtime occurs, technicians will have to start manual recording of results. I would recommend periodic "fire drills" in which the manual report system is practiced by every technologist and clerk at unscheduled

---

^{R} Filesafe is a registered trademark of Digital Equipment Corporation

intervals.

Building Flexibility into the Laboratory Computer

Philosophies on implementing a laboratory computer system vary from hospital to hospital. Our intent was not to build the laboratory around the computer, but to model the habits we already had-the habits of all 80 lab employees, 125 doctors, and 900 nurses.

With the Clinical Lab-12 system, a laboratory can retain its own individualities. Since programs are modular, the user can define his own system. Let me describe some of these modular elements.

The Requisiton Entry program allows the user a choice of arranging the enteries individually or in problem oriented test groupings, Figure 17.

The pickup or specimen collection lists also have various options. As shown in Figure 18, the pickup list contains specimen requirements such as serum, plasma, and a variety of anticoagulants. We also have a choice of dividing collection into patient subgrouping such as inpatient and outpatient.

The organization of the work bench, Figure 19, is probably the most individual characteristic of any laboratory. For example, workbench organization for a Technicon SMA 12/60 is entirely different than the schedule for a single or dual-channel auto-analyzer. The Clinical Lab-12 provides a wide variety of worklist formats. The system also allows the worklist to vary during the week, on weekends, and on holiday shifts.

It is my contention that even labs that operate only manual tests can benefit from a system such as ours. Our original interest was not in the on-line auto-analyzer feature of the system, but rather in better organization of the patient record. The on-line and quality control features are a bonus.

As previously shown, the Patient Summary Printouts, Figure 20, may be printed in a variety of formats. Tests may be organized in clinically oriented groupings tailored to the desires of the user. With the Clinical Lab-12 system, changes are easy to make.

Billing, reagent inventory, and quality control information are prepared for management through the billing report, the quality control routines, and the daily test census, as shown in Figure 21. Quality control reports include a printed control chart. Also, the test program allows the user to set up his own patient categories: surgical, maternity, outpatient, etc.

Getting the Most from a Laboratory Computer System

What makes a computer system work in the laboratory? The arch in Figure 22 is built on hardware and software on the one hand, and service and software support on the other. The keystone, however, is the user. The user himself must be motivated, and he must desire to motivate his doctors and the entire laboratory staff.

But even more important, to implement the system effectively, he must "learn his laboratory"--study and understand its hour-by-hour and day-to-day operations. Only then will he be able to use the computer to model these operations and complement them to its fullest capability.

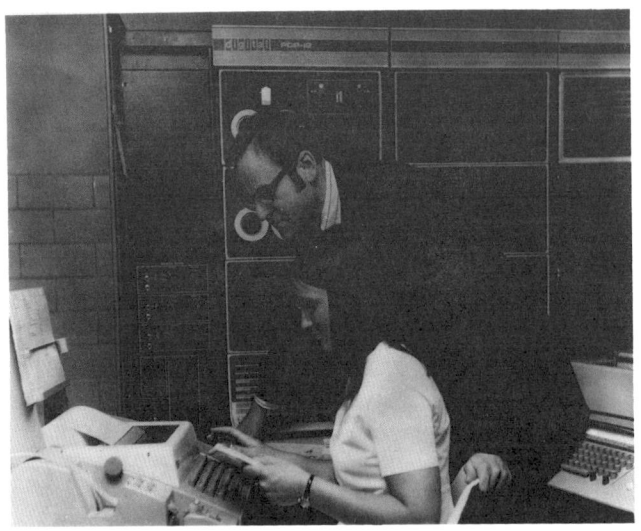

Figure 1

```
Administrative Update      (AD)
Requisition Entry          (RE)
Work Sheet Generator       (WO)
Master Work Sheet          (SU.M)
Accession Number Entry     (AC)
Setup Analysis             (SE)
Update Test Results        (TE)
Patient Summary Printouts  (SU)
System Inquiry Program     (IN)
Delete Data                (DE)
Billing Routine            (SU.B)
Control/Schedule Block Gen (CS)
Daily Test Census          (DA)
Display Channels           (DI)
Calculations               (CA)
Print Test Results         (PR)
```

Figure 2. Clinical lab 12 program list

DOCUMENTATION OF LABORATORY DATA

PATIENT SELECTION / Report Type	Subgroup	ALL PATIENTS IN FILE			SPECIFIED PATIENTS		
		N NUMBER	W WARD	A ALPHAB.	I* INDIV.	name NAME	ddddd NUMBER
S	(Cumulative Summary)	S,N,	S,W,	S,A,	S,I,	S,Name	S,pat#
I	(Incomplete Test Report Summaries)	I,N,	I,W,	I,A,	I,I,	I,Name	I,pat#
C	(Complete Test Report for Today)	C,N,	C,W,	C,A,	C,I,	C,Name	C,pat#
M	(Master Worksheet, Tests for Today)	M,N,	M,W,	M,A,	M,I,	M,Name	M,pat#
W	(Ward Reports Specific Day)		W		W,I,	R,Name	R,pat#
R			W,m,d		W,I,md	R,Name m,d,	R,pat# m,d,
B	Billing Reports	B B,m,d					

Options are as follows
   a * Name
   b * pat #
   c * D, doctor code
   d * W, ward
   e * Carriage Return

Figure 3. Clinical lab 12 summary report program codes

```
AD

E M OR S: E
NAME (L F MI): SULLIVAN GEORGE H
PATIENT # : 1464698
N.S.: 6E
DR: SIL
ROOM #: 618
SEX: M
DATE OF BIRTH: 07/17/1940
CHANGES ? Y

NAME (L F MI): SULLIVAN GEORGE H *
PATIENT #: 1464698 * 1454698
N.S.: 6E *
DR: SIL *
ROOM #: 618 *
SEX: M *
DATE OF BIRTH: 07/17/1940 *
CHANGES ? N

NAME (L F MI):
```

Figure 4. Administrative update

RE

ENTER REQUISITIONS AS:
TIME, PATIENT #, TEST TYPE(S), ACC #

* 1:13P, 1493821, GLUC, 325
  GREENBAUM NORMAN *

* 1:20P, 1605326, VITA, 326
  EASTMANN, TERRANCE B *

* 1395720, LABC
  (PKG) WINCHELL SUSAN

NEW PKG OK? Y OR N *
   TEST,   TIME,   ACC #   TYPE I TO IGNORE A TEST

   CBC   *   6:20P   4732
   OK ?   Y

   DIFF   *   I

   GLUC   *
   #4733   OK ?

   BUN   *   2:10P   328
   OK ?   Y

   RPR   *
   #329   OK ?

   URIN   (6:25A, #6918)

   CL   *
   #331   OK ?

END OF PACKAGE

* STOP

RE DONE.
TTY IS FREE.

Figure 5. Requisition entry

DOCUMENTATION OF LABORATORY DATA

```
WORKSHEET FOR GLUCOSE                         PAGE 01
8-31-70      11:30AM
SELECTION 1

CUP    ACC #   NAME                    PATIENT #

...     1     ANNIN  LOUIS              6145      **B
...     4     BATT  SYLVIA              2367      **B
...     6     BOEHM  MARY              18694      **B
...     7     BROWN  ROSE               4567      **B
...     8     CASANUEOVO  JOHANN       17073      **B
...     9     CLARK  WILLIAM  L         9090      **B
...    12     DAVIDSON  MARTIN  M      10568      **B
...    14     EVANS  DIANNE  E          3452      **B
...    15     ASHBURNHAM  MAX  G      784163
...    16     BROOKLINE  MARGARET    2005673
...    17     CLINTON  DIANE  B       5605621
...    18     LOWELL  HERBERT         4509887
...    19     MEDFORD  WILLIAM  X     4503612
...    20     PENNINGTON  THOMAS  J   4503458
...    21     REVERE  ROBERT  M       3075021
...    22     WAKEFIELD  MARGARET     4447098
...    23     WELLESLEY  HARVEY       5883176
WORKSHEET COMPLETE
```

Figure 6. Work sheet

WORKSHEET FOR ELECTROLYTES 1   PAGE 1
5-18-71   1:35PM
SELECTION 1

CUP	ACC #	NAME	PATIENT #	NA	K	CL	CO2
...	7B	BYERS HAROLD	548389		*		
...	8B	ALEXANDER D	541108	*	*	*	*
...	10B	GREUNWALDT PETER A	44	*	*	*	*
...	16B	SONNE GLADYS C	545599	*	*		
...	47B	EWING WILLIAM A	548114			*	
...	48B	ELLIS HARRY F	548045	*	*	*	*
...	49B	DIETZ JACK L	547556			*	*
...	52B	ANDERSON ARTHUR C	2208715	*	*		
...	54B	BARNARD HILLIARD S	1093422		*	*	
...	97B	BAGBY TONIA L	548089	*	*		

WORKSHEET COMPLETE

Figure 7

DOCUMENTATION OF LABORATORY DATA

```
PR
RETYPE RESULTS FOR * LYTS
PLATE 2, CUP6 IS LAST
START AT PLATE, CUP * 1,23
STOP AT PLATE, CUP * 1,38

10:23 HRS      11/16/70
```

CUP	ACC#	NA	K	CL	CO2	BAL
PLATE 1						
23		183V	MP	389V	120V	NC
24		248V	MP	366V	147V	NC
25	STD	312V	167V	342V	190V	NC
26	STD	380VD	251V	322VD	238VD	NC
27	STD	447V	343V	298V	324V	NC
28		MP	436VD	203V	374V	NC
29	MP					
30	VEAA	155#	3.0C	110C	26.0C	NC
31	....	142	3.2	103	29.6	145
32	2014	138	3.8	97	31.9	141
33	2020	138#	4.2	96	32.6	141
34	2018	140	4.0	104	27.5	143
35	2017	138	3.8	100	30.1	142
36	2014	137	4.8	106	23.5	141
37	....	135	5.3	94	22.7	129
38	....	139	5.1	99	21.9	133

```
NA
PLATE 1
 30 0111111
 33 0111111
```

Figure 8. Print test results

QUALITY CONTROL CHART FOR POOL, ALK. PHOS   FROM 06/01 TO 06/14

	63.0	64.0	65.0	66.0	67.0	68.0	69.0
06/01	.	X	.	*	.	.	.
06/02	.	.	.	*	.	.	X
06/03	.	.	.	X	.	.	.
06/04	.	.	.	*	.	.	>
06/05	<	.	.	*	.	.	.
06/06	.	.	.	*	.	.	X
06/07	.	.	X	*	.	.	.
06/08	.	.	.	X	.	.	.
06/09	.	.	X	*	.	.	.
06/10	.	.	.	*	.	.	X
06/11	X	.	.	*	.	.	.
06/12	.	.	.	*	.	X	.
06/13	<	.	.	*	.	.	.
06/14	X	.	.	*	.	.	.
	-3SD	-2SD	-1SD	MEAN *	+1SD	+2SD	+3SD

Figure 9. Quality control

DOCUMENTATION OF LABORATORY DATA

TE
E M OR S * E
TECH CODE * 12
TEST/WORKSTATION NAME * WSAD

ACC # * 31   FAWCETT MICHAEL D   Y

   11/23   NA   :   137.

   11/23   K   :   4.1

   11/23   CL   :   102.

   11/23   CO2   :   24.2

   11/23   PH   :   6.8

ACC # * STOP

TTY IS FREE

TE
E M OR S * M
TECH CODE * 12
TEST/WORKSTATION NAME * GLUC

PAT # * 1343378

ACC # * 5364   CANNARD ALLISON H   Y
   11/23   GLUC   168.   :

PAT # * STOP

TTY IS FREE

Figure 10. Update test results

GREENWALD PAUL A   44   58 /272-2   PG   08/04/78   13:05   PG 01

ELECTROLYTE UNIT

	ACET MG/DL	GLUC MG/DL	BUN MG/DL	CRET MG/DL	NA MEQ/L	K MEQ/L	CL MEQ/L	CO2 MEQ/L	PH	PCO2 MM HG	OSMO MOSM
08/01 07:56A	RTF	110.	12.	1.0	NEW	NEW	NEW	NEW	7.4	40.	Q
08/02 08:14A	RTF	112.	14.	1.1	141.	3.8	99.	27.	7.5	42.	292.
08/03 08:00A	RTF	104.	11.2	1.4	142.	3.8	104.	26.	7.6	CONT	292.

ENZYMES

	ACID PHOS	ALK PHOS	GPT UNITS	GOT KARMEN	LDH WACKER	CPK I.U.	AMY UNITS	LIP UNITS
08/01 02:00	7.5	Q	Q	Q	52.	67.7	122.	SRL
08/02 03:26P	7.3	36.	14.	39.	36.	50.0	118.	SRL
08/03 02:00P	7.9	38.	14.	36.	33.	45.2	102.	SRL

LIVER FUNCTION

	TSP G%	ALB G%	GLOB G%	AG	BILT MG/DL	BILD MG/DL	CEPH	THYM UNITS	CHOL MG/DL	UROB EH.U.	BSP %	NH4 MCG%
08/01 08:22A	5.6	4.4	2.8	INC	.5	.12	INC	7.	223.	.9	2.1	81.1
08/02 09:22A	NEW	NEW	NEW	INC	NEW	NEW	NEW	NEW	NEW	NEW	2.4	76.
08/03 09:00A	7.1	4.2	2.8	INC	.6	.13	INC	4.	212.	1.0	2.6	72.9

RENAL FUNCTION

	PSP	CREA CLEAR	UREA CLEAR	ADIS COUNT	FISH BERG	MOS ENTHAL
08/01 25:26P		INC				
08/02 03:44P		INC				
23:44P			INC	INC	INC	INC

HEMATOLOGY 1

	RBC MILL	HGB G%	HCT %	WBC THOU	MYEL %	META %	BAND %	SEGS %	LYMP %	MONO %	EOS %	BASO %
08/01 10:40A	5.3	14.5	55.	6.2	0.	0.	2.	36.	40.	4.0	2.	.2
08/02 11:24P	5.2	17.3	62.	5.3	0.	0.	3.	44.	40.	5.0	4.	.4
08/03 11:00A	4.6	15.6	48.	6.2	0.	0.	4.	42.	37.	6.7	3.	.3

HEMATOLOGY 2

	SED MM/HR	RETC %	MCH	MCV	MCHC	DIR COOMBS	IND COOMBS	SICK CELL	LE PREP	ANAB
08/01			NEW	NEW	NEW					
08/02			29.0	86.2	36.4					
08/03 03:00P			28.	88.	32.6					

SEROLOGY

	TYPH H	TYP O	PARA A	PARB B	BRUC ABORT	OX19	OX2	OXK	MON SLIDE	HET TITER	DAV G.PIG	DIF BEEF
08/01 02:00P	INC	INC	INC	INC	INC	INC						
08/02 22:00P	INC	INC	INC	INC	INC	INC						
08/03 01:00P	INC	INC	INC	INC	INC	INC						

SEE SEE REPORT
QNS QUANTITY NOT SUFFICENT
CONT CONTAMINATED SPECIMEN
NSS NO SPECIMEN SUBMITTED
Q   QUESTION OF INTERFERRING SUBSTANCE
NEW REQUEST NEW SPECIMEN
RTF REPORT TO FOLLOW
SRL SENT TO REFERENCE LAB

Figure 11. Cumulative summary report

DOCUMENTATION OF LABORATORY DATA

```
         WARD REPORT            07/29/70      12:18

NAME                 PAT. #          N.S./ROOM #
WAYNE SALLY G        267534          3E/341        DATE REQUESTED 03/29

ACC #      TECH      TEST            RESULT              TIME

7229       12        GLUCOSE (FASTING)  92. MG/100ML     7:20A
           12        UREA NITROGEN      23. MG/100ML     7:20A

7230                 ELECTROLYTE UNIT                    7:20A
           12        SODIUM           138. MEQ/L
           12        POTASSIUM        4.1 MEQ/L
           12        CHLORIDE         110. MEQ/L
           12        CO2 CONTENT      22. MEQ/L
           12        PH               7.1
           12        PCO2             46. MM HG
           12        OSMOLALITY       24.7 MOSM

7230                 PROTEIN UNIT                        9:00A
                     TOTAL PROTEIN   INCOMPL.
           12        ALBUMIN          1._ GM%
                     GLOBULIN        INCOMPL.
                     A/G             INCOMPL.

105                  CBC                                 9:00A
           4         HEMOGLOBIN       13.4 MG%
           4         HEMOCRIT         42. %
           4         WBC              10.4 M/CU.MM.
105                  DIFFERENTIAL CNT                    9:00A
           4         BANDS            46. %
           4         SEGS             10. %
           4         LYMPS            35. %
           4         MONO             4. %
           4         EOS              2. %
           4         BASO             3. %
           4         DESCRIPTION      0.

7340       14        GLUCOSE          142. MG/100ML      11:10A

7341                 CALCIUM          INCOMPL.           11:10A

7341                 PHOSPHORUS       INCOMPL.           11:10A
```

Figure 12. Ward report

SIDNEY A. GOLDBLATT

BILLING REPORT
PATIENT NAME   PAT. NUMBER   N.S./R.N.

GREUNWALD PAUL A   2963420   6E /634-A   DATE 08/01
                    GLUC,BUN   4.00
                    ELECTROLYTE UNIT   27.00
                    ACETONE   1.00
                    CREATININE   3.50
                    LIV FUNCTION   27.50
                    BSP 45 MIN   2.00
                    ENDOCRINE TESTS   14.00
                    PROTHROMBIN TIME   3.00
                    CBC   8.50
                    RBC   3.50
                    FEBRILE AGGLUTIN   8.00
                    ACID PHOSPHATE   9.00
                    LDH   8.00
                    CPK   15.00
                    AMYLASE   3.00
                    LIPASE   9.00

                                                    148.00

Figure 13. Billing

DOCUMENTATION OF LABORATORY DATA

DAILY TEST CENSUS

DATE 11/10/1970

	TEST	COUNT		TEST	COUNT
1.	GLUCOSE	121	2.	UREA NITROGEN	93
3.	SODIUM	97	4.	POTASSIUM	104
5.	CHLORIDE	97	6.	CO2 CONTENT	97
7.	PH	29	8.	PCO2	18
9.	OSMOLALITY	7	10.	SGOT	44
11.	SGPT	37	12.	ALK PHOSPHATASE	34
13.	TOTAL PROTEIN	44	14.	ALBUMIN	33
15.	GLOBULIN	33	16.	A/G	31
17.	BILIRUBIN, TOT	45	18.	BILIRUBIN, DIR	19
19.	CHOLESTEROL TOT	25	20.	CEPH FLOC	8
21.	DIFFERENTIAL CNT	57	22.	URIC ACID	22
23.	MCH	19	24.	MCV	21
25.	MCHC	21	26.	PRO TIME, SEC	46
27.	PRO TIME %	46	28.	PBI	11
29.	BLOOD TYPE	18	30.	RH FACTOR	18
31.	DU FACTOR	4	32.	PHENOTYPE	5
33.	PHOSPHORUS	35	34.	URINALYSIS	33
35.	VITAMIN A	3	36.	MAGNESIUM	7
37.	CALCIUM	38	38.	PROTEUS OX 19	8
39.	RPR	7	40.	HEMOCRIT	54
41.	HEMOGLOBIN	49	42.	WHITE BLOOD CNT	46

END

EXIT - TTY IS FREE

Figure 14. Daily test census

IN

LIST OF ALL PATIENTS 11/06/79 1:30 PM PG 01

PATIENT NAME	NUMBER	N.S.	ROOM #	DR.	DATE OF BIRTH	SEX
ALDERMAN ROBERT S	1562024	OPD	001	ALD	3/22/1941	MALE
ALDRICH HENRY U	2340961	5S	501	ALD	UNKNOWN	MALE
ALTSCHULE ARMAND C	1012569	7Y	722	2AE	9/15/1936	MALE
ANDERSON ARTHUR C	2208715	4E	401	B2W	1/14/1934	MALE
ANNINE LOUISE B	6145220	WE2	2487	FAM	5/61/1941	FEMALE
ASHBURNHAM MAX G	7841631	17D	1738	52A	8/14/1921	MALE
BALDWINSON ROBERT F	7707731	3E	338	BL	6/06/1949	MALE
BARNARD HILLIARD S	1093422	2S	213	CCC	2/26/1932	MALE
BATHESON JOHN R	1044356	3K	341	2E4	12/16/1934	MALE
BEALIER MIRIAM D	5503671	3E	331	E6	4/30/1929	FEMALE
BECKETT PHILLIP M	2332451	4W	404	BEC	4/15/1944	MALE
BEECH DWIGHT J	3474940	8N	882	BEA	4/09/1937	MALE
BISHOP ANDREW B	4680932	5S	512	BFG	2/14/1929	MALE
BLANDT SYLVIA S	2367091	OPD	005	EW7	4/22/1938	FEMALE
BOEHMGARTEN MARTIN S	1869423	43E	18-34	GRU	10/10/1940	MALE
BOTWARD HAROLD G	8017332	2N	230	BOT	1/11/1937	MALE
BREITER GEORGE W	6606752	7W	712	FOF	10/04/1926	MALE
BROOKLINE MARGARET D	2005673	12W	1204	5ET	12/16/1934	FEMALE
CASANUEVO JORGE M	1707322	2A	7-108	GGG	6/17/1925	MALE
CLARK WILLIAM L	9090122	23W	234W	GHJ	7/56/1956	MALE
CLINTON DIANE B	5605621	6S	666	M67	5/12/1947	FEMALE
COFFLIN KENNETH B	2234095	5N	512	COF	5/13/1912	MALE
COOPER NORMAN S	4639043	5S	529	COP	6/12/1932	MALE
CORNELIUS HERMAN S	4666124	2N	292E	JON	4/22/1925	MALE
COTELAND BRADSHAW T	1003456	4E	4-4	COP	12/12/1912	MALE
CROMLEY LEO P	1027743	6H	6-114	CRO	2/06/1938	MALE
DAVIDOWITZ MARTIN M	1056811	OPD	412F	SMI	5/83/1934	MALE
DAWSSON JOCELYNE T	3467022	OPD	003	EW4	12/16/1944	FEMALE
DISILVIO THOMAS N	1026985	6E	698	DIS	UNKNOWN	MALE
DUBLIER EZRA M	1034667	5B	50	DUB	8/22/1921	MALE
EILROD MAXWELL U	1043885	4W	42	FIL	4/23/1929	MALE
ELTON WILLIAM J	3035926	23W	2352	ELT	1/12/1940	MALE
EVANS DOROTHY F	3452113	22	123W	COP	12/15/1941	FEMALE
EVERETT RONALD A	3609532	5N	501	EVR	5/12/1941	MALE
FARGO HUMPHREY L	1335269	2W	206	FAR	5/15/1932	MALE
FINLETTER PAUL D	1054409	4D	47	FIN	6/23/1935	MALE
FISHER ANDREW W	1092341	4E	403	AND	UNKNOWN	MALE
FLLOYD DAVID T	5122809	5W	522	DAB	UNKNOWN	MALE
FORD FRANKLIN E	3099032	9W	990	FOR	9/26/1938	MALE
FOSSBERG ERIC N	4527100	4E	480	FOS	UNKNOWN	MALE
FRANKLIN DELORES D	2202215	WE2	3412	2-A	12/23/1941	FEMALE
FRANNDEL RICHARD W	5850991	4W	411W	MEN	4/24/1940	MALE
FURUYAMA MAKATO N	2341093	6S	627	TOD	3/07/1937	MALE
GABRIELE JENNIFER B	8809441	16E	1623	GAB	12/12/1938	FEMALE
GAMBOLINO THOMAS R	1078236	4W	66-4	GAM	6/06/1932	MALE
GARCIA MANUEL P	2033021	6N	621	GAB	3/19/1940	MALE
GEILLER SAMUEL G	6709832	OPD	002	EW3	5/23/1924	MALE
GILBERT ROGER K	6793475	8T	802	GIL	8/03/1945	MALE
GILLIUND DANA G	4536094	7W	773	GIL	10/04/1942	FEMALE
GLOVIER HENRI D	2109942	3W	355	GLO	5/04/1927	MALE

Figure 15. Inquiry

DOCUMENTATION OF LABORATORY DATA

1. PATIENT INFORMATION RECORDED ON TAPE
   a. AFTER REQUISITION ENTRY
   b. END OF DAY
2. RESULTS RECORDED ON CARDS
3. EDIT-CHECKING OF PATIENT FILES
4. MANUAL REPORTING

Figure 16. Preventing data losses

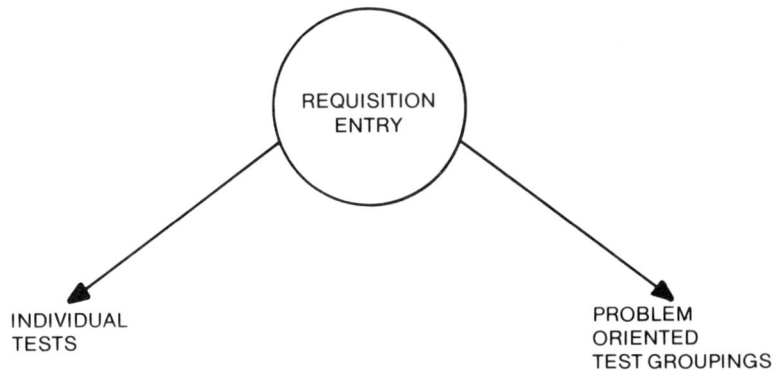

Figure 17. Requisition choices

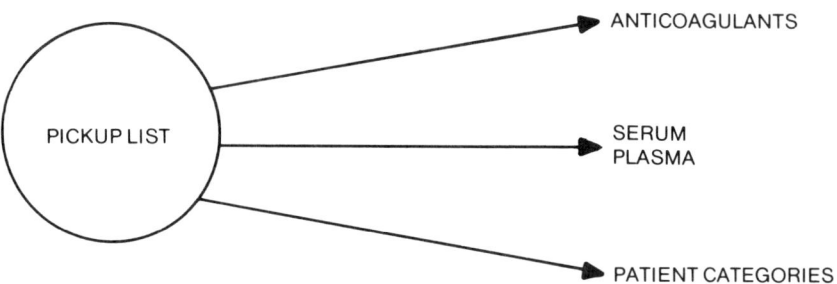

Figure 18. Pickup list options

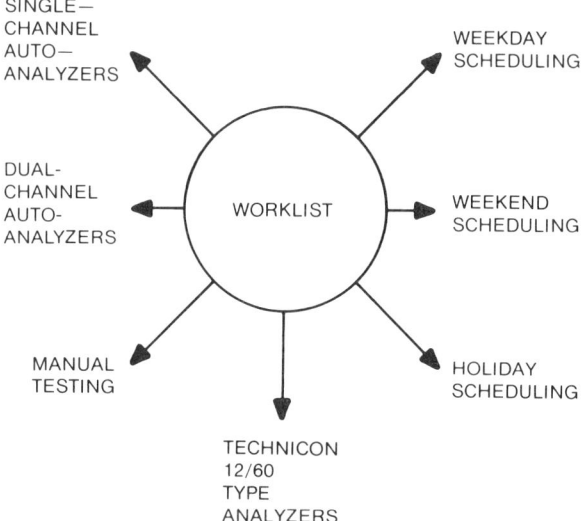

Figure 19. Organizing the workbench

DOCUMENTATION OF LABORATORY DATA

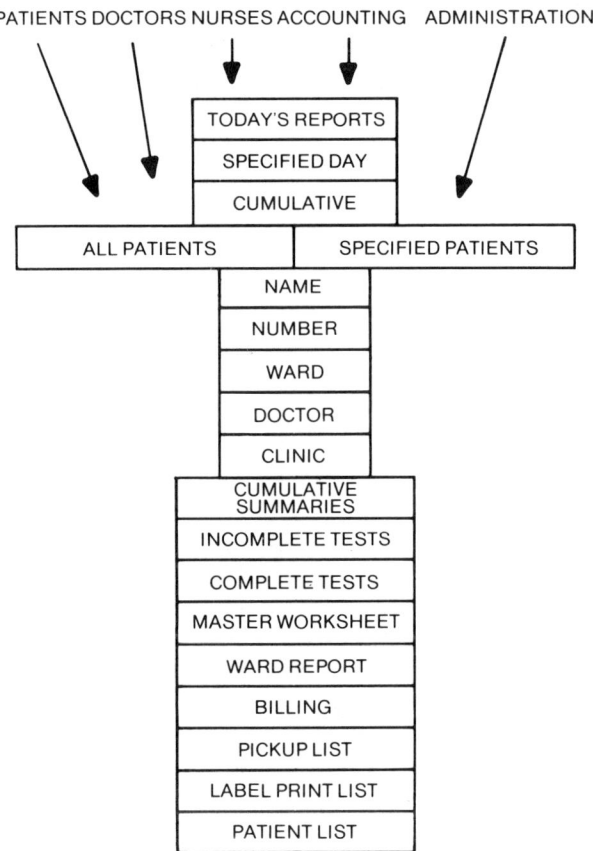

Figure 20. Report flexibility

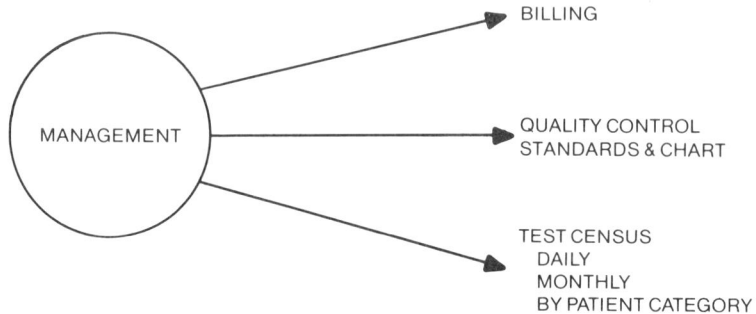

Figure 21. Management reports

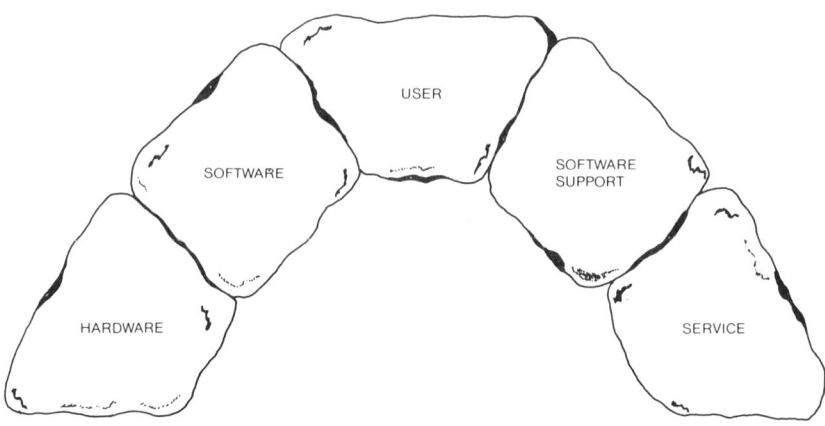

Figure 22

EVALUATION OF CLINICAL LABORATORY SYSTEMS
Infotronics CL-II System

L. E. Loveless, Ph.D.

The data processing system in Clinical Laboratories is currently undergoing the third hardware and software modification in five years. Each of these changes has been handled by Infotronics personnel. The system is discussed here as it will be at the completion of this current modification.

The CL-II system in our laboratory is dedicated to the laboratory - to gathering, calculating and correcting, collating, editing, and reporting of data from the clinical laboratory. Since we are not a hospital laboratory we do not have the problem of updating and presenting summary information daily or weekly on the same patient. Likewise, our system is not used for accounting, payroll, and/or inventory functions. The control of the system is completely in the hands of the medical technologist.

General Operation of the System

As specimens arrive at the laboratory (through the mails, courier service or our own patient laboratories) they are logged into the computer at a Patient Information Terminal. The patients' name, address, attending physician, pertinent information about the patient (age, sex) and the condition of the specimen (lipemia, icterus, or hemolysis), and tests to be performed are entered by a secretary. At this time the system assigns an accession number to the specimen and labels containing the accession number and patient information are printed for various aliquots of the specimen.

Upon request by the technologist at each particular work station a work list for that station is compiled and printed. For AutoAnalyzer^R stations this work list designates the content for each cup of a tray. In the case of PBI determinations an Edit must be performed before a Work List can be generated. This Edit eliminates all specimens that are contaminated and contain more than 20 µg I/100 ml.

After the analyses have been performed the data are retained on disc until the technologist performs certain checks to insure validity and accuracy of the data. Upon completion of these checks and upon command of the technologist a report is printed on a line printer and, if applicable, transmitted via a data phone set to a remote terminal, e.g., a rural hospital 100-150 miles from the main laboratory. Data are stored on magnetic tape.

Various statistical programs allow us to calculate quality control information monthly and to correlate results of analyses with other information - normal values, test results, disease conditions, etc.

Hardware

The hardware of the CL-II system consists of a PDP8 Computer with 16K of core and a 256K Disc. This allows us to have 1000 incomplete or unreported tests in the system at one time. There are 2 DEC - tape units - one for patient results and one for the monthly standards and control serum values. The digitizer A-D converter contains 36 ports for analytical stations. Three manual entry stations, two of which have calculator capabilities, are used for entering results of off-line tests such as T-3 uptake, urea clearance, and endocrine assays.

^{R}Trademark: Technicon Corporation

DOCUMENTATION OF LABORATORY DATA

There are three patient information teletypes and one label printer for entering specimen information and a line printer and a RO 35 Report Writer for printing of final reports. Two communication teletypes allow the technologists to communicate with the computer. There is the capacity for a dial-up network for remote transmission of reports to 64 rural or remote terminals.

The analytical system which is on-line with the computer consists of 16 channel AutoAnalyzers and 2 Model R 110 Beckman Densitometers (capability of 4). An oscilloscope display is provided to allow visual observation of the serum electrophoresis tracing and the marking of the various protein fractions by the technologist.

Instrumentation Capabilities

The basic programs for gathering and handling data include AutoAnalyzer and Electrophoresis capabilities. Interfacing for SMA 12, Hycel Mark 10, Coulter S, and gas chromatographs are available but not a part of our system.

The CL-II AutoAnalyzer Program is a system of routines which use digitized chart position data to evaluate the results of a continuous flow AutoAnalyzer's chemical reactions. Both Beer's law and linear %T versus Concentration signals are processed by the program.

The program is designed to establish dynamically each test's baseline and make drift correction throughout the duration of a run, calibrate each test according to known standards and calculate and remove the effects of sample interaction. The program provides quality control checks, replication checks on patient serum and the detection and notification of questionable peaks which might require dilution or rerun. For these peaks, answers are calculated which are usually reliable. The technician has the option of accepting or rejecting these values.

The seven types of specimens allowed for processing are:

1. Interaction standards
2. Calibration standards
3. Drift standards
4. Quality control standards
5. Replication checks
6. Blanks
7. Patient serum

Patient electrophoresis patterns are stored by the system in the course of automatic system operation. At the technologist's convenience, the desired control or patient pattern is recalled by accession number and displayed visually at the Protein Analysis Station. The technologist may then electronically interpolate the trace, visually eliminating those portions of the curve which are not desired in the analysis. Statistical analysis of the traces is then begun by integrating the exact curve peaks desired by the technologist performing the analysis. The integration results are visually displayed for verification. If results are not judged acceptable, she may recall the original trace for review and repeat the entire process. Total protein values previously entered in the system are used to report protein weights and protein percentages.

Software Programs

Various programs offer features which we have found necessary in our operation. These include:

1. A Loading Sequence Generator modifies existing sample tray configurations, changing cup definitions within trays for a particular test or set of tests from an automatic analyzer.

2. A Processor Table Modifier allows changes in calibration, concentration, tolerance figures and other parameters used in the system's test analyses.

DOCUMENTATION OF LABORATORY DATA

3. A System Regenerator Procedure is used following the Processor Table Modifier to incorporate new test parameters on the permanent system tape.

4. A Patient Information Procedure enters vital statistics of the patient and lists the doctor's name and the tests he requested. Accession numbers are assigned and listed automatically by the system.

5. A Work List Procedure provides the technologist a listing of all samples in the order in which they are to be analyzed. For patient samples, the work list indicates the patient's name or specimen number, cup number and accession number. Control or standard samples do not require accession numbers. However, replicate samples are listed with the correlated original cup numbers for the approval of the technologist.

6. A PBI Edit Procedure enables the technologist to eliminate specimens that have excessive I levels which would contaminate the System.

7. A Dilution Response Feature notifies the technologist with an audible call and prints the accession number, the test that is out of range, and the questionable value. The test may then be accepted, rejected or rerun as a dilution. If a dilution run is selected, the system requests dilution factors and reschedules the test.

8. A Statistical Evaluation Feature provides computer assisted statistical evaluation of specified patient data or standards and control data. Special options allow specification of time periods, patient age limits, test type, etc., for the analysis.

9. An Impunge Procedure allows adding test requests to those already scheduled for a specimen in the system.

10. An Expunge Procedure deletes specific tests for

any particular patient. An added feature of this procedure also allows deletion of specified tests for all patients currently in the system.

11. A Delete Procedure is a simple method which eliminates any or all patients from the system without any loss of data.

12. An Inquiry Feature enables the listing of incomplete tests without interrupting those tests in progress.

13. A Partial Results Feature ensures that immediate information is available to the staff when necessary. Results of partially completed test batteries need not wait for a scheduled report printout. The technologist has direct control and quick access to all test information in the system.

14. A Report Generator Program prints laboratory reports automatically when all requested tests are complete. The system can accomodate 2 such report generator stations, in the laboratory and in remote locations, with each remote printer receiving selected patient reports. After a patient's report is generated, the complete patient information on file is stored on a permanent magnetic tape.

15. An Information Retrieval Feature provides, upon request, a report of all previously reported patient information.

16. A Directory Generator provides by date an alphabetic directory of patient data which has been stored on magnetic tape and includes the patient's name, tape record number and requestor's name.

17. An important feature is the Equipment Failure Program which prevents the loss of current data and recovery when a power failure occurs, a pump tube

DOCUMENTATION OF LABORATORY DATA

breaks, a colorimeter bulb fails, a recorder pen sticks, or any number of the many daily malfunctions that do happen routinely in the laboratory.

Summary

The development of any system in a new area is exceedingly time consuming. In the development of these programs the contractor and we grossly underestimated the time and expense involved. For the past eighteen months this effort has been justified for we are handling a much larger volume of work without additional personnel. Without this system we would currently need two additional secretary-typists and two to three additional medical technologists. The value of the system can only be appreciated when the computer is inoperable because of hardware failure or equipment modification or changeover.

The major disadvantage to this system is that it is programmed in machine language, and an extremely unusual programmer who is knowledgeable with the laboratory work as well as the computer is required to make major modifications to the program. This handicap can put us at the mercy of "specialized specialists" who appear to be inherently a mobile migratory work force.

THE B-D SPEAR CLINICAL LABORATORY AUTOMATION SYSTEM IN A COMMUNITY HOSPITAL LABORATORY:

A CASE REPORT

William W. McLendon, M.D.

Introduction

One of the major decisions facing most clinical laboratory directors today is the one concerning the role of a computer system in his laboratory. Once he has made the decision that he should use a computer he is faced with the even more difficult choice of determining which of the many approaches to the computerization of the clinical laboratory he should follow.

Those of us in the laboratory, as well as physicians generally, have often approached the problem of the role of computers in medicine in the same way we approach the problem of the patient who is chronically ill with a disease we don't understand and can't cure. Such a patient is frustrating to the conscientious physician and we try to refer him to someone else, but he keeps coming back to haunt us. Similarly the computer keeps coming back to frustrate and challenge us.

In dealing with problem patients we can often benefit from others who have documented their experience with similar problems. I would like to present my discussion of our experiences with a laboratory computer system in the form of a case report, utilizing the same approach one would use as a physician approaching a new patient.

I. HISTORY. In medical school we were taught to begin our questioning of the patient by asking, "What brought you to the hospital?" When we ask this question of the computer, we find that it has a very long history, even though our contact with it in medicine has been relatively brief. Calculating machines in the form of the abacus have been used in the Orient for several thousand years, while workable mechanical calculating machines were designed and made in the 1600's. The punched card --that symbol of the alienation of modern youth from our computerized society--was first used in France in 1801 to program the pattern for an automatic loom and has had ever expanding applications in data processing since its use by Hollerith to tabulate the 1890 census in America. Much of the theory of modern computers was developed by Charles Babbage and Lady Lovelace, the daughter of Lord Byron, in the early 1800's in England, but it took the technological advances of the early and mid-1900's to translate their theories into the working computers which became generally available in the 1950's.

The LINC computer, the ancestor of the present SPEAR computer, is a small digital computer with analog-to-digital conversion capabilities. It was developed by Dr. Wesley Clark and his group at MIT in the early 1960's under an NIH grant[1] and modifications were later made available commercially by SPEAR and DEC. The LINC computer was primarily designed for bio-medical research purposes and was used for this purpose by most of the early users. Dr. Phillip Hicks and his group in the Clinical Chemistry laboratory at the University of Wisconsin Hospital foresaw the potential for this type of computer in the clinical laboratory and published a paper on such a use in the JAMA in 1966.[3]

The development of the SPEAR Clinical Laboratory Automation System (CLAS) began in the mid-1960's through collaboration between Dr. Glenn Fellows and

DOCUMENTATION OF LABORATORY DATA

others of SPEAR with Dr. Hugo Pribor and his staff in the Laboratory of the Perth Amboy General Hospital in Perth Amboy, New Jersey, and has evolved through cooperation between the company and many other clinical laboratories. Our system at Moses Cone Hospital was the third system which SPEAR installed and at present there are over 25 systems operating or being installed in community and university hospitals and private laboratories in the United States and Canada.

Our own involvement in the laboratory computer field began in the mid-1960's when we came to realize that automation was breaking the bottleneck of doing laboratory tests, but that we would soon be faced with a greater bottleneck in information handling. The first seminar I attended on this topic was sponsored by one of the large computer manufacturers. The presentations left me enthusiastic about the potential in this field, but completely frustrated because of their armchair approach to the problem and the tremendous monthly rentals involved when one used the conventional computers. The need for a large staff of programmers to develop a laboratory computer system also seemed out of the question for us at that time.

I returned from that seminar in the fall of 1966 to attend the annual meeting of the American Society of Clinical Pathologists in Washington, D. C. In the corner of the exhibition hall at that meeting I discovered SPEAR's first exhibit and met Dr. Glenn Fellows. In contrast to all the speculation about numbered computers and peripherals with large rental figures I had heard the previous week, I saw a small computer actually processing data from an attached single-channel AutoAnalyzer, and I found a man who knew his computers and was willing to live in the clinical laboratory to promote this marriage of the laboratory and the computer. That chance meeting in September, 1966, led to several visits by myself and our clinical chemist to the SPEAR plant and to hospitals which were then using computers. After a presentation by representatives from SPEAR at our hospital, our Trustees approved the purchase of a SPEAR Clinical Laboratory Automation System.

During 1967-68 our laboratory was busy with the introduction of the SMA-12 and other automated instruments and with preparations for the coming computer installation. That installation was much longer in coming than we had originally expected. When our computer did arrive in April, 1968, it was a completely redesigned and greatly improved computer from the one we had ordered. We have had other delays in delivery during the years we have been working with SPEAR, but in each case we have received far more for our investment than we were originally promised.

Computer use in our laboratory has gone through two stages. The first one was a long and trying one and reflected the fact that both we and SPEAR were exploring new territories. I would not want to live through this period again, but I would not give anything for the experience since it has resulted in a system which is working well with ever increasing dividends in terms of service to our patients and our laboratory. This first or developmental phase of our computer operation began when we received our computer in April, 1968. We gradually went into a parallel operation during the summer, and in October, 1968, shifted to the use of the computer alone for much of our clinical laboratory work. In spite of the fact that we had many problems, we were able to struggle along with this system until September, 1969, when we made the decision to shift back to a parallel operation while needed improvements were made in both our hardware and software.

During 1969-70, SPEAR made major and quite significant improvements in the software. From our standpoint, the addition of the ward report and abnormal value

DOCUMENTATION OF LABORATORY DATA

reports were of major importance, along with the complete re-working of the cumulative reports to eliminate problems which had been encountered. Numerous other improvements resulted in increased efficiency of operation and many additional functions. The addition of the line printer and card reader eliminated two of the other major bottlenecks of the first phase of our operations.

During the summer and early fall of 1970 we profited by our previous mistakes and make a slow and orderly transition from the parallel manual operation back to the complete reliance on the computer operation. We planned this implementation step by step; first, making a listing of all the necessary steps (Fig. 1) and then putting these in graphic form (Fig. 2). We had an extensive orientation period for all the involved hospital staff and physicians. A display showing the computer system with a step-by-step progression from requisition to reporting was found very useful for orientation purposes. We started using the computer reports on one nursing division at a time in order to be sure that the personnel were thoroughly familiar with the system. After all divisions were receiving the reports, we eliminated the duplicate manual reports.

Since the fall of 1970 we have been completely operational with our system in the clinical laboratory, where it is used for all areas except bacteriology. During the last 6-8 months we have been operational in this second stage, we have had the usual small problems that one would expect with any operation this complex, but we have had no major down-time and the computer is now well accepted by both our laboratory and hospital staff.

II. EXAMINATION. After completing the history we shall now examine the computer system. The original computer system installed in 1968 consisted of the SPEAR micro-LINC 300 computer with a 4 K memory and 4 tape units. Input to the computer was by the conversational mode using the keyboard and cathode ray tube and by on-line connections to the automated laboratory instruments. The Teletype initially was our back-up printer with the Kleinschmidt printer being the primary printer. In addition to its slow speed and frequent breakdowns when used as a primary printer, the latter was quite noisy. The noise was eliminated by using a soundproof enclosure. The addition of the Data Products Line Printer in the spring of 1970 as the primary printer was a welcome relief after all of the difficulty we had had with the Kleinschmidt printer. This line printer can print up to 1200 lines per minute and has been virtually trouble-free during almost a year of continuous use. At the time the line-printer was added, we also added the Hewlett-Packard card reader and had the computer modified so that it could later be expanded to an 8 K memory. The card reader can read either mark-sense or punched cards and is being used daily without difficulty for entry of all urinalysis and differential results. In the near future we hope to add other card entries, including test requisitioning.

Our present computer still has a 4 K memory and uses the 4 tape drives as the primary memory storage. We find this satisfactory for our present volume but plan to increase the core memory to 8 K and add the disc in the fall of 1971 in order to more efficiently handle the ever increasing volume of work and to handle the bacteriology reporting which we hope to start in early 1972.

In medicine we realize that cell biology has real meaning only in relation to the biology of the individual; and the individual is increasingly being studied in relationship to his environment. Similarly, the electronic computer components have meaning to the computer user only in relationship to the total system of hardware and software. Just as importantly, the computer system must be examined in relationship to the environment in which it functions and the people who use it.

DOCUMENTATION OF LABORATORY DATA

Our computer is located in the environment of a privately-endowed, general community hospital which was established on paper in the early 1900's by Mrs. Moses Cone as a memorial to her late husband and as a gift to our community. Planning for the hospital began at her death in 1947 and the hospital was opened in 1953. There have been several expansions since and it is now a 425-bed hospital with approximately 15,000 admissions and discharges a year.

The clinical laboratories and pathology department are located in approximately 15,000 square feet of space on one floor of an original hospital wing and in a two-story addition which was completed in 1965. The laboratories are supervised by four pathologists who share the anatomic pathology and who have individual responsibility for the various clinical pathology areas. There is a staff of over 60 technical and clerical personnel, including approximately 30 registered medical technologists and cytotechnologists.

In keeping with the current interest in "management by objectives" we have attempted in recent years to formulate general goals for the laboratory, while at the same time setting more specific goals and deadlines for meeting those goals in each area of the laboratory. We find that our general goals can be grouped into three areas:

1. We share with other members of the hospital staff and the medical staff a commitment to be a vital part of a hospital dedicated to providing the finest possible scientific medical care in an atmosphere of genuine personal concern for each patient served and of mutual respect for each of our co-workers in this endeavor.

2. Our unique commitment in the laboratory is to provide the physician with the most information possible about his patient in order to facilitate his diagnosis and

treatment. We have a further obligation to make this information as accurate and precise as possible; to make it available in the appropriate quantities and at the appropriate times; and, to provide it at the lowest possible cost to the patient.

3. Our hospital is committed by its charter to be concerned with education and this is manifested by our affiliation with the University of North Carolina School of Medicine for house staff and medical student training and by the various programs for allied health personnel which are based at the hospital or at one of the local universities or technical institutes and use the hospital facilities. Within the laboratory we have a School of Medical Technology with 10 or 12 students annually. We also have an approved residency in anatomic and clinical pathology with both full-time residents in our program and senior residents from the medical school pathology program taking a four-month elective rotation in clinical chemistry and clinical pathology.

As I will point out in the discussion that follows, we feel that our laboratory computer system makes a very significant contribution toward meeting each of these three general goals.

The people involved with the laboratory computer system are, of course, the essential ingredient (Fig. 3). The central person is the patient himself and his welfare must be a paramount consideration in all of our activities.

Our approach to the staffing of the computer operation has evolved over the past several years (Fig. 4). Initially, I naively assumed that the technologists at night could enter the test requisitions and that the technologists during the day had time to enter all their own data and prepare reports. This approach simply added to the clerical burden of the technologists. It also overlooked the many other functions that are performed by the computer and the absolute necessity for continuity of operation if essential steps in the processing of the daily work are not to be overlooked. We thus trained two of our existing clerks to share the day computer clerk duties and added several part-time clerks for evening and night. We have more recently added a person on the midnight shift in order to put in data done at night and in order to get an earlier start on the next day's routine operation. All of these persons have been trained on-the-job in a relatively short time. Although typing skill is an asset, previous computer experience is not needed. We have found a ready source of willing workers for the evening and right shifts among the high school, computer school and university students in the community.

Initially, I tried to handle all of the immediate supervision of the computer operation, although our chief and senior technologists were involved in the planning and supervision. Last year we added the supervision of the computer operation to the duties of our clinical chemist. Since the computer is physically located adjacent to the chemistry section and since the chemistry operation is so intimately connected with the computer operation, this supervisory arrangement has functioned very well and has improved our entire operation.

On the basis of our experience I think it is essential that the laboratory director or his associate and at least one of his senior technologists be intimately involved in the initial planning and in the long-range supervision of the computer operation. The choice of the persons would, of course, vary from laboratory to laboratory. It goes without saying that success in any venture such as this also involves getting the entire laboratory staff and the affected hospital staff in on the initial planning as well as on the subsequent modifications. The laboratory director and the computer supervisor play a major role in coordinating all of these activities, including the planning for software and hardware maintenance, the assurance of the availability of supplies, and communications with areas such as the admitting office and business office.

III. FUNCTION TESTS. After a physician has taken a history and examined his patient he usually will perform various tests of the patient's functions, such as EKG, neurological testing, laboratory determinations, etc. To carry this analogy along with our analysis of the laboratory computer system, let us now see how it functions during a 24-hour period in the life of the clinical laboratory.

The file structure of the laboratory computer is patient oriented. When the patient is admitted to the hospital we receive a duplicate copy of admission data which is then fed into the computer through the keyboard. Once this basic information is entered, the patient's administrative or laboratory data can then be simply retrieved, corrected or added to by use of the patient's six digit unit number. When the physician writes an order for laboratory work, the ward clerk or nurse prepares the lab requisition using the patient's addressograph identification plate. We are temporarily continuing to use conventional lab requisition slips, the last copy of which is used for billing by an off-site IBM 360 at a service bureau. The SPEAR computer now has the ability to dump billing data directly to such a business computer and we hope to by-pass this duplicate handling in the near future. If the test request is for routine work the next morning, the computer clerk on the evening or night shift simply has to enter the patient's unit number and the test number(s) requested. After the night computer operator has entered all of the tests requests for the next day, he calls for the pick-up program, which results in typed labels for all patients who have had requests. These are arranged in order of ascending room number. These labels are used by the technologists to identify their blood samples when they are drawn the next morning.

DOCUMENTATION OF LABORATORY DATA

Requests for emergency laboratory work are made on the same slips; the technologists perform the work and reports it back to the physician on the top copy of the slip which is placed in the chart as a preliminary report. The information on the lab copy of the request and report slip is later entered in the computer and appears on the patient's next cumulative report.

The day computer operations begins with the preparation of various administrative reports for use during the day, including a list of the unfinished procedures which serves as the log for the day's work.

When the technologists return from the floors in the morning with their blood samples, the worklists sorted by test or test groups are available so they can immediately begin their work. The night clerk also has labeled all of the cards for data entry of the differentials, so that the technologist in hematology has only to fill in the various percentages. In the case of the automated procedures, the technologist places the samples on the sample plate in the same order as they are on the worklist and indicates to the computer that the run is beginning by flipping a single switch at the analyzer. At the end of the run the technologist goes to the computer to inspect the data and make any necessary corrections in the data such as the results of dilutions. She can also at this time make any comments to be filed with a patient's data. We have continued to send a copy of the SMA-12 chart to the patient's chart, using the computer label for identification. This represents some duplication of effort, but both we and the physicians on our staff feel there is value in having such a graphic presentation of the data. The same data appears in digital form on the various reports to be described below. In the case of both the manual and on-line data, a checklist showing the data actually in the computer for each patient is printed; the technologist must check this against her original data and must initial that the computer data is correct. At this time she can very simply make any corrections in the data before it is distributed to the patient's file in the computer, if this is necessary.

Current laboratory data is reported to the floors twice during the day by means of ward reports, which list the patients and their data by wards. We profited from our mistakes during our first phase of operation and have these reports printed on a grey-bar paper to distinguish them from the white cumulative report which go on the charts. The ward reports are placed on a clip board at each nursing station, where they stay until they are replaced the next day. We have found the ward reports to be a very valuable feature of this system. They have eliminated many telephone requests. The nurses feel that it is "their report", since it gives them in one place a complete summary of all the laboratory reports on their patients. They particularly like having all of the prothrombin times in one list so that they can make all the necessary calls about dicumarol therapy at one time.

The calculation and generation of reports for electrophoretic studies has been a particularly time-saving feature of the computer operation. These can be printed either with or without a listing of the diagnostic considerations.

Late in the afternoon we print cumulative reports on all patients who have had new data since their last report. The cumulative reports show a range of "normal values" for most tests; these ranges can be automatically selected on the basis of the patient's age and sex from the 12 available age-sex groupings of normals for each test stored on the computer tapes. When the patient has additional data the next day, an updated cumulative report is printed and replaces the original one on the patient's chart. In the first phase of our operation, this simple step almost wrecked our entire system, since the clerks had always been taught never to throw away anything.

Half the physicians seemed to understand the system and criticized the clerks if they didn't remove the old reports, while the other half criticized the clerks if they did! The results on many floors was chaotic with the charts overflowing with paper. This situation has been completely eliminated by color coding the various types of reports and by the consolidation of all reports on one cumulative (originally there were A, B and C cumulative reports, with resulting confusion). Most importantly, each ward clerk has been given orientation concerning the entire computer operation and has seen how a duplicate report can be generated in less than 60 seconds should she ever mistakenly discard a report.

When the patient is discharged, a discharge cumulative report is printed on three-part green paper. The original copy goes to Medical Records, where it replaces any previous white copies in the chart. The second copy is kept in the lab (the same data is also available on magnetic tapes). The third copy of the discharge report is sent to the physician for his office file.

One of the most valuable by-products of the computer operation in the laboratory from my standpoint, has been the abnormal value report, which we print out each afternoon before the cumulatives are printed. Each day one of the pathologists and/or the clinical pathology resident checks this report. This gives us one additional point where the laboratory data can be checked for errors of transcription or for results that don't appear to fit with the other data. More importantly, it allows us to be aware of every patient in the hospital with interesting abnormal laboratory findings. Not only does this improve the quality control for the laboratory, but it has been an invaluable teaching aid. We use this report and cumulative reports of patients with interesting data as a basis for informal abnormal rounds each afternoon. These rounds are made by one of the pathologists, the clinical pathology residents, and sometimes by the clinical pharmacist. Once a week the medical technology students attend and have the opportunity to obtain a better insight into the importance of their work in the laboratory. We usually pick several cases from the abnormal report and then review the charts, x-rays, etc. in order to correlate the laboratory results with the total clinical picture. Although we don't routinely see patients on these rounds, we have found that a valuable by-product of the rounds is the daily contact with many of the nurses, ward clerks, clinical house staff and attending physicians that results because of our interest in their patients and our presence on the wards. Not only do we learn from such contacts, but we frequently receive valuable feed-back about problems or potential problems concerning our laboratory service.

Another recent addition to the standard CLAS software is the trend report. This allows one to plot on the cathode ray tube (or plotter, if available) a graph of the results of up to three tests on a patient on the y-axis against time on the x-axis. For example, the enzyme changes in myocardial infarction or the relationship of calcium to the BUN in a patient with renal insufficiency can be studied using actual laboratory data from our own patient population. This again is an extremely valuable by-product of the computer operation for educational purposes and for use when a physician comes to the laboratory to discuss a particular patient problem.

The PALI plot is still another plotting technique available to CLAS users. Although we have not yet made use of it, we are greatly impressed with it and hope to start using it in the next year. The PALI (or Progressive Accelerated Laboratory Investigation) was conceived by Dr. Charles Altshuler of St. Joseph's Hospital in Milwaukee. When a physician requests a PALI, the laboratory does over 20 routine determinations including routine hematology and urinalysis, SMA-12, PBI, etc. Guidelines have been set up in the laboratory so that an abnormality detected on this portion of the testing automatically results in the performance by the laboratory of a more definitive test; for example, any abnormalities of the SMA-12 protein determinations would be followed by a protein electrophoresis (and immunoelectrophoresis, if indicated); an elevated LDH results in an LDH isoenzyme electrophoresis, etc. Additional tests may be done after the pathologists reviews the data before reporting. The CLAS is used to accumulate all this data, which appears on the usual reports as I have described above. In addition, a graphic presentation of the same data is available from the computer using a plotter. Unlike the printed SMA-12 charts with one "normal value" range for each test, the PALI plots show an age/sex specific "normal range" drawn in a color different from that used for the data plot. The graphic presentation of laboratory data, the potential for improved and more rapid diagnosis, and the effect that this type of definitive investigative activity has on the laboratory staff represents one of the most exciting developments in laboratory medicine in recent years in my opinion.

IV. DIFFERENTIAL DIAGNOSIS. In order to understand a disease, one should know its natural history and the various ways in which it might present. Similarly, an understanding of the natural history of a computer installation and some of the syndromes which may result from such an undertaking may be of value to the person entering the field.

Based on our experience during the first phase of our computer use, one can graphically depict the history of a computer installation using an arbitrary enthusiasm/performance index on the y-axis and time on the x-axis (Fig. 5). The graph has two peaks of enthusiasm--first, when the decision to order a computer is finally made and, secondly, when the computer actually arrives at the laboratory. Following the installation there is usually a downward trend as the parallel operation is begun and the staff is doing twice the work with few immediate benefits. We experienced a sharp drop in our enthusiasm and performance during our first phase but only a very slight drop during our second or operational phase due to better planning and the tremendous advancements that had been made in both the hardware and software in the interval. We are now far above the "status quo" point with our computer installation and seem to realize new benefits from our investment almost daily.

During our installation, the most difficult time came during the parallel operation in our first phase. Although no one beginning today would need experience more than 5 to 10% of the problems we had 3 years ago, still it is worthwhile to recognize this stressful period and be prepared for it.

It was during this period of stress that we recognized two syndromes, which I am told by others are not unique to our environment in North Carolina. The first of these resembles the "The Middle of the Way Syndrome" (Fig. 6), which is described so well by Dr. Paul Tournier, a very humane and perceptive physician from Geneva, who writes about his patients who become anxious midway on their journey from the security of their home to the security of his office.[4] Tournier generalizes this experience to cover the many situations in life where we leave a secure place to begin a new adventure. The laboratory and hospital personnel pass through a similar period of anxiety as the transition is made from the old, well-established routine to the new system and this should be expected.

The second syndrome I have labeled "The Syndrome of the Savage and the Epileptic." In less sophisticated times it was not unusual for man to place the blame for some unexplained event such as an epileptic fit on a "devil" or "spirit". (Fig. 7). We found that the modern physician may also use this same thought process-- the only difference being that he blames everything that went wrong in the laboratory or hospital on "that damn computer"! (Fig. 8)

V. CLINICAL IMPRESSION. After our analysis of this 5 year exposure to the problems of clinical laboratory computerization, what are the conclusions?

First, we might begin by honestly asking, "did the computer have any enemies?" The answer to this question would have to be "yes." Yet when we made a survey of our staff in December, 1970, (Fig. 9) I was surprised to find a high level of acceptance of the new system in view of the fact that we had only been operational in our second phase for several months and that the mistakes and problems of the first phase were still clearly in most minds. As mentioned earlier, the ward reports were most appreciated by the nursing personnel with 73% of the nurses and 86% of the ward clerks finding them "useful" or "very useful". The daily cumulative laboratory reports on the patient's charts were found useful or very useful by 76% of the physicians with only 8% expressing a dislike for these reports. In our hospital both the physicians and the nurses expressed strong approval of the computer generated "normals" on each report. Our medical records librarian has been particularly pleased with this feature, since the HAS (Hospital Activities Survey) forms now require listing of certain abnormal laboratory results and the number of blood transfusions for each patient-both of which are now clearly summarized (with abnormals flagged) on our cumulative discharge laboratory report.

On the other hand, automation is certainly not the only answer to the problems of the laboratory or other areas in the hospital. The potential for error and harm, however, is no different than that which faces us in other areas of medicine when new and powerful drugs or techniques are introduced, such as the antibiotics, open-heart surgery and cancer chemotherapy. The greater the potential for good, the greater the possibility of harm if the technique is misused. The challenge to see that these new techniques are used to benefit the patients we serve is one I believe we must accept if we are to provide the type of laboratory services that are needed for the future.

The potential dehumanizing effect of the computer is also one that has concerned all of us. I do not see this as a necessary result, for as Dr. John Gardner has reminded us in one of his thoughtful books,[2] it is we and not science nor technology that design our organizations and institutions. In our own system we have insisted that the patient be identified by both a name and a number on all printed materials, even though internally the computer is sorting and processing by numbers. This serves not only to assure proper identification but constantly reminds us that we are working with materials from a human being rather than from the production vats of some chemical factory. We carry this further in insisting that our technologists and technicians all share in the blood collecting routine in the mornings in order to be constantly reminded of the patients they are serving, even though we realize that a phlebotomy team approach is probably a more efficient one.

The problems of a laboratory computer operation can be summarized in terms of the personnel involved, the hardware and software, and the necessity for both a psychological and financial commitment on the part of the laboratory and the hospital. During the early phase of our system, the hardware and software problems were considerable, but in the past year these have been negligible. This, I think, reflects the fact that the SPEAR organization is in the fairly unique position of having both the hardware and software responsibilities under one roof, in addition to having over 5 years experience in actually working in over 20 laboratories of various types.

DOCUMENTATION OF LABORATORY DATA

The necessity for a psychological commitment cannot be overemphasized. If a student tells me, "I think I might want to be a physician," I am very reluctant to encourage him to continue in that direction. The same thing applies to the computerization of the laboratory. If the laboratory director doesn't want to get involved in the details of the operation of his laboratory and doesn't want to get out of his office and get involved in the hospital, then I can't recommend such a course.

The laboratory and the hospital must also be well aware of the cost of such an undertaking. The components of the cost include the depreciation, lease or rental costs; the direct costs for personnel and supplies and for hardware and software maintenance; and the indirect or overhead costs. For 1971 we estimate that our total annual cost for the computer operation will be approximately $43,000 (Fig. 10). This includes $14,000 depreciation ($70,000 capital investment with a five-year depreciation), $18,000 personnel costs, $3,000 for supplies, and $8,000 for maintenance contracts. This figure represents 6.3% of our budgeted operating costs for the entire laboratory and pathology department for 1970-71. These costs must be evaluated in relationship to the estimated savings of personnel time and the value of the added services. We have not attempted to derive any firm figures for our saving, but I would think that now our added costs are almost balanced by the resulting savings. When we begin using our laboratory computer to handle the inital billing activity, I think there will be no question concerning the savings. On the other hand, I would strongly advise against justifying a laboratory computer solely on the basis of saving money. You might well run into the same response from your Trustees that I received from my father when I went to him as a pre-med student and told him I had decided to get married then rather than wait until later "since two can live as cheaply as one." In both situations, the intangible benefits far outweigh any tangible savings!

The seemingly large cost of a "turnkey" laboratory computer system such as described here (that is, with the hardware and software furnished as a package by the manufacturer) must be evaluated in relationship to the high developmental costs one hospital would have if it attempted to do all of the system planning and programming itself. Knowledgeable computer experts who have seen our system or heard it described have estimated that conservatively we would have had to spend at least a quarter to a half million dollars just for the programming had we done it ourselves. Because these costs of development can be shared by dozens of laboratories which are using or will use a system such as the one described, the initial cost of the system is much more reasonable. Furthermore, all users benefit from the corrections of mistakes and "bugs" found in the earlier systems and from the continuing developments that are made in response to specific needs of other users. On the surface, such a commonly developed system would seem to imply an extreme degree of rigidity. In practice, however, we have found that the modular programming used in this system allows us a wide range of options at most all steps in the system and thus we have never felt that we were unduly restricted by any lack of flexibility.

The specific things we have been able to accomplish with our system can best be listed in reference to our initial goals. Within the laboratory the computer performs most clerical tasks and calculations; assists with the quality control and on-line monitoring of automated equipment; and is available for storage and retrieval of patient data and for derivation of population data. The computer generates ward reports, cumulative reports and discharge reports for the physician and medical records.

One of the most important benefits of the system in my estimation is the fact that the pathologist and the supervising technologists now have a tool for constant monitoring of both the technical quality and the administrative function of their laboratory operation. Although one physician commented that the printed computer reports "looked as if they were never touched by human hands," in practice the technologists and pathologists with the help of the computer are involved at multiple stages in the processing and checking of each piece of information to assure accuracy of reporting. The unfinished work reports, the statistical and census reports and other reports are by-products of the operation which for the first time furnish meaningful management tools with no additional clerical effort. Just as importantly, the abnormal reports, the trend plots and the ready availability of cumulative reports on individual patients give the pathologist invaluable information for his consultative and educational functions in the hospital. All of these cited benefits might best be summarized in the words of Mesthene taken from a recent article concerning the role of computers in our society:

> The more machines take over what we do,
> The more we are freed to do what machines cannot do.

In spite of what has been accomplished to date we have long-range plans to continue a gradual evolution of our system (Fig. 11). As mentioned before, this includes the addition of a disc and one or more remote terminals within the laboratory for data entry and inquiry during 1971-72. We hope to implement the programs for bacteriology reporting in early 1972 and also to use our computer for transmitting the billing data directly to the business computer. In the future we are considering the possibility of using the laboratory computer in conjunction with a multiphasic screening operation in our proposed ambulatory care facility. We are also looking forward to the prospect of interfacing our laboratory computer system to a larger, medically-oriented hospital computer system during the next several years.

Many of the things we propose to do in the next year or so could be the initial part of a new laboratory computer system installed at this time due to the striking advances which have been made since our system was first installed. The beauty of such a system as this is that one can start with a simple system and gradually modify and add to it as one's needs and applications grow. I no longer feel a compulsion to accomplish everything overnight. At one time the visiting pathologist who had nothing more than a desk calculator in his laboratory caused me concern by his disappointment that we didn't have a direct print-out of laboratory results to the bathroom in the doctor's lounge, but I am much more philosophical about these matters today! I would strongly advise that fairly complete planning for all possible computer uses be done early, but that the actual implementation be done in stages, beginning internally with each laboratory area involved. This can be followed by a gradual introduction of the computer reports in parallel to the old system and then by a complete change to the new system. Such a planned, orderly approach will avoid many of the anxieties and mistakes we experienced in the first phase of our operation.

In conclusion, we might summarize this case report of our experiences with laboratory computer system as follows: A marriage was entered into by two well-motivated, but relatively inexperienced teenagers of different ethnic backgrounds--one from the world of computers and one from the world of the clinical laboratory. As is usual, conception occurred with ease, but delivery followed a prolonged period of gestation characterized by morning sickness and false labor. The offspring suffered a period of colic, but is now healthy and thriving with prospects for a long and ever more useful life. Although the parents have matured considerably as a result of their experiences together, they, like other parents, find it difficult to be completely objective about the accomplishments of their offspring and invite the reader to make his own evaluation.

References

1. Clark, W. A. and C. E. Molnar, A Description of the LINC, in Stacy, R. W. and B. Waxman, Editors, "Computers in Biomedical Research," Volume II, pp. 35-66 Academic Press, New York, (1965).
2. Gardner, J. W., "Self-Renewal," p. 57, Harper & Row, New York (1963).
3. Hicks, G. P., et al, Routine use of a small digital computer in the clinical laboratory, J. Amer. Med. Assoc.: 973-978 (1966).
4. Tournier, P. "A place for you," 157-169, Harper & Row, New York, (1968).

ACKNOWLEDGEMENTS. An undertaking of this complexity could never have succeeded without the support of numerous persons and special appreciation is extended to the following: The medical, nursing, supportive and administrative staffs and the Trustees of the Moses H. Cone Memorial Hospital for their patience and cooperation; the manfacturing, programming, and field service staffs of B-D SPEAR Medical Systems for their continuing interest and support of all our efforts; the entire staff of the Laboratory Department of the Moses H. Cone Memorial Hospital for their skill, dedication, and continuing support; Miss Marue Summerlin, MT (ASCP), Chief Medical Technologist, and Mr. T. A. Weisner, MT (ASCP), Clinical Chemist and Supervisor of the Laboratory Computer Operation, for their unfailing leadership and support; and to my wife, Anne, my family, and my professional associates for their understanding and support during these several busy years. I am also most grateful to the late Edward K. Atkinson of Greensboro for many of the cartoons which illustrated this presentation and to Miss Anna Trogdon for typing of the manuscript.

Step No.	Description of Steps	Required Prior Steps	Time Weeks	Week of Completion Anticipated	Actual
1.	Order and receive new computer paper 1-part white--cumulative reports(daily) 2-part green--interim discharges; discharges; out-patient reports (Following paper already available: 1-part gray bar-ward reports Gummed label paper--pick-up lists	--	4	May 4	
2.	New A Tape (Program) Received & Implemented	--	1	April 13	
3. a.	Line Printer Received and Installed	--	1	April 20	
	(1) Paper Holder Constructed	--	1	April 27	
b.	Keyboard-Scope Received & Installed	--	1	April 20	
4.	Software for SMA-4 On-Line	--	4	May 4	
5.	Laboratory Organization				
a.	All slips with date, time and lab # lab # on all worklists	--	1	April 13	
b.	Review and up-date normal values in computer; pediatric normals	2	1	April 20	
c.	Prepare detailed schedule and log sheets of computer operation	2, 3	1	April 27	
d.	Review and document back-up procedure	2, 3, 5c	1	May 4	
6.	Prepare Display on Laboratory Computer system for use in instruction of Medical & nursing staffs	1	4	May 4	
a.	Photographs of system (for use in steps 7 & 8)	1-6	2	May 11	
7.	Meeting with staff on Trial Division (4500)	1-6	1	May 11	
8.	Meeting with Nursing & Medical Staffs a. Nursing-Head Nurses & Supervisors b. Medical Full-Staff Meeting c. Surgical Full-Staff Meeting d. Pediatric Full-Staff Meeting e. OB-Gyn Full-Staff Meeting	1-6	1	May 11	
9.	IMPLEMENTATION OF FULL REPORTING ROUTINE FOR TRIAL DIVISION (4500)	1-8	1	May 18	

Figure 1. Implementation schedule

WEEK #	1	2	3	4	5	6	7	8	9	10	11	12	13	14	15	16
WEEK OF	Apr. 13	20	27	May 4	11	18	25	June 1	8	15	22	29	July 6	13	20	27

1. Computer Paper
2. New A Tape
3. a. LinePrinter
    3a)
    3.b Keyboard-Scope
4. SMA-4 On-Line
5. a-d Lab Organiz.
6. Educational Display
7. Meetings (div. 4500)
8. Staff Meetings
9. Test-ward Reporting
10. Discharge Reports
11. Ward Reports
12. aCardread.
    12bDiff and Urin. Entry--Card Reader
13. REPORTS TO ALL WARDS
14. Back-Up Implementation
    Discontinue Parallel

Simultaneous Special Projects:

1. Reporting and Requisitions for WE Lab work
2. SMA-12 Reporting
3. Cumulative Reporting for Out-Patient Prenatal Screening Tests
4. Cumulative Reporting for Out-Patient Prothrombins

LONG-RANGE GOALS FOR LABORATORY COMPUTER SYSTEM

1. Additional Quality Control and Statistical Programs
2. Card Design and Programs for Card Reader Input of:
   a. Test requests
   b. Admissions & Discharges
   c. Bacteriology Data
3. Bacteriology Data on Reports
   a. Sensitivity statistics
   b. Infections Dis. Committee
4. Transmission of billing data to Business Computer
5. Terminals for Counting and Automated Entry of Data from Differentials
6. Ultimately: On-line with hospital Computer for Test Requisition, Reporting and Billing

Figure 2. Graph of implementation schedule

PEOPLE

and the

LABORATORY COMPUTER SYSTEM

The people who design, build, program, sell and maintain it

The people who use it in the laboratory

The people who are served by it:

THE PATIENT

The Physician, Nurse, Clerk

The Laboratory Staff

Figure 3. People and the laboratory computer system

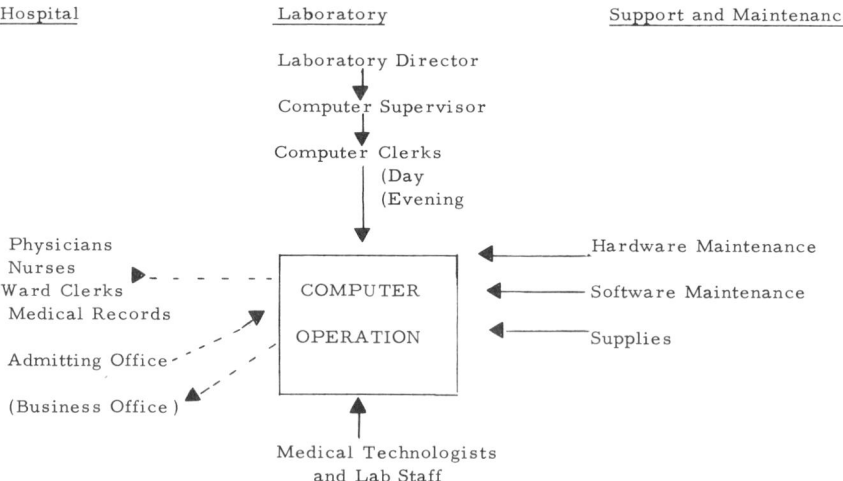

Figure 4. Staffing for the laboratory computer operation

DOCUMENTATION OF LABORATORY DATA

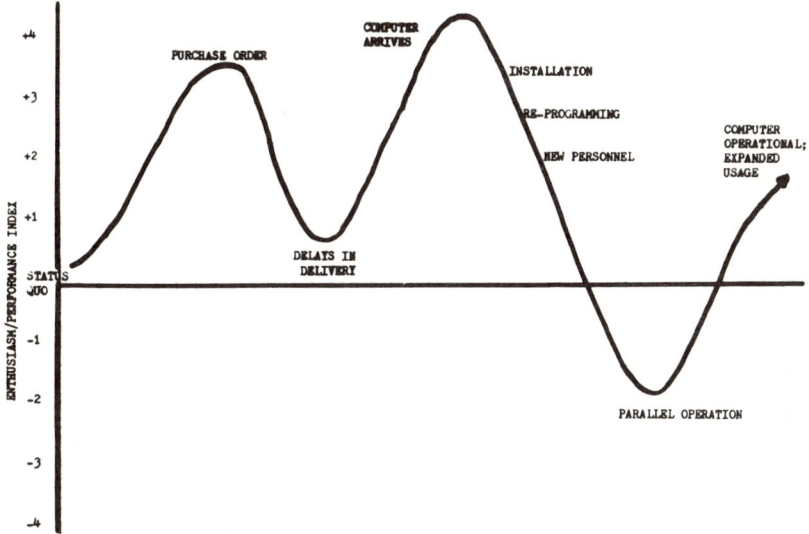

Figure 5.   Natural History of a computer installation

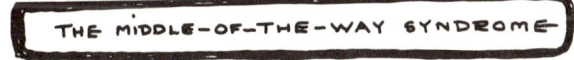

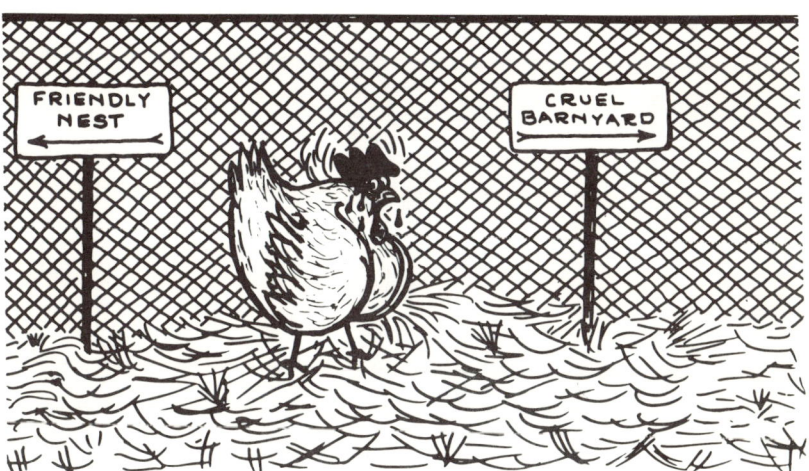

Figure 6.   The middle of the way syndrome (After Dr. Paul Tournier)

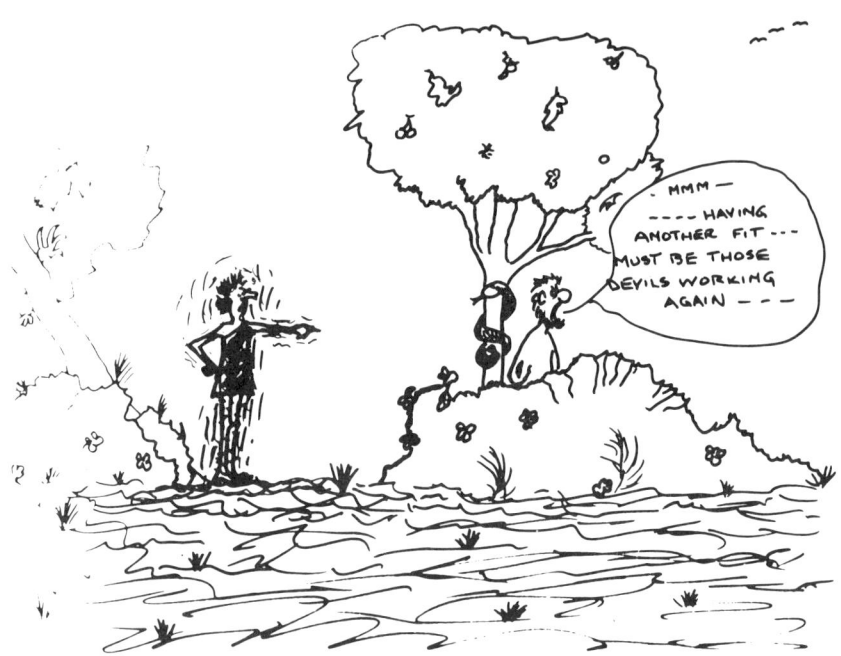

Figure 7. Syndrome of the savage and the epileptic Part I

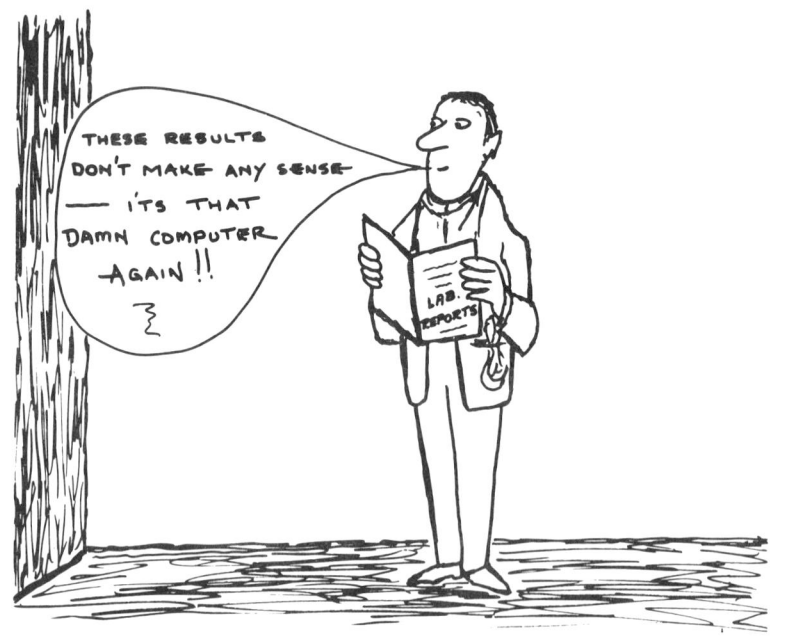

Figure 8. Syndrome of the savage and the epileptic Part II

DOCUMENTATION OF LABORATORY DATA

LABORATORY COMPUTER SYSTEM QUESTIONNAIRE
Moses Cone Hospital--December 1970

	VERY USEFUL	USEFUL	DON'T LIKE	NO OPINION or NO ANSWER

I. WARD REPORTS

```
MD(59)----------------28%------35%-------17%------20%------MD
RN(19)----------------47%-------26%------- 5%------22%------RN
CLERKS(14)----------50%-------36%-------       ------14%------CLERKS
```

II. DAILY CUMULATIVE LAB REPORTS FOR PATIENT CHARTS

```
MD(59)-----------------39%------37%------- 8%------16%------MD
RN(19)----------------- 32%------47%-------15%------ 6%------RN
CLERKS(14)-----------36% ------29%-------14%------21%------CLERKS
```

III. CUMULATIVE DISCHARGE REPORTS

```
MD(59)---------------- 42%-------27%------ 5%------26%------MD
MED. RECORDS
LIBRARIAN(1) -------------100%
```

IV. NORMAL VALUES BY AGE/SEX ON REPORTS

```
MC(59)---------56%---------23%-------- 7%--------14%------MD
RN(19)--------78%--------- 15%--------        --------7%------RN
CLERKS(14)----36%--------- 14%-------- 7%-------- 43%------CLERKS
MED RECORDS
LIBRARIAN(1)-------100%
```

Figure 9. Staff reaction to laboratory computer system

LABORATORY COMPUTER SYSTEM:
Estimated Costs for 1971
Moses Cone Memorial Hospital, Greensboro, N. C.

I. Depreciation on Equipment

Computer system, peripheral equipment and
software ($70,000/5 years) $ 14,000

    Subtotal: Equipment $14,000

II. Personnel

Computer Clerks (Range: 375 to 430/month)

1.4 Positions @ $400/month (day)   6,720
1.5 Positions @ 400/month (evening) 7,200
1   Position @ 400/month (night)   4,800

    Subtotal: Personnel   18,720

III. Supplies

Computer Tapes, Printer Ribbons,   2,000
Cards (Spear)
(Actual 1969-70: $1560)
Stock computer paper for reports   1,000
and imprinted computer paper for
discharge reports
(Actual 1969-70: $774)

    Subtotal: Supplies   3,000

IV. Maintenance

Software (Zapping) @ $250/month   3,000

Hardware   4,970
   Main frame (4K) (Spear) @ 250/month
   Card reader (Spear) @ 35/month
   Line printer (Spear) @ 100/month
   Kleinschmidt (Kleinschmidt) @ 350/year

    Subtotal: Maintenance   7,970

    TOTAL ANNUAL COST $ 43,690

Note: 1) For budget year, 1970-71, estimated total
direct operating expenses for clinical laboratory and
pathology: $698,216
    Estimated computer operating expenses of
    $43,690 represent 6.3% of total operating
    expenses.

    2) These cost estimated do not reflect the estimated savings in clerical and technologist time resulting from the use of the computer.

Figure 10

DOCUMENTATION OF LABORATORY DATA

SUGGESTED LONG-RANGE OBJECTIVES FOR LABORATORY COMPUTER SYSTEM
Moses H. Cone Memorial Hospital

YEAR:	1970	1971	1972	1973-75
GOALS:	1. Fully operational lab computer system for chemistry, serology, hematology, urinalysis.	1. Faster requisitioning, processing, reporting; faster inquiry; improved specimen receipt and delivery to lab areas. 2. Improved automation in hematology.	1. Add bacteriology to lab computer system. 2. Admission & discharge data to lab computer on cards or on-line; lab computer to dump billing data to business computer 3. Offer PALI; have ability to graphically plot lab data. 4. Sample identification system for all specimens. 5. Remote printouts of reports to other labs or hospitals.	1. Computer processing of multiphasic testing data and data for patients in ambulatory care center. 2. Laboratory computer center integrated with total hospital information system with direct request & reporting capability at each floor and clinic.
PREREQUISITIES:	1. New Programs 2. Line printer 3. Card reader with cards for data input.	1. a. Remodel & enlarge space for lab computer; build adjacent specimen receipt station for all lab specimens. b. Add disc and increase computer core memory. c. Add remote terminals for input and inquiry. d. Design machine readable requisition forms and new request and report form for stat work. 2. Hemalog in hematology on-line to computer.	1. Bacteriology programs and data entry devices. 2. New programs and interfaces for lab and business computers. 3. Add plotter and PALI programs. 4. Availability of reliable sample identification system. 5. Dataphone interface.	1. Completion of proposed ambulatory care center and multiphasic testing facility with appropriate communication network. 2. On-site or shared hospital computer system interfaced with lab computer system.

Figure 11

AN APPROACH TO AUTOMATED DATA COLLECTION AND PROCESSING*
(1130 SYSTEMS)

David Seligson and Donald McKay

Over the past five years we have developed a data processing system for the clinical laboratory. Five years ago we installed a small-general purpose digital computer in the Clinical Chemistry laboratory which we now consider the basic tool of the laboratory. In this regard I am not talking about an IBM #1130 System as the title implies but the use of a general purpose computer to do what we want it to do. It is a tool for our use. I must emphasize the general purpose part and that it is our servant.

We have some simple goals for it. The first purpose of the computer is to function as an extension of each analytical instrument in the laboratory. When the computer is used in this way it allows the analytical instrument to remain quite simple. For example, the electrical signal from our photometers is a voltage proportional to transmittance. After this analog signal enters the data system, it is processed to a clinical result. The digital processing of the voltage eliminates from our laboratory a vast amount of analog-processing electronics from each instrument and eliminates numerous recorders, all of which together, I estimate, would cost a fair share of a computer. Furthermore, if carryover of sample or reagents occur in our automatic machines, a correction is automatically applied. For example, the correction for urea is 1.8 per cent. We have found the digital pro-

*Computer Grant # HS-00075

cessing of the voltage taken as close to the transducer as possible is more accurate and reliable than the analog processing we used to do with analog computers and servo-driven systems. To avoid wasting the capabilities of the computer we multiplex our instruments into the data system so that they can operate independently and asynchronously. In this first goal we consider automatic data collection a sine qua non for success. While we enter some data by hand (key punched), more than 90% of 1.5 million entries per year are automatic.

The second purpose of the computer is to generate the many reports necessary for use by physicians in the practice of medicine and the reports needed by the laboratory personnel for operating the laboratory. Since the analytical value has been logged into the computer for processing to a clinical result and since this information is accompanied by the necessary identifications it is relatively easy to file it and format it into reports.

We have numerous other such goals which relate to:

1. Accuracy in the processing of data and use of the computer to improve methodology accuracy.
2. Speed in producing reports which affects the turnover of patients and reduces hospital stay.
3. Convenience to the laboratory; it is centrally located and always available.
4. Economy; it should provide a real saving per test, which it does.
5. Availability; the computer should function day and night.
6. Versatility; the computer should be able to process data as you wish it to do.

Our clinical laboratory computer is the IBM #1130 model which includes:

1. 1131 Model 2B Central processor. It has 8192-16

bit word core memory. (3.6 usec. access time).
2. Single disk drive with replaceable disk packs (each pack can hold up to 512,000 words of programs and/or data files).
3. Console keyboard printer.
4. 1442 Model 6 Card-read-punch that reads up to 300 cards/min. and punches at a minimum of 50 cards/min. It reads the requisition card which contains the accession number, the patient's name, hospital number, ward name, and enters the requested tests and corresponding specimen information into appropriate files in the bulk memory. The card is then sent to the business office for setting up charges by the hospital's accounting computer.
5. 1132 line printer that is programmed to print up to 110 lines per minute (120 characters per line).

This computer hardware and several IBM card punches rent for less than $20,000 per year. For cost accounting purposes if we add $16,500 for labor and supplies our annual operating cost is $36,500 or $100 per day. The cost for processing a measurement (1.5 million measurements), if we were using the computer for this function alone, is 2.43 cents. If we consider that our blood bank inventory and many other functions carried out on this computer is worth half the cost, the cost per test measurement falls to about 1.2 cents per measurement. These are operational costs and not development costs.

Our system starts with a tube of blood and a machine readable requisition, which is a Port-A-Punch Card listing 60 tests for constituents in blood, urine, cerebrospinal fluid or other material. A physician or nurse on the ward requests the desired tests by pushing out one or more pre-scored holes in the card. One hole can be used to request the liver function battery of tests. When the card and sample arrive in the laboratory, it is accessioned by giving it a four digit number (in chronological sequence).

After preparation of the sample, it is placed in a machine and analyzed automatically, or it is preprocessed manually. In any event the instrument reading goes into the computer for data processing. Our automatic machines read 120 samples per hour, each machine has one or more analytical channels. Our manual photometers (attached to the computer) read up to 250 samples per hour. The manual mode backed up by the computer is capable of great speed.

Figure 1 diagrams the operation of the laboratory. The computer is in the center of the laboratory. A1, A2 etc. are analytical stations. A1 may be a manually operated station that reads the final reaction mixture and produces a voltage proportional to transmittance or it may be a fully automatic machine.

The analog signal is picked up by the data logger (DL) (also shown in Fig. 2) and is converted to 4 characters of information. A fifth character is generated by a digital volt meter in the data logger to indicate the decimal point for the voltage, thereby preserving four significant figures for all readings whether high or low. The analytical station also presents two digits that identify the test; a four digit accession number that identifies the patient and one digit indicating a dilution for a very high concentration of the test substance. A station, therefore, generates 12 characters of information for each analysis. The buffer register of the data logger receives this information and drives a coupler for a paper tape punch for backup. Simultaneously the 12 characters are printed on paper. The paper tape is read into the computer automatically. In this manner, the laboratory is on line with the data logger and virtually on line, but not completely, with the computer. We have the capability to run short or long off-line programs while collecting data. When the computer is used for the blood bank inventory, the blood bank disk is inserted and the new data are entered and processed. The chemistry data are collected all the while in the data logger. When the computer or its components is serviced or repaired we continue to collect data. The data is automatically read into the computer when it is put back up. While station Al might be manually operated A2 might be an automatic instrument. The various instruments are multiplexed so that all instruments can read data into the system without loss of data. The technologists use the console typewriter for interactive communication with the computer.

About 98 per cent of the tests in our busy university hospital laboratory are performed and entered as I have indicated. The raw data for a few tests which require numerous calculations are key punched onto cards which then are entered off line into the computer. Isotope measurements, such as T_3 uptake, Thyroxine, Vitamin B_{12} and radio-immunoassays, are collected on punched-paper tape or key punched and entered into the computer for calculation. Use of the computer for many off-line calculations saves many hours and eliminates errors.

We use the computer to improve our laboratory work. For example, every analysis is accompanied by a fresh set of standards (usually six) and a set of quality control serums. The computer automatically computes the data for the standard curve and indicates the deviations of each point from the theoretical curve obtained by a least squares fit procedure and lists the control values. The computer in an interactive mode asks the technologist if the information is acceptable. If it is the technologist types in "YES" on the keyboard and the computer prints out the results on all the patients in the run and files the data. Each sample is analyzed in duplicate. Duplicates which do not agree within defined limits are starred for repeat. If the standard curve is unsuitable the technologist will answer "NO". The computer will then ask for the standard point to be deleted which might reflect a deteriorated standard. If such is the case the deletion (which is marked by the computer) is made and the standard curve recalculated. (See Table 1). Most frequently if recalculation is needed it is because of one bad standard. Aside from increasing accuracy, the wastefulness of redoing large numbers of samples is avoided.

Not infrequently we have 1600 results for a single constituent filed in our computer on the patients in the hospital over a 14 day period. Fig. 3 shows a frequency distribution of creatinine. Such a study is helpful to us in evaluating the quality of our work. Fig. 4 shows the distribution of 18 tests.

We believe the computer should not only increase our data processing accuracy but also increase our methodology accuracy. For example, the measurement of total protein in serum is seriously affected by the presence of lipidemia, bulirubinemia or hemolysis. We have built a machine that measures total protein, albumin, turbidity (which is a measure of lipidemia), bilirubin and hemaglobin. The turbidity correction is applied by the computer to the other four channels for correction. The hemaglobin and bilirubin measurements are entered into simultaneous equations for their corrections and then subtracted from the total protein and albumin levels. The calculations required for the operation of this machine cannot be done by hand because they are too time consuming; a computer is necessary. Furthermore, the machine measures these proteins (5 measurements per serum) at the rate of 120 per hour. It needs a computer too for its operation. Fig. 5 shows the computations for a single analysis (see legend). Table 2 shows the adverse effect of jaundice on the protein measurements and Table 3 shows the adverse effect of turbidity. It is our belief that these data are more accurate than laboratories are now getting.

An added bonus is that the turbidity measurements are an indication of the level of triglycerides and worth reporting to physicians. The bilirubin and hemoglobin values are worth knowing too. While these three constituents have clinical value they also are important to know for technical reasons because they cause errors in the measurement of other constituents. The computer could be used to make many corrections similar to those described for protein.

Fig. 6 shows an electrophoresis report designed for easy interpretation by physicians.

We have numerous goals of which the following are some:

1. Get good data out so that clinicians can make decisions.
2. If a doctor asks a question (by requesting a test) it is our desire to answer it, to help him. By doing so we can help him ease suffering, treat disease, operate and so on. By helping him respond faster we can reduce costs and days in the hospital. Our hospital stay is less than that in community hospitals even though we deal with the most difficult clinical problems.
3. Our Blood Bank inventory saves blood. It is problem oriented.
4. Use the computer to collect data, process it, improve it, and give doctors good reports to read that are well formatted and easy to interpret.
5. Now that we know how to do that we want to, integrate the data, make it meaningful, extract more information than we put in, that is, make $1 + 1 = 3$.
6. Help the rest of the hospital get the essential data into a computer, merge it with ours and interpret it. Experience with a laboratory computer aids the whole hospital and its non-laboratory personnel to think "Computer."

The computer is relentless in its ability to follow through on an assigned task. It will help us answer problems we detect, help us structure our functions.

I thought at first to apologize to Dr. Weed because I was not able to rise to his challenge. I do not think I will because we have used the computer to provide better data for physicians to think with. I think we have had a salutary effect on him and we know how to move up to a new system which will have a much greater effect on medical care. We also have a list of problems of the patient that only we know about. Some are, for example, the hyperglycemias, the hyperlipidemias, the anemias, the uremias and a host of other findings that we now call to the attention of the physician if they are unknown to him. Furthermore, we will make this part of our system so that certain clues lead us to work up a facet of patient before the physician knows about it. For example, one of my colleagues in our laboratory performs a B_{12} and folic acid analysis on all patients whose M.C.V.s detected in the laboratory are above 115. He is discovering pernicious anemia and folic acid deficiencies unknown to the attending physicians. They are now able to establish diagnoses and initiate therapy faster with consequent savings in the cost of medical care. When we enlarge our data base in the computer it will detect automatically such clues and request the necessary laboratory tests.

Given the support we will jump to a whole new level of intellectual function and computing and we will have a great salutary impact on physicians, the hospital and patient care.

TABLE 1A

Nominal	Calculated	%Error
1	1.10	10.15
2	1.68	-15.87
4	4.81	20.28
6	5.26	12.32
8	7.82	2.18

TABLE 1B

Nominal	Calculated	%Error
1	0.99	-0.35
2	2.01	0.56
4	*5.57*	*39.46*
6	5.97	-0.35
8	8.01	0.17

Table 1A lists the nominal values of the potassium standards in meq per liter, the calculated values derived from a standard curve established by the computer using the nominal values and flame photometer voltages. "% Error" indicates the % deviation of the calculated value from the nominal value. The technologist perceives this to be a very bad curve and indicates to the computer to delete the 4 meq/liter standard and recalculate the curve.

Table 1B shows the recalculated curve. The bad value is starred indicating it is listed and computed but not used for establishing the curve. The analytical curve is now an excellent one and all the patient values in disk behind it are calculated and put into file. The technologist knows that the aberrant standard needs replacement.

TABLE 2

Bilirubin	Total Protein		
	Uncorrected	Corrected	Kjeldahl
30	7.1	6.3	6.5
31	6.3	5.5	5.4
30	6.2	5.5	5.4
6	6.3	6.1	5.8
30	7.4	6.6	6.6
3	9.0	8.8	8.6
36	7.4	6.4	6.5
36	6.4	5.8	5.7
26	6.4	5.8	5.7
15	7.6	7.1	7.0
20	6.7	6.2	6.2
36	5.0	4.1	4.4
26	6.6	6.0	5.8

Table 2 shows the total protein values determined in jaundiced patients before correction and after correction. The corrected values compare favorably with the total proteins determined by Kjeldahl analysis. Errors as large as 1 gram in 7 occur if no correction is made.

TABLE 3

Turbidity	Total Protein		
	Uncorrected	Corrected	Kjeldahl
14	7.9	7.5	7.4
21	6.1	5.8	5.8
30	7.6	7.2	7.0
14	6.6	6.3	6.2
15	6.9	6.6	6.4
26	6.6	6.0	-
10	8.1	7.8	7.7
58	7.9	7.0	7.0
134	8.6	6.6	7.3
51	7.6	6.9	6.7
32	6.3	5.7	5.8
14	7.5	7.3	7.4
113	5.3	3.6	3.6
33	5.8	5.3	-

Table 3 lists the total protein values determined in serums with small and large amounts of turbidity or lipemia. Less than 10 turbidity units is normal. Uncorrected values are too high by as little as 0.2 g and as much as 1.7 g in this series.

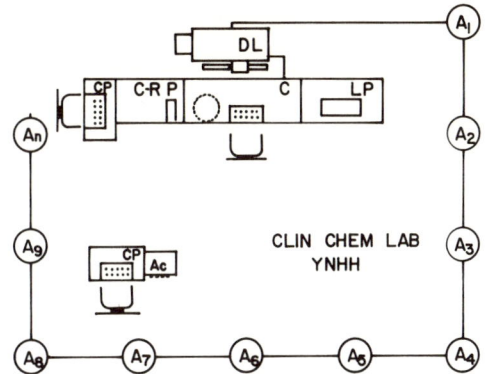

Fig. 1. This diagram indicates the data acquisition and processing system. A1, A2 etc. represent analytical instruments. DL is the data logger which contains a multiplexer that accepts data from all the stations in a random on demand basis. (See Fig. 2.) CP is a card punch. CRP is a card-read punch. C is the computer. LP is the line printer.

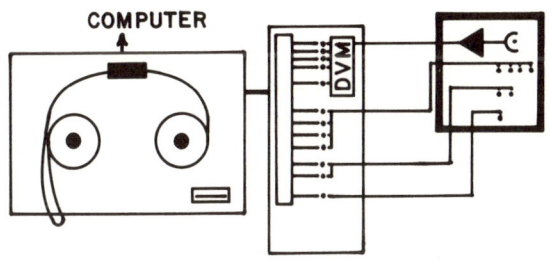

Fig. 2 is a diagram of one analytical station connected to the data logger. The analog signal is sent via the multiplexer to the digital volt meter where it is converted to 4 binary coded digits. The digital signals for accession number or patient identification; the instrument number and dilution character are sent to the data logger simultaneously. This information is sent to the paper tape punch and a 12 digit line printer for hard copy. When the computer is available it automatically reads the tape. When it is not the tape accumulates. The tape provides an almost infinite back-up for the computer. The laboratory is on line with the data logger and essentially on line with the computer.

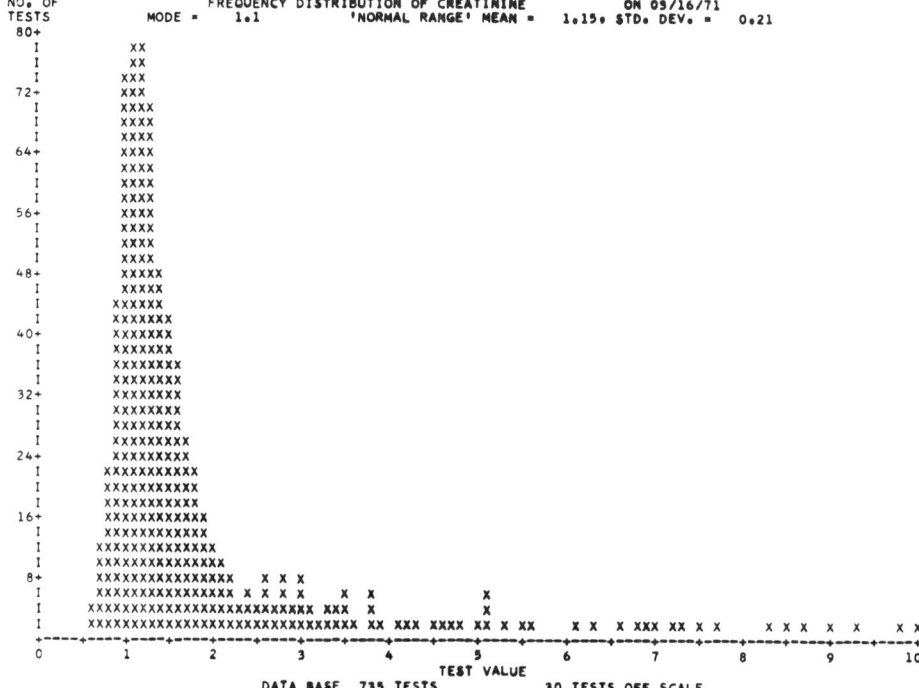

Fig. 3 shows a frequency distribution of all values in file on the computer at any one moment. It is generated periodically in order to study the quality of work.

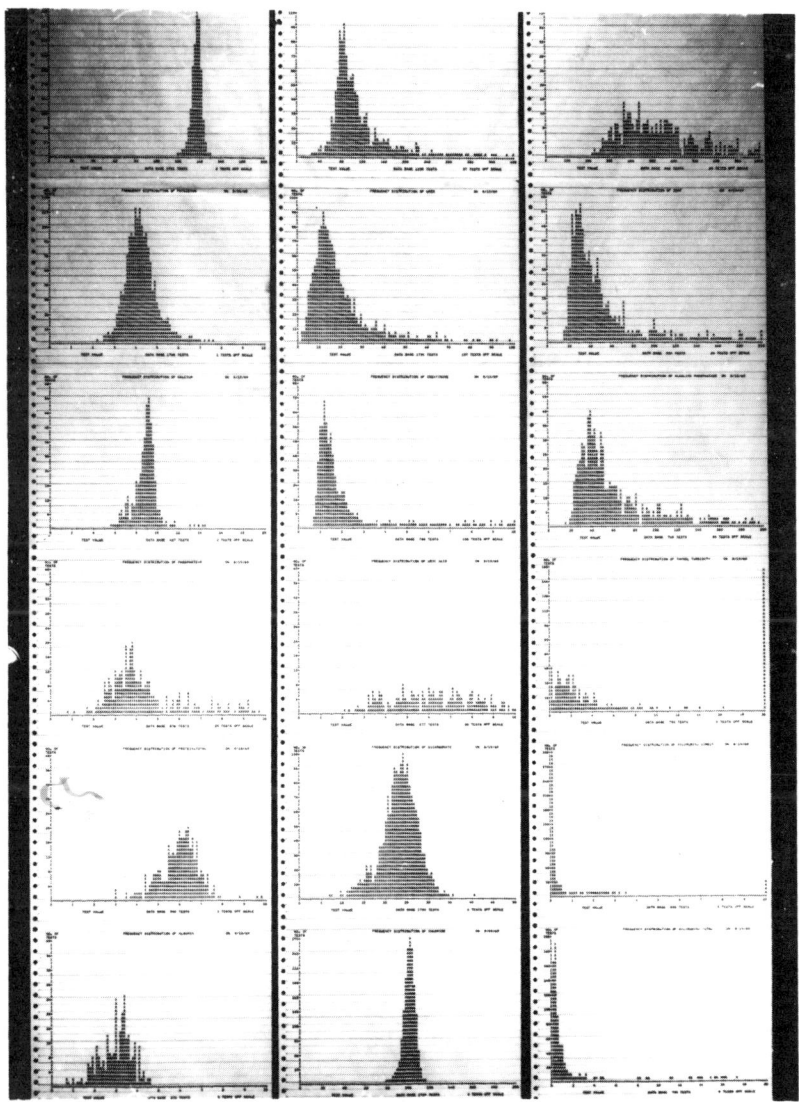

Fig. 4 is a frequency plot of 18 tests periodically issued for our quality control evaluation.

```
SAMPLE                              CHANNEL DATA      04/13/71         PAGE 13        UNCORRECTED
NUMBER        LIPIDS    HEMOGLOBIN  BILIRUBIN    TOTAL PROTEIN  ALBUMIN      TOTAL PROTEIN   ALBUMIN

3059  VOLTS    0.47        8.82        4.17         3.69         1.34
      ABSRB                0.0173      0.3417       0.3387       0.8728        5.4           2.4
UNCORRECTED                94.88       31.62        6.10         1.57          6.11          1.57
LIPID CORRECTIONS         -22.28       -0.37        -0.11        0.01
LIPID CORRECTED            72.59       31.25        5.99         1.58
HGB CORRECTIONS                        -0.06        -0.02        0.00
BILI  CORRECTIONS         -62.37                    -0.62        0.93
CONCENTRATIONS  7.43       10.22       31.19        5.35         2.52


3059  VOLTS    0.46        8.83        4.17         3.61         1.34
      ABSRB                0.0168      0.3417       0.3482       0.8728        5.4           2.4
UNCORRECTED                92.43       31.62        6.28         1.57          6.28          1.57
LIPID CORRECTIONS         -21.85       -0.36        -0.10        0.01
LIPID CORRECTED            70.58       31.26        6.17         1.58
HGB CORRECTIONS                        -0.05        -0.01        0.00
BILIP CORRECTIONS         -62.42                    -0.62        0.93
CONCENTRATIONS  7.29       8.16        31.21        5.53         2.52
```

Fig. 5 shows the computer printout of a protein analysis (in duplicate). In the first analysis the total protein by biuret analysis is 6.11 g%. The lipid correction is -0.11, the hemoglobin correction is -0.02 and the biliburin correction in this jaundiced patient is -0.62. The corrected value is therefore 5.35 which compares favorably with the Kjeldahl analysis which was 5.4.

The uncorrected albumin is 1.57. The lipid correction is -0.01, the hemoglobin correction is 0.00 and the bilirubin correction is +0.93. The corrected value is therefore, 2.52 which compares favorably with the electrophoresis value of 2.4

DOCUMENTATION OF LABORATORY DATA

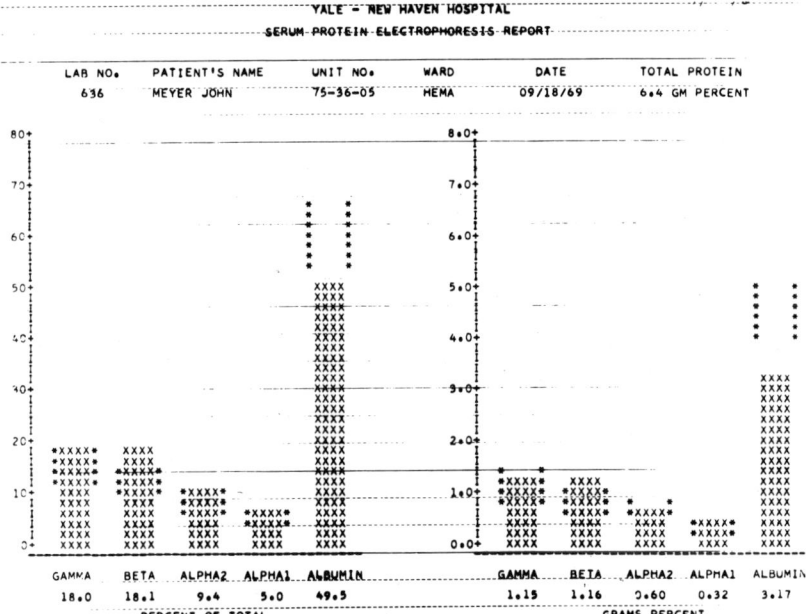

Fig. 6. The electrophoresis report is generated by the computer from dye eluted from the electrophoretogram. The protein fractions are shown and listed by per cent of total protein and by weight. The total protein is listed. Normal values are shown by stars.

USE OF THE IBM 1800 UNIVERSITY OF KENTUCKY MEDICAL CENTER HOSPITAL LABORATORIES

Wellington B. Stewart, M. D.

We assume that the advantages of data acquisition and processing equipment would be improved accuracy, alleviation of heavy workload, and improved turnaround time for report generation. These should be the results of a proper data acquisition and control system. Disadvantages would include some increased rigidity in the functioning of the laboratory and perhaps additional expense.

The IBM 1800 is illustrated in Figure 1. The layout of the system at the University of Kentucky is as follows: we connected the data acquisition equipment to a series of autoanalyzers; in actuality we had as many as eight or nine on-line simultaneously. In addition we had connected a Coulter Counter Model S to the digital input part of the 1800.

Figure 2 gives a generalized description of the overall system as it evolved. Methods for reporting manual as well as automated procedures were included. The italicized letters in bold type are the names of programs that performed certain functions. These program names have changed, but the general overall functions remain the same.

Figure 3 illustrated the general format of the request cards. The number of cards used depended on the particular section of the laboratory involved. These cards were designed in such a way that they could be prepared external to the laboratory, however in the recent past they were still being punched in the laboratory. The source documents were the normal laboratory requisitions (Figure 4). These cards were read by machine and various types of "logs" or documents were prepared for the different sections of the laboratory depending on the information required.

Interfacing the Coulter Counter to the 1800 was not difficult. The Coulter Counter produces digital information which includes the sequence number of the patient. This sequence or log number was entered into the computer and associated with the patient record number, name, and location. The digital output of the Coulter Counter comes in a known sequence of values and the machine gives a pulse to the computer which allows it to know that the Coulter Counter is ready to deliver data. These data can then be collected, temporarily stored in core and when a set is collected, transmitted to a disc file. They are later associated with the patient and ultimately appear on the laboratory report form.

Interfacing with the autoanalyzers was somewhat more difficult. At the time the system was designed we did not have any SMA-type autoanalyzers. When using these machines we had to sample at frequent intervals and decide when a peak had been reached. The peak-picking program which we devised recognized the maximum or minimum and had a number of programmed steps in it which served as smoothing functions and noise filters. The peaks were picked in sequence, the technologist's only constraint being that she run the correct number of standards as the first set of peaks. The computer at the time it prepared the log also printed a list of patients and the sequence in which the technologist should place the samples in the trays. Various facilities were provided for the technologists to change the sequence of patients if necessary. The general overall system allowed the technologists to inform the computer which test was being performed on which autoanalyzer and then the computer would pick the peaks. When the test was finished the technologist would inform the computer of this fact, the results would be calculated and subsequently be associated with the individual patient.

The device we chose to use for technologist interface with the computer was an IBM 1092 matrix keyboard (Figure 5) and a nearby typewriter (IBM 1053). The general layout was that the device number was entered in the first two columns, the particlar test code in the next several, and then one column was reserved for various manipulations. After an entry the typewriter makes an appropriate response.

At the time the technologist starts a test, she enters her own code in the last two columns on the 1092. The code number was subsequently transformed to her initials at the time a report was generated.

It became apparent as we went along that we had to give the technologist considerable freedom in communicating with the computer. We ended up with ten different types of messages she could send through the 1092. She could indicate to start a test or stop a test. The continue function allowed a restart without the necessity of rerunning standards or satisfactory peaks in case some untoward event occured. The delete function permits elimination of selected or all of the results in case of necessity. It was possible for the technologist to instruct the computer to exchange the values of certain peaks, and in case this was done wrong, she could take that out and re-do it. The sixth function was to list which particular devices were currently running. The next function --to count the peaks-- allows the technologist to enter device and test code to instruct the machine to inform her of how many peaks it had actually collected. This is important sometimes in case of certain problems and for correction of difficulties. It was also possible to obtain a list on the nearby 1053 as to what exchanges had been ordered to facilitate making corrections if necessary or to check that they were correct. The last function allowed the technologist to do an on-line calculation. This was useful in case of emergency requests, and also to check that the known or "pool" values had come out correctly, among other things.

The general reporting method was to wait until the late afternoon when most of the work had been performed and to produce a single page report for the patient chart (Figure 6).

Since the results tended to be locked up in the machine until reporting time, several times during the day we would generate an alphabetic list of all the patients who had laboratory requests that day and distribute this to the various nursing stations. This had the advantage of allowing a physician to look up his patient no matter where he was in the hospital.

In addition a simple on-line inquiry was provided in the laboratory. This used a telephone dial and one need only dial the patient's number and a convenient 1053 typewriter would type out what results had been obtained as well as indicating those which had been ordered and were not yet complete.

In addition to the system described above there is also an extensive blood bank system on the 1800. This system was largely developed by Dr. R. A. Stewart. The earliest version of it has been described in TRANSFUSION: subsequent to that description an on-line system was developed using an 1816 typewriter-keyboard. This permitted the technologists to enter information into the machine as they performed the work. The program was written so that certain errors were detected and reported back to the technologist; it also kept a continuous summary of the inventory with a description as to where each unit of blood could be located.

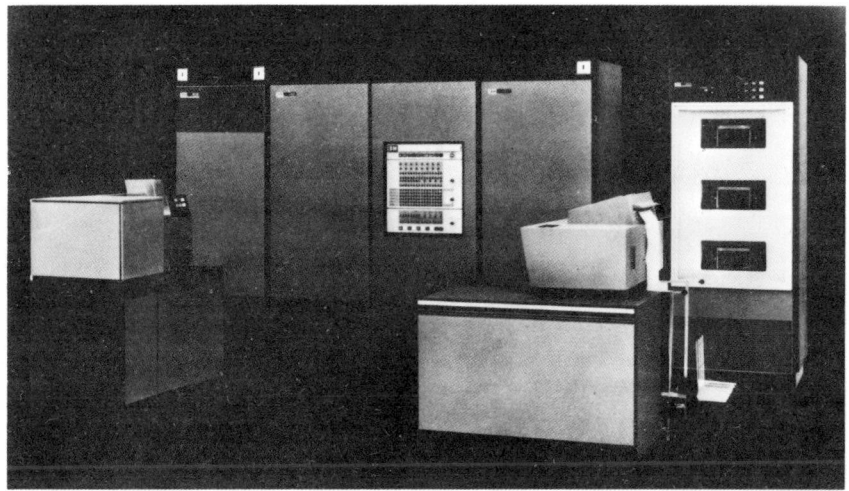

Figure 1

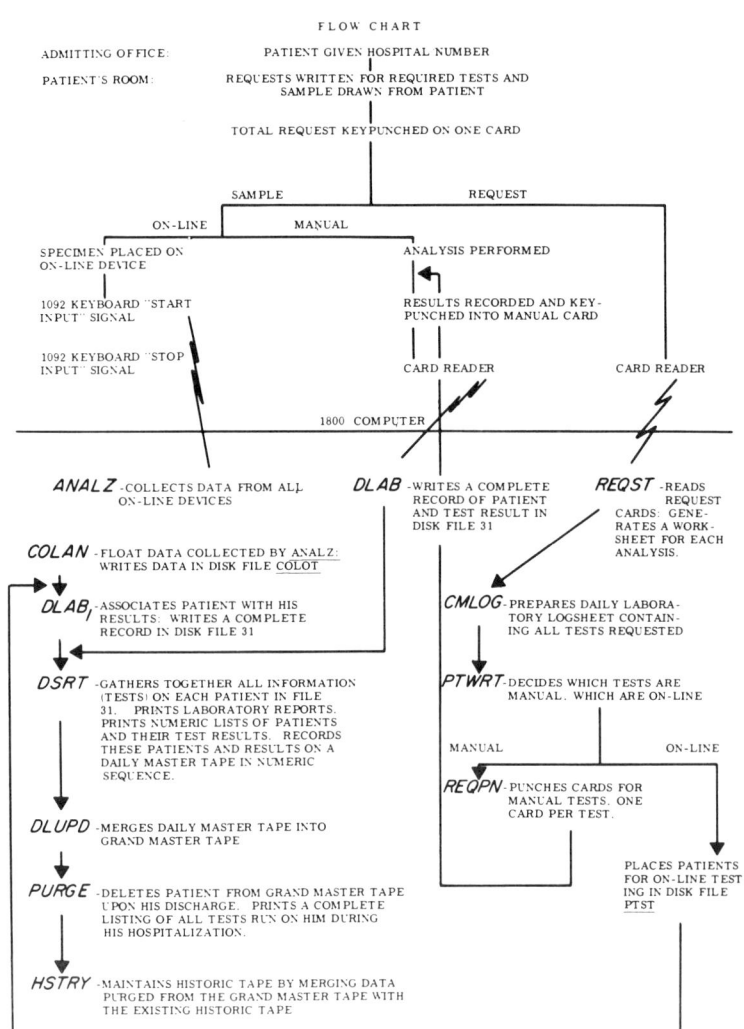

Figure 2

DOCUMENTATION OF LABORATORY DATA

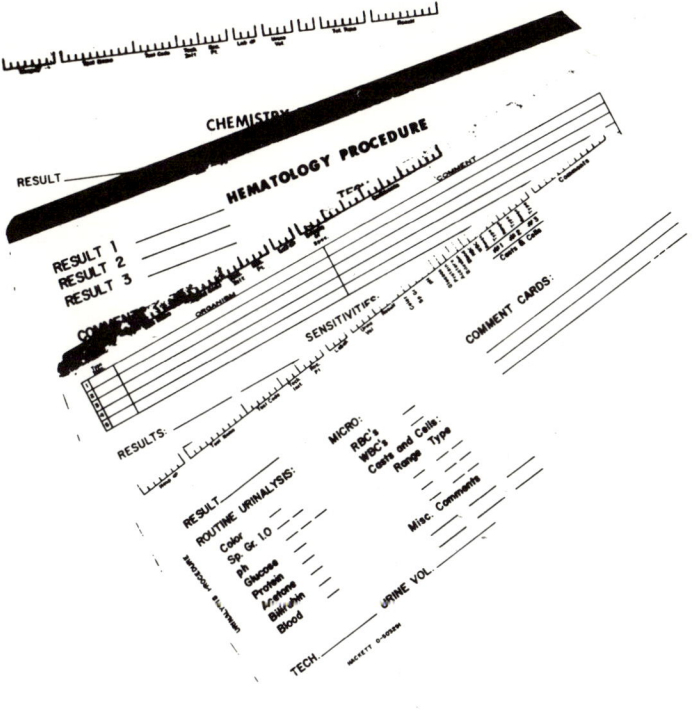

Figure 3

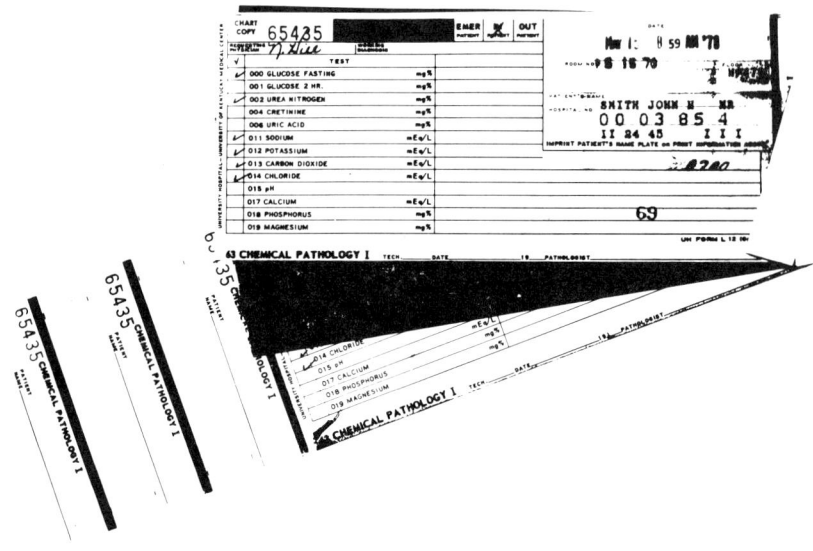

Figure 4

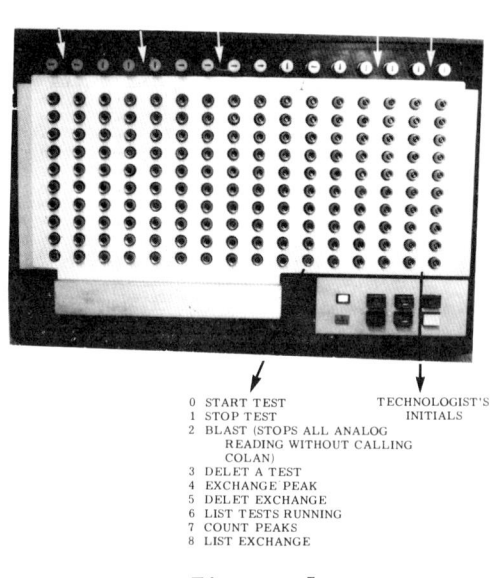

```
0 START TEST                TECHNOLOGIST'S
1 STOP TEST                 INITIALS
2 BLAST (STOPS ALL ANALOG
  READING WITHOUT CALLING
  COLAN)
3 DELET A TEST
4 EXCHANGE PEAK
5 DELET EXCHANGE
6 LIST TESTS RUNNING
7 COUNT PEAKS
8 LIST EXCHANGE
```

Figure 5

DOCUMENTATION OF LABORATORY DATA

CLB, TRICK LD XQ

SUMMARY REPORT
QUANTITATIVE LABORATORY DATA
02/27/69 - 03/05/69

118432 DOE JOHN   SW

TEST	02/27	02/28	03/01	03/02	03/03	03/04	03/05	UNITS
BLD GLUC	110.			104.				MG/100ML
BUN	12.		9.5	13.		10.		MG/100ML
CREATININE		.5	.6		.8		.6	MG/100ML
SODIUM	140.			140.			140.	MEQ/L
POTASSIUM	4.5			4.4			4.8	MEQ/L
CO2	27.			26.			26.	MEQ/L
CHLORIDE	101.			102.			101.	MEQ/L
CALCIUM	4.8			4.9			4.7	MEQ/L
PHOSPHOR	3.7			4.2			4.0	MG/100ML
HEMOGLOBIN	14.6		14.6	14.8	14.4	15.0	14.8	GMS/100ML
HEMATOCRIT	42.		43.	43.	42.5	44.	43.	%
WBC	6000.		7000.	7100.	6600.	5500.	6900.	/CMM
RETIC	.8			.8			.8	%
SED RATE	12.							MM/HR
SR-CORRECT	9.5							MM/HR
DIFF								
SEG NEUT	70.		69.	65.	70.		68.	%
STAB NEJT	3.		2.	3.	3.		3.	%
EOSINO	2.		2.	2.	2.		2.	%
BASO	1.		0.	1.	1.			%
MONOCYTES	5.		6.	8.	5.		3.	%
LYMPHS	18.		19.	18.			21.	%
ATYP LYMP	1.		2.	3.	1.		2.	%

Figure 6

265

EVALUATION OF CLINICAL LABORATORY COMPUTERS

Diversified Numeric Applications

Thomas O. Swallen, M. D.

North Memorial is a 553 bed acute care community hospital located near the northwest corner of Minneapolis. Most of the hospital, including the laboratory facilities, is less than seven years old. Proximity to the freeway system engenders an active emergency room, with 40,199 patient visits in 1970. Average length of patient stay at North Memorial is 6.1 days.

In the hospital laboratory, workload has grown annually at a rate of about 15% per year. In 1965 we did 198,853 tests, in 1970, 354,890 tests.

Since late 1969, the laboratory has had a DNA (Diversified Numeric Applications) Clinical Laboratory System. Selection of this system followed several years of interest and investigation of laboratory computer systems by the hospital pathologists. The DNA computer system was installed in December 1969. This paper will describe the DNA system and its implementation and operation at North Memorial Hospital.

GENERAL DESCRIPTION OF THE DNA SYSTEM
DEFINITION

The DNA laboratory computer system is a "turnkey" or package system for the laboratory. This simply means that the system includes both hardware and programming. The "package" can be modified in many respects to meet the individual user's needs. Thus individual systems, while having the same basic makeup, will vary with respect to hardware (disc storage capacity, number of remote terminals, number of analog inputs, etc.) and with respect to programming (names and numbers of tests, normal limits, formats for reports, etc.)

DNA systems are currently installed in the following locations: Hennepin County General Hospital, Minneapolis, Minnesota; North Memorial Hospital, Minneapolis, Minnesota; Lutheran General Hospital, Park Ridge, Illinois; St. Joseph Mercy Hospital, Pontiac, Michigan; Centre Hospitalier Universitaire, Sherbrooke, Quebec, Canada; St. John's Hospital, Detroit, Michigan.

HARDWARE COMPONENTS:

The central processor in the DNA System is a Raytheon 703 Computer with 8K core memory (16 bit word length). Mass memory fixed-head discs store patient files and results, as well as the computer programs.

The central processor is connected to the following peripheral components:
    1. Special desk top terminals for requesting tests, for inquiry, and for result entry.
    2. A master console keyboard.
    3. Card reader.
    4. High speed line printer.
    5. Magnetic tape system.
    6. Small label printer.

At North Memorial the SMA-12 and three dual channel autoanalyzers are connected on-line to the computer, via an analog to digital convertor. Special autoanalyzer terminals are on the bench to provide for technologist control of autoanalyzer runs. The Coulter-S is also on-line via a special control terminal.

A distinguishing hardware feature of the DNA system

is its specialized terminals for input of laboratory results. Each is specially designed for its particular section of the laboratory. Thus the panel of keys on an input terminal is in a format and in language appropriate for its specific laboratory division. The terminals are used for result input by all laboratory personnel, no computer operators being required. All terminals include a printing head, providing a permanent printed record (audit trail) of every transaction with the computer.

Terminals in the North Memorial System are:
1. Request/Inquiry, with auxiliary keyboards (2).
2. Chemistry.
3. Hematology and Auxiliary.
4. Urinalysis and Auxiliary.
5. Bacteriology and Auxiliary.
6. Autoanalyzer (2)
7. Coulter-S

OPERATION:

All interactions with the computer are through the special terminals. Laboratory personnel do not perform operations directly on the computer control panel. The computer contains a real-time clock and automatically keeps track of the date, hour and minute.

All of the patient information in the computer is on the fixed-head disc storage. Thus, there is immediate access to all patient information at any time. Programming is such that all operations may be conducted simultaneously. Thus results may be entered from various laboratory divisions at the same time that inquiries are being made, and while reports are being printed. The technologist entering results, or the clerk inquiring as to results on a patient need not be concerned with what others may be doing at that moment.

REPORTS:

Reports are requested through the master console, and are produced at the line printer. The output array includes specimen collection lists, worksheets, ward reports, cumulative patient chart reports, unfinished work reports, labels, and patient census. The feature of immediate access to all patient information in the computer files makes it possible to obtain any of the reports at any time, with no delay. For example, one may obtain an individual patient's cumulative summary report, containing all of his laboratory work (up to 7 days prior) at any time.

The exact report formats may vary somewhat from one user to the next. Details are worked out by the individual laboratory to best meet their needs.

DISTINGUISHING FEATURES:

The DNA system is like other laboratory computer systems in its use of a small dedicated computer with peripheral terminals, and with programming specifically designed for the clinical laboratory. It differs, to greater or lesser degrees, from other systems, in several features:

1. The specialized terminals for result entry have been mentioned. These have been developed with the technologist in mind, specifically for entry of laboratory data.
2. A printed permanent record (audit trail) is generated for every transaction with the computer. A printing head is an integral part of each terminal.
3. The random-access fixed-head disc memory provides immediate access to all information in patient files. This is in contrast to systems which have current patient information on disc and older patient information on tape, and which require special "merging" or "meshing" pro-

cesses before all patient information is available.

4. Specimen numbers are assigned automatically by the computer, as requests are made.

THE DNA SYSTEM AT NORTH MEMORIAL HOSPITAL
BACKGROUND

In considering the possibilities of computerization for the laboratory at North Memorial, criteria were developed which we felt a system should possess.

1. It must operate full time, 24 hours a day, 7 days a week. The laboratory operates on this basis. If the computer system were to do otherwise, we would need two separate functioning systems for requesting and reporting laboratory work.

2. It must be simple, meaning that existing laboratory personnel can operate the system. We felt that the system should be an integral part of the laboratory, operated by the technologists as part of of their regular laboratory work process.

3. It must be reliable. 24 hour test availability and prompt reporting have always been stated goals (admittedly not always met) in our laboratory. Both first-line reliability and fail-safe backup were deemed essential.

4. The system must be flexible enough to allow for reasonable changes after initial experience, and for updating as laboratory procedures change.

5. Finally, we felt that the system should, within reason, approximate our then-existing conventional requesting/reporting system. We wanted a system which we could understand and explain in narrative and flow design in comparison with our conventional system.

Prior to installation of the system, there were several months of preparation, during which we developed and modified report formats, decided upon test names and units, and set normal limits and result reject limits. Decisions as to terminal placement, and wiring modifications were made prior to installation. Computer equipment was installed Dec. 10, 1969.

BREAK-IN AND ORIENTATION

Over a 5 month period we converted, by stages, from our conventional system to the computer system. A technologist orientation program included group lectures and individualized instruction at terminals. About 1-1/2 hours of individual orientation was required for each technologist (this "individual" orientation was often conducted in groups of two or three).

Operation manuals were written for each terminal. These manuals provide step-by-step instructions for entering results and obtaining reports, as well as backup and trouble-shooting information.

Conversion to the computer system required communication with nursing services and with staff physicians. Our first outside-the-laboratory output was March 1, 1970, when we began sending ward reports to the nursing stations. About this time we also switched completely to using computer-generated blood drawing lists.

On June 1, 1970, we began sending out patient cumulative chart reports. For one more week we ran entirely parallel systems (retaining the lab. slips in the laboratory however), and doing tallied comparisons of all computer reports with lab. slips. The tally was 100%, and writing of results on lab slips was then discontinued. Since June 1, 1970, all requesting and reporting has been via the computer system.

During the break-in period we underwent one major hardware modification. By February, it had become apparent that a single mass memory disc would soon be inadequate for our patient load. In March, 1970, therefore, a second disc was added to the system.

DOCUMENTATION OF LABORATORY DATA

OPERATION

The operation of the computer system at North Memorial will be described in the following sections: Admitting patients to the computer files; requesting laboratory tests; organization of laboratory workload; entering test results; reports; daily schedule.

ADMITTING PATIENTS TO COMPUTER FILES:

The computer must have in its memory the names of all patients in the hospital. Outpatients, or patients seen in the emergency room who have lab work must also be in the computer's files. Our "file" of information on a patient includes:

>account number
>patient name
>hospital number
>room
>age
>sex
>doctor

The account number in our system has 8 digits. The number is unique to a single hospital admission, or a single outpatient visit. The DNA system uses a check digit (Modulus 11) to detect random or transposition errors in account numbers. It detects 91% of random errors, 100% of transposition errors.

When a patient enters the hospital, we must tell the computer his account number, his name, and the other information mentioned above. Entering this information into the computer is called "admitting the patient" or "doing an admit". There are two ways in which we may admit a patient:

a) manually via a keyboard terminal
b) via a card reader with Hollerith cards

To admit a patient manually, the Request/Inquiry terminal is used with its auxiliary keyboard. The clerk types in the account number, patient name, and other identifying information. A printed audit trail of this input is produced by the Request/Inquiry terminal, as the clerk types it. It takes a clerk 15-30 seconds to type in this information.

Where do we get the information (account number, name, etc.) on patients being admitted? Our hospital admitting department assigns the account numbers to patients as they come in. We receive from them a card with the necessary patient information printed on it.

The other method of admitting patients is via the card reader. This requires a Hollerith card with machine-readable information, meaning punched holes. We receive a stack of cards each morning from our hospital's data processing department. There is a card for each patient who has been admitted, discharged, or transferred from one room to another in the past 24 hours. The card's punched information includes all of the items in our patient file, i.e. name, account number, age, etc. We read these cards each morning at about 6:00 a.m. and this serves to keep our files updated with respect to discharges and transfers, and is a check on admissions.

Our system has room for 1024 patients, using 101,000 words of the disc storage for patient files. North Memorial has 553 beds, but computer file space is needed for outpatients and for the lag period of 24-48 hours from the time a patient leaves the hospital unit his file is removed from the computer.

In summary, patients may be admitted either manually via a keyboard, or via a card-reader. Our practice is to use the keyboard to admit patients as they arrive through the day and evening. Every morning we update our patient files by reading a stack of Hollerith cards with admissions, discharges, and transfers of the past 24 hours.

REQUESTING LABORATORY TESTS

Our laboratory test request forms include a Hollerith card. The nurse uses a Standard Register punch machine to punch the patient's account number in the card. She then marks the test to be done, before sending the request form to the lab. When we receive a request, it includes:

1. Patient name, account number, hospital number, etc. printed in the upper right hand corner.
2. Patient account number punched in the card in machine-readable form.
3. An X in the box corresponding to the test requested.

The computer is notified of the test requested by either using the punched card, or manually via a Request/Inquiry terminal.

In the lab we use the Standard Register punch to punch a test code (eg. 053 for BUN) in the card. The card then may be used to enter the requests into the computer via the card reader. The card is also used by the data processing department of our hospital to charge the patient for the test. For manual entry of a test request, the technologist or clerk enters the patient's account number and the three digit test number. Thus tests may be requested either manually at the Request/Inquiry terminal, or via the card reader. Our practice is to use the card reader for the batch of routine AM tests, and the manual request procedure for tests ordered at other times.

ORGANIZATION OF WORK

The computer has now been told what tests are ordered on what patients. With this information, it can give us various documents useful in organizing the laboratory workload.

1. A specimen collection list (blood drawing list) may be produced which lists by nursing station and room each patient with blood to be drawn. It includes computer generated specimen numbers, names of tests to be done, and the types of vacutainer tubes needed. In our laboratory a specimen collection list is produced each morning at 6:30 a.m.

2. Labels may be printed. They include patient name, room, specimen number, etc. These are taken to the station along with the collection list. When a tube is drawn the label is immediately stuck to it.

3. Worksheets may be produced. These have various formats designed for use at the bench where the test is done. They include the patient's name, the specimen number, and spaces for the technologist to write in data as she performs the test. These worksheets are printed while the technologists are out on the stations drawing blood. They are kept in binders at the permanent laboratory workbooks.

4. An inventory of work ordered but not yet completed may be obtained at any time. Division supervisors use these reports to check on the status of work in their departments.

ENTERING TEST RESULTS

Results from manual procedures are written in the workbook by the technologist. Results are then entered into the computer by the technologist at the appropriate terminal (i.e. chemistry, bacteriology, etc). The result as entered is printed out at the terminal for visual checking by the technologist. If correct, she presses a

DOCUMENTATION OF LABORATORY DATA

"verify" key, and the result goes to the patient's file.

The SMA-12 and Autoanalyzers are connected on-line to the computer via an Analog to Digital converter. The computer calculates specimen values in comparison to standard lines obtained from standards at the beginning of each run. The technologist may add or remove specimens from a run, make dilutions as necessary, or otherwise modify a run. She notifies the computer of changes thru the autoanalyzer terminal which is on the bench adjacent to the analyzer.

The Coulter-S is also on-line to the computer. Specimens may be run in a "stat" mode, with results printed out immediately at the terminal; or a series may be run in the "summary mode. Results from a series of specimens may be printed out when desired. The results are then sent to computer files using the verify key.

In all result entry transactions a number of checks are made by the computer. Before a result is accepted the computer determines that such a test has actually been ordered on the particular patient, and that the specimen number is correct. It also checks to see if the answer is within acceptable limits. If all is in order, the printer head at the terminal will print the name of the test (e. g. serum glucose), the specimen number, and the answer entered. The technologist visually checks this and if correct sends it to the patient's files by pressing the verify key.

REPORTS

Ward reports are printed each morning at 10:00 a.m. and sent to the nursing stations. These include all work done and entered so far that morning. Our policy is to have the morning electrolytes, glucose and BUN, transaminases, CBC's, prothrombin times, bilirubins, urinalyses, and culture and sensitivity reports completed and entered into the computer by 10:00 a.m.

Cumulative patient chart reports are printed at 6:30 a.m., 3:30 p.m., and 10:00 p.m. A cumulative chart report will print only when a patient has had some new result entered into his file since the last cumulative chart report. Once daily, at 2:00 p.m., we print 7-day cumulative chart reports. These include patients on their 7th, 14th, 21st, etc. hospital day, and patients discharged since the previous day. The 7-day and discharge reports are printed on blue paper, daily cumulative reports on green paper.

The cumulative chart reports contain up to seven days results. Days are arranged horizontally across the top of the page, test results are listed vertically beneath the appropriate date.

Unfinished work reports provide an up to the minute inventory of tests requested by not yet answered. We routinely obtain an unfinished work report at 12:30 p.m., 3:00 p.m., and 9:30 p.m.

DAILY SCHEDULE

We have evolved a daily schedule for computer functions. Copies of the schedule are kept in a loose leaf notebook by the master console, and the schedule is initialed as each function is carried out. This Daily Computer Procedure Schedule provides control and serves as a checklist, assuring that all necessary functions are performed. The schedule which we use was developed over several months of actual operation with the computer system.

Between 5:00 a.m. and 7:30 a.m. the routine test requests are entered, patient files updated, specimen collection lists and labels printed, 6:30 a.m. cumulative chart reports printed and worksheets are printed. At 10:00 a.m. ward reports are printed and sent to stations.

Additional cumulative reports are printed at 3:30 p.m. and 10:00 p.m., and unfinished work reports obtained at 12:30 p.m., 3:00 p.m. and 9:30 p.m.

Four times a day, at 7:30 a.m., 10:30 a.m., 3:25 p.m. and 9:55 p.m. we copy the entire disc contents onto magnetic tape. This is strictly a precautionary measure, preserving the disc contents in case of an electrical failure which might cause loss of some information on the disc. The magnetic tape system is used solely as a protective device, a form of insurance against loss of patient files, results, and programs.

SUMMARY AND CONCLUDING REMARKS

Since December, 1969, North Memorial Hospital has had a DNA Clinical Laboratory Computer system. Since June 1, 1970, all test requesting and result reporting (with the exception of blood bank procedures) has been through the computer system.

Successful implementation of the system entailed a rigorous planning stage prior to installation, a formal program of orientation for laboratory personnel, and continued re-evaluation during the break-in period This system has been fully operational and successful for 11 months. Modifications since installation have included addition of a second mass memory disc, minor report format changes, addition of a cathode ray tube inquiry terminal, addition of the Coulter-S terminal, programming changes resulting in a more rapid terminal response time, and addition of a motor-generator power supply and a magnetic tape system.

Benefits to the laboratory have been in the area of improved control of workload and decreased reporting errors. Benefits to patient care are in the area of faster and more coherent reporting of laboratory results.

MEANING AND POTENTIAL CONTENT INFORMATION OF LABORATORY STUDIES: PROBLEMS OF CLINICAL MICROBIOLOGY

Erwin Neter, M. D.

The documentation of laboratory data represents an indispensable part of medical care. The information obtained in the laboratory must be accurate, should become available to the physician without delay, and should be rendered suitable for easy and rapid retrieval. In addition, it is highly desirable that the laboratory data be comparable from hospital to hospital and from community to community. Obviously, a computer-assisted communication system represents the ideal mechanism to this end.

Microbiology presents special problems which must be kept in mind when devising an effective communication system.

A meaningful communication system begins with the request for laboratory tests by the physician. Clear identification of the purpose of the examination and of the clinical problem at hand are indispensable to make certain that needed laboratory tests are carried out and that unnecessary procedures, adding to the cost of laboratory services, are avoided. To illustrate, if it is of clinical import only to learn whether a given subject harbors hemolytic streptococci in the throat, it is unnecessary to identify all other organisms present in such a throat culture. On the other hand, serotyping of Escherichia coli in a fecal specimen obtained from an infant with diarrhea is necessary for the microbiologic diagnosis of enteric infection, but, usually, unnecessary when dealing with specimens from adults. Many other examples could be cited to indicate the importance of clear and meaningful communication by the physician with the laboratory.

The receipt of a specimen by the laboratory should be communicated to the physician; too often, a time-consuming search for laboratory reports is being made on specimens that never reached the laboratory or were not even procured from the patient! Once clinically significant information becomes available in the laboratory, a preliminary printed report should be transmitted. Such preliminary reports fulfill two purposes. (1) They provide helpful information to the clinician, such as the presence of streptococci in a blood culture, and (2) they afford him the opportunity to request additional tests at a time when a particular culture is still available. Alternatively, this system of continued two-way communication can be utilized to eliminate tests no longer required. Needless to say, these preliminary reports must be followed by final reports. A printed communication system has the obvious advantage of avoiding time-consuming contact by telephone and the transmission of misunderstood or incomplete information.

The printed information system and computer storage are of help also to the epidemiologist or to the infection-control committee. Perusal and retrieval of reports may alert the responsible individual to the existence of an incipient epidemic or of hospital-acquired infections. It is obvious that this computer-stored information can be of immense value also to researchers.

An effective computer-assisted communication system in the field of diagnostic microbiology presents certain problems which have to be met, if meaningful interpretation and retrieval are to be accomplished. Among these problems are the following. (1) All too often, the specimens submitted to the microbiology laboratory are not standardized, rendering quantitation difficult, if not impossible. It is only necessary to mention specimens such as sputum and feces. Even when the relative preponderance of a pathogen is being assessed on a semiquantitative basis, a uniform, generally accepted reporting system is not available. (2) Specimens taken from mucous membranes present the additional problem of the presence of a distinct normal microbial flora, differing from area to area and influenced by numerous factors, such as age. The existence of this normal flora at times complicates the search for a given pathogen and, in addition, renders a uniform reporting system difficult. Some laboratories submit a report of "normal flora", others report only the presence or absence of a given pathogen, and still others identify the particular microorganisms, both normal and abnormal. The report of a "normal" flora is particularly hazardous when one keeps in mind that the presence of a given microorganism, such as staphylococcus, can be "normal" in a newborn and distinctly "abnormal" in an older child. Additionally, incomplete identification of a microorganism as Neisseria in a culture from the upper respiratory tract must not be interpreted as necessarily indicative of Neisseria meningitis colonization. (3) The third problem in the meaningful interpretation of laboratory findings is related to lack of information on the methods used for the isolation of certain pathogens, and without this information conclusions may be in error. To illustrate: if a report on a specimen from the upper respiratory tract of a child with croup does not mention the absence of Haemophilus influenzae, it does not follow that this pathogen was not present in sufficient numbers to be isolated unless an appropriate culture medium (such as chocolate agar) was used. Thus, it becomes imperative to relate the report to the methods used in any one laboratory at any one time. Otherwise, data may not be comparable from laboratory to laboratory and from one year to the next. (4) With certain specimens submitted for microbiologic examination the care used in their procurement may profoundly affect the laboratory findings, and yet the relevant information is not always available and incorporated into the record. Merely labeling a urine specimen as "clean catch" is not sufficient to indicate that it was, in fact, properly obtained. (5) Uniform methodology, such as the determination of antibiograms, becomes an indispensable part of a hospital-to-hospital and community-to-community comparable system. Whenever a change in methodology or in reporting is put into effect, this information must become part of an effective computer-assisted retrieval system. Suffice it to mention, in the Kirby-Bauer method the zone of inhibition must exceed a certain minimum (say 21 mm) to indicate susceptibility of the microorganism to certain antibiotics. A 15 mm zone, then, indicates resistance. Previously, many laboratories reported the identical finding of a 15 mm zone as indicative of susceptibility or slight susceptibility. (6) Care must be taken in the utilization and recording of laboratory data to avoid misinterpretation. A communication system that identifies all urine cultures with bacterial counts of 10^5 or higher as "significant" and all cultures with lower counts as "insignificant" may lead to errors in diagnosis and of therapy as well.

In summary, the goal of a generally acceptable, computer-assisted communication system of laboratory data is meritorious beyond question, and every effort must be made to attain this goal on as broad a basis as possible. To render such a communication system truly effective, careful attention must be paid to the special problems of a two-way communication system in the field of diagnostic microbiology.

COORDINATED COMMUNICATION BETWEEN CLINICIAN AND LABORATORY FOR DIAGNOSIS AND THERAPY OF URINARY TRACT INFECTIONS

Alf M. Tannenberg, M. D.

Rapid progress in the last few years in biomedical research has given greater insight into disease mechanisms, and has provided in many instances better diagnostic aides and increasingly more powerful therapeutic capabilities. However, this laudable evolution has also created a new problem in clinical medicine, namely a rapidly growing gap between the expanding front lines of knowledge and bedside medicine. Therefore, new means must be found for efficiently channeling pertinent new information selectively to the bedside. The purpose embodied in the concept of a computer assisted program for therapy of urinary tract infections is to eliminate this informational gap or barrier between expanding medical research and bedside medicine with respect to this particular clinical problem.

The area of urinary tract infection as found in the hospital setting has been looked at from the standpoint of systems analysis. Accordingly three major phases have been identified as illustrated in Figure 1. The first phase is the initial interaction of patient and physician elucidating the signs and symptoms that logically lead to a presumptive diagnosis of urinary tract infection. The second phase illustrates microbiologic laboratory sequences required to establish the exact etiologic agents and their sensitivities to specific therapeutic drugs. Finally, the third phase is an amalgamation and interaction of the first two phases, and is directed towards the overall therapeutic plan. This is the area on which we will now concentrate.

The urgency for instituting the therapeutic plan is governed mainly by the clinical picture or Phase 1. It is a general clinical rule to wait for the bacteriologic results prior to beginning therapy if a delay is feasible. Whether or not empiric therapy is begun, Phase 2 or the input of the Bacteriology Laboratory starts to become available within 24 hours. The therapeutic decision then is of a higher order representing the amalgamation of available clinical and laboratory data. In deciding on an antibiotic, the clinician must take into consideration what we call unique modifiers. As can be seen from Figure 2, the unique modifiers directly influence the choice of drug. Table 1 lists some of the unique modifiers. One category of unique modifier pertains primarily to host physiologic factors or the clinical status of the patient. These factors, the host factors, can be considered in terms of patient age, kidney function, liver function, whether or not pregnancy is involved, and known allergies.

The other category of unique modifiers pertains mainly to drug factors or the known toxic effects on the major organ systems of a therapeutic agent. As can be seen from the unique modifiers, drug host interaction must be kept in mind in determining drug dose, frequency of administration, and duration of therapy. In addition, the unique modifiers may preclude the use of a certain drug because of allergy or because of pregnancy since for example the possible deleterious effects of Tetracycline in the third trimester outweighs its therapeutic effects.

From the clinician's standpoint, with the ever increasing number of antibiotics and unusual clinical situations such as the anephric patient on chronic hemodialysis, a major information barrier exists in terms of available utilizable information on unique modifiers. It is true that the information is available if the clinician has the time to spend searching for it. But for all practical purposes this information is not readily available for utilization in terms of "real time", and this is where the barrier exists. To eliminate this information barrier, a data bank for antibiotics to be used in urinary tract infections has been designed taking into account the unique modifiers in determining appropriate dose, frequency of administration, and required laboratory monitoring. In this design, the final urine culture report as seen by the clinician contains the pertinent drug data amalgamated to the specific bacteriology. The final form of the report has three parts: clinical data, bacteriology results, and dosage information with monitoring tests as is illustrated in Figure 3. This design also eliminates the information barrier between the clinician and the bacteriologist since the clinical data which may be of use to the bacteriologist is readily available to the bacteriologist. The form, therefore, implements a bi-directional information flow rather than the old style unidirectional information flow with its built-in barriers to information flow between the different segments of the health team.

The first part of the report form as illustrated in Figure 3 gives the pertinent clinical data in terms of the type of urinary tract infection, the sequence of the urine culture, the time that it was collected, whether it is a routine or urgent request, and the source from which the urine was obtained; plus whether or not the patient is presently on antibiotic therapy and if antibiotic allergy exists. The second part gives the pertinent bacteriology data such as the microscopic results of the urine examination, the testuria or quantitative culture results, the organisms found, and their antibiotic sensitivities. The key for the number antibiotics shown in Part II is normally found on the back of the report, but for illustrating purposes the key is now shown in Table 2.

The third part as seen in Figure 3 is the clinical pharmacology section giving dosage information with monitoring tests. This section lists the antibiotics to which the organism or organisms showed sensitivity as well as the unique modifiers to be considered. With respect to the unique modifiers, a No. 4 represents a major consideration while a No. 1 represents a minor consideration. The loading dose and the frequency of administration depending on the degree of renal impairment as estimated from the blood urea nitrogen or serum creatinine is also specifically noted. Lastly, the necessary monitoring laboratory tests are shown for each antibiotic listed on the report form. The effect of the antibiotic on the infecting organism is monitored by the instruction for repeat cultures 48 hours after starting therapy and 1 week after finishing the antibiotic course. Consequently, the clinician receives a concise and easily interpretable report containing all the necessary data for initiating and following through on a given therapeutic regimen with attention already having been focused on the possible drug side effects.

As we have eluded to already, the therapeutic program does not end with the selection of a proper drug and its appropriate dosage. This is only the start of the therapeutic regimen. Whenever a drug is administered, the side effects or toxic effects must be monitored periodically until the drug is discontinued. Part of this has already been illustrated in Part 3 of the report form. In addition, the clinical effect of the drug must also be monitored periodically. These two important monitoring systems are illustrated by the laboratory loop and the clinical loop illustrated in Figure 2. This illustration helps to convey the idea of a continuing process. The laboratory loop, not shown in detail here, includes the various specific monitoring profiles for the hemopoietic system, for liver function, and for kidney function. Included as well is the provision for automatic periodic urine cultures such as two days after the initiation of therapy and 1 week after completion of therapy. In a similar fashion the clinical loop includes the clinical parameters of signs and symptoms to be periodically monitored and fed back to the original diagnostic impression, emphasizing a continuing dynamic state during therapy.

With this design, information barriers are eliminated with the subsequent bi-directional flow of pertinent information between the clinician and the Bacteriology Laboratory. For the bacteriologist, he immediately knows the source of the urine culture and the time it was collected. He also knows the sequence of the culture, that is, whether this is an initial culture or a repeat culture with its implication of efficacy of therapy. Furthermore, the bacteriologist knows whether or not the patient is presently on therapy and, therefore, is better able to interpret the colony count. For example, for colony counts less than 100,000, on a patient who has an initial culture and is not on therapy, sensitivities are not routinely done. However, if this is a repeat culture and the colony count is less than 100,000 but not negative, this would dictate doing sensitivities. Furthermore as the system exists at our institution, this design streamlines the whole process of obtaining the bacteriologic data. In the past, two separate reports were required. One for cultural results and one for sensitivity results. Furthermore, each organism, if multiple organisms were found, demanded separate reports. All of this is hereby eliminated.

For the clinician, all of the pertinent information for a rational use of a therapeutic agent is made immediately available to him in terms of the clinical pharmacologic part of the report. A report such as this stressing the clinical pharmacology, of course has never existed in the past. The same holds true for the section stressing monitoring.

This program as outlined has been instituted on a trial basis on three different wards at our institution. Two of the wards are Urologic wards and one is a General Surgery ward. This also somewhat defines the type of patient. The patients tend to be in the older age group and especially on the Urologic wards, constitute elderly men with various types of urinary outlet obstruction with associated chronic urinary tract infections. The acute urinary tract infections therefore, are superimposed upon chronic urinary tract infections, and of course represent a more difficult therapeutic problem in which more potent antibiotics are utilized with their concomitant more toxic side effects. The General Surgical ward is a female ward and, therefore, also constitutes a pool of chronic urinary tract infections with superimposed acute urinary tract infections.

The concise tripartite urinary tract infection form was explained to the appropriate personnel who handled the form. Part 1 of the form, as noted previously, refers primarily to the clinical data section. This information is filled out by the ward personnel, either the physicians, nurses, or aides. It constitutes a simple check off form with 7 different categories. The ward personnel were instructed only to focus on Part 1, and thereby not become overwhelmed by the total form.

The personnel in the Bacteriology Laboratory were instructed in how to fill out Part 2 of the form which pertains to the bacteriologic results. Once again this is a check off type of form which makes for rapid processing. At this point, the interaction between the clinical data of Part 1 and the Bacteriology Laboratory was pointed out so that the information in Part 1 could be utilized if desired by the bacteriologist.

Finally the house staff physicians were instructed in how to deal with Part 3 of the form, the clinical pharmacologic report. The point was stressed that by focusing on the information in all three parts, all of the pertinent information necessary for making logical choices and decisions with respect to therapy could be made without hunting through the chart for added data. For example, for what is considered a "sensitive" E. coli as illustrated in Figure 3, a recommended list of antibiotics is found in Part 3. This list does not necessarily include all of the antibiotics to which the organism showed sensitivity, but it includes those which are thought to be best and also gives the opportunity to utilize either oral or parenteral routes as well as alternatives if allergy is a problem. The house staff physician then selects the antibiotic from the recommended list in Part 3, and at one time is able to order the antibiotic with its specific loading dose, the followup dosage tailored for renal functional status, the appropriate lab tests for toxicity monitoring, and the followup cultures to determine the effectiveness of the overall therapeutic program.

For each of the commonly found urinary pathogens a recommended group of antibiotics was selected. This selection was based on an overall survey of the antibiotics to which the organisms at our institution showed susceptibility. Once this survey was completed for each organism antibiotics were selected which would offer if possible both oral and parenteral choices, plus different classes of antibiotics in case allergy to one type existed. Obviously for certain organisms a rather complete list in all categories could be recommended, while the other organisms such as pseudomonas the list of recommended antibiotics was quite constricted. For example, a "sensitive" E. coli allowed a choice of 5 antibiotics as noted in Table 3. A "sensitive" E. coli was defined as an E. coli which showed susceptibility to at least 2 of the 5 recommended antibiotics. Otherwise the E. coli was considered a "resistant" organism with the recommended antibiotics as shown in Table 4. The same process was used for all the other common gram negative urinary tract pathogens.

The initial analysis of the results of this pilot study were quite interesting. A given form is only worthwhile if the data requested is obtained in an accurate way. We will first concentrate on Part 1 of the form which represents the clinical data base. Table 5 lists the 7 categories for which data was expected. It should be kept in mind that this is the part that was usually filled out primarily by the ward personnel other than physicians. For each of the 7 categories, at least in 75% of the instances, the data was provided. The major exception, however, was in the first category, the type of urinary tract infection, in which the data was available only in 50 out of 129 cases or 38.5%. The next category, the sequence of culture, was somewhat better in that in 100 out of 129 cases or approximately 75% of the instances, the requested information was provided. Of particular interest, is the fact that in 100% of the cases, information on antibiotic allergy was correctly given.

At this point it would be worthwhile to consider the reasons for this particular pattern of results. The excellent results with the last 2 categories, antibiotic allergy and present antibiotics, is attributed to the fact that this information is readily available on the nurse's cardex where the original order for the urine culture is also found. The same reasoning also holds true for the urgency of the culture and the source of the culture. The individual who collects the urine sample from the patient marks in the time of the culture so that this is usually accurately and efficiently done. The major hangup, the type of urinary tract infection and the sequence of culture, relates primarily to the fact that this information usually is not available on the nurse's cardex. This, therefore, would necessitate checking the patient's hospital chart. This, of course, is impractical and probably accounts for the poor showing in these 2 categories.

Part 2, the bacteriology results, provided very few surprises and was accurately filled out. However, it was noted that the bacteriologist did not take advantage as much as he could from his release from isolation into the mainstream of information flow. For example, in most instances the information of a repeat culture with a patient on antibiotics was not utilized in terms of doing sensitivities for organisms with a colony count less than 100,000 . However, we expect that this problem will be soon overcome as soon as the bacteriologist's vision adjusts to the glare of the new light.

We now come to Part 3 or the clinical pharmacology section. This most intriguing part, as anticipated, provided the most problems. If we first focus on the problem of matching the specific recommended antibiotics with the actual sensitivities noted in Part 2 of the form, we find that there is almost, as noted in Table 6, 50% complete agreement with the master list of recommended antibiotics when taken as a whole. The expected diversity of agreement of the recommended antibiotics with the actual sensitivities is noted in Table 7 which is broken down as to the specific organisms involved as well as the number of antibiotic choices available per organism. As would be expected the more antibiotics to choose from, the smaller percentage of complete agreement with the actual sensitivities. The organisms with the most constricted list of recommended antibiotics, such as the pseudomonas and the "resistant" proteus, as would be anticipated have the best percentage match with actual sensitivities. If we compare the results as noted in Table 8, with complete matches plus those that match all except for 1 of the recommended antibiotics, we find almost complete matches in approximately 75% of the cases. When one considers the population involved and that most of the circumstances were that of a chronic urinary tract infection with or without superimposed acute urinary tract infections, I think these results are very encouraging. When the antibiotics are listed in Part 3, those antibiotics from the master lists which do not match the actual sensitivities are deleted.

The frequency in which the house staff physician followed the recommendations of Part 3 that is, the clinical pharmacology section, provided the most disappointing results. It became apparent that it is difficult to break old habits even in young physicians. But again the disappointing results may just be due to the novelty of the situation. I think with more emphasis on the overall concepts, the problems of this area will be overcome. In Table 9, we find that the house staff had 18 opportunities in which to follow the recommendations of the clinical pharmacology section of the report. The recommendations were followed only approximately 1/3 of the time. All of the reasons for not following the recommendations are unclear at this time, but certain possibilities exist. For instance, certain patients were already on antibiotics and were found to have a satisfactory clinical course with respect to fever and other clinical signs, and therefore the antibiotic was not switched even though as noted on the right hand side of Table 9, in 6 cases the organism showed resistance to the antibiotic. In other cases it was apparent from perusal of the clinical chart that the physician only wished to have suppressive therapy, and was not interested in a bacteriolgic cure because of the nature of the clinical situation such as indwelling catheters or chronic hydronephrosis. Table 10 reveals that we still have not gotten the message across that the therapeutic program is a dynamic continuing process requiring monitoring of both cultural results as well as the toxicity factors. Followup cultures again were only ordered in approximately 1/3 of the cases, and unfortunately no monitoring tests were ordered in any of these cases. Unfortunately the 1/3 of the group that showed an understanding of the concept of the followup culture did not realize that the antibiotic, the followup cultures, and the toxicity monitoring laboratory test could all be ordered at the same time.

In conclusion, although initially there have been disappointments, I think the results to date certainly are encouraging so that ultimately this approach will be found workable; and the dual goals of better information flow and better therapeutic programs will be attained.

DOCUMENTATION OF LABORATORY DATA

TABLE 1

UNIQUE MODIFIERS

HOST FACTORS	DRUG FACTORS
AGE	LIVER TOXICITY
PREGNANCY	RENAL TOXICITY
KIDNEY FUNCTION	HEMATOPOIETIC TOXICITY
LIVER FUNCTION	NERVOUS SYSTEM TOXICITY
ALLERGY	ETC.
ETC.	

TABLE 2

NUMBER KEY FOR ANTIBIOTICS
FROM PART II

1 AMPICILLIN   7 STREPTOMYCIN
2 CHLORAMPHENICOL   8 SULFISOXAZOLE
3 COLISTIN   9 TETRACYCLINE
4 GENTAMICIN   10 NITROFURANTOIN
5 KANAMYCIN   11 CEPHALOGLYCIN
6 CEPHALOTHIN

TABLE 3

E. COLI - "SENSITIVE"

RECOMMENDED ANTIBIOTICS

AMPICILLIN
CEPHALOTHIN
SULFISOXAZOLE
TETRACYCLINE
NITROFURANTOIN

TABLE 4

E. COLI - "RESISTANT"

RECOMMENDED ANTIBIOTICS

CHLORAMPHENICOL
COLISTIN
KANAMYCIN

TABLE 5

PART I CLINICAL DATA RESULTS

CATEGORY	# NOTED/TOTAL CASES
TYPE OF UTI	50/129
SEQUENCE OF CULTURE	100/129
TIME OF CULTURE	119/129
URGENCY OF CULTURE	112/129
SOURCE OF CULTURE	113/129
ANTIBIOTIC ALLERGY	75/75
PRESENT ANTIBIOTICS	71/74

TABLE 6

MASTER MATCHES

TOTAL REPORTS WITH SENSITIVITY	46
TOTAL COMPLETE MASTER MATCH	21
% COMPLETE MASTER MATCH	46%

TABLE 7

MASTER MATCHES BY ORGANISM

ORGANISM	# ANTIBIOTIC CHOICES	A COMPLETE MATCHES No.	%	B MATCHES - 1
E. coli, "sensitive"	5	3/10	30	2/10
E. coli, "resistant"	3	3/5	60	0/5
Proteus, "sensitive"	3	3/5	60	2/5
Proteus, "resistant"	2	4/4	100	0/4
Kleb. Aerobacter	4	4/13	31	6/13
Pseudomonas	2	4/5	80	1/5
Enterococcus	3	0/4	0	2/4

DOCUMENTATION OF LABORATORY DATA

TABLE 8

MASTER MATCHES BY ORGANISM

ORGANISM	# ANTIBIOTIC CHOICES	A & B COMBINED No.	%
E. coli,"sensitive"	5	5/10	50
E. coli,"resistant"	3	3/5	60
Proteus,"sensitive"	3	5/5	100
Proteus,"resistant"	2	4/4	100
Kleb. Aerobacter	4	10/13	74
Pseudomonas	2	5/5	100
Enterococcus	3	2/4	50

TABLE 9

CLINICAL PHARMACOLOGY RESULTS

FOLLOWED RECOMMENDATION		ON INEFFECTIVE ANTIBIOTIC	
YES	NO	YES	NO
6	12	6	3

TABLE 10

CLINICAL PHARMACOLOGY RESULTS

FOLLOWUP CULTURES ORDERED		TOXICITY MONITORING	
YES	NO	YES	NO
7	11	0	12

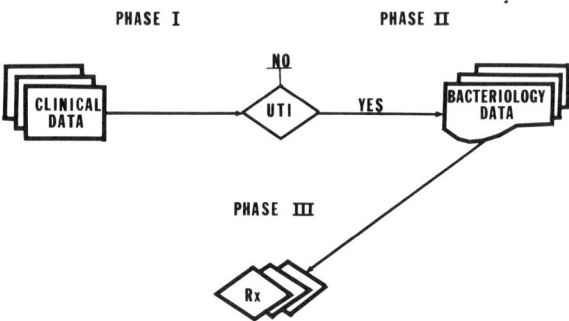

Figure 1. Schematic representation of the basic steps involved in the diagnosis and treatment of urinary tract infections

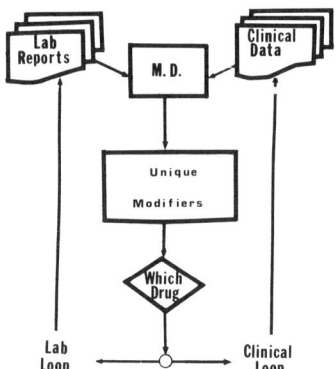

Figure 2. Schematic representing the dynamic continuing process plus the direct influence of unique modifiers on drug choice

DOCUMENTATION OF LABORATORY DATA

PART I

CLINICAL DATA URINE CULTURE		Addressograph

*Asymptomatic UTI ☑
Acute UTI ☑
Chronic UTI
*Initial Culture ☑
Repeat Culture
*Time Collected **9** AM, PM   Source: ☑ Catheter / ☐ Clean Voided / ☐ Other
*Antibiotic Allergy: SPECIFY Penicillin
*Present Antibiotics: SPECIFY None

*Routine ☑
Urgent
*AFB

BACTERIOLOGY LAB # **5/42**

PART II   *TIME REC'D IN LAB: **10 AM**   REPORT DATE: **5/11/71**

BACTERIOLOGY RESULTS:
*Urine Exam: gram +☐; -☑; bacillus☑; coccus☐; WBC: few☐; mod☑; many☐
*Testuria: 0-2 (<10,000)☐; 3-25 (10,000-100,000)☐; >25 (>100,000)☑
*Organism: ① E. Coli   3 Proteus   5 A. Aerogenes   7 Pseudomonas
           2 Interm. coliform 4 Enterococcus 6 Klebsiella   8
*Sensitivity: Circle Appropriate Antibiotics

Organism # **1** ① ② 3 ④ ⑤ ⑥ 7 ⑧ ⑨ ⑩ ⑪ 12 13 14
Organism #   1 2 3 4 5 6 7 8 9 10 11 12 13 14
Organism #   1 2 3 4 5 6 7 8 9 10 11 12 13 14

NOTE: Key for Antibiotics on Back

PART III

CLINICAL PHARMACOLOGY
CR = serum creatinine
BUN = blood urea nitrogen
KP = CR, BUN
LP = SGOT, SGPT, LDH
HP = CBC
NT = specific nerve test
LD = loading dose

ANTIBIOTIC	AGE	PREGNANCY	LIVER	KIDNEY	BLOOD	NERVES	ADULT LOADING DOSE	DOSAGE TAILORED FOR LEVEL OF RENAL FUNCTION			LAB MONITORING TOXICITY				
								CR <2	BUN <30	2-5 30-75	>5 >75	Q	L	H	Q5D
												10	P	P	
												D	P	P	
												N	K	T	
1 Ampicillin	1	1	1	1			500 mgm	LD QID	LD QID	LD QID					
6 Cephalothin	1	1	1	1			500 mgm - 1gm	LD QID	LD/4QID	LD QID					
8 Sulfisoxazole	4	4	4	1			4 gm	X	X	X				X	
9 Tetracycline	4	4	4	1			500 mgm	LD Q2H	LD Q2H	LD Q72H	X	X			
10 Nitrofurantoin	1	1	4	1	1		100 mgm	LD QID	X	X	X	X			

REPEAT CULTURES: 48 Hrs. after start of Rx and 1 week after end of Rx.

Figure 3. Urine culture report form illustrating its three integral parts

BEDSIDE ASPECTS OF MICROBIOLOGY

Martin E. Plaut, M. D.

Introduction

Even in the best run microbiology laboratory, accurate identification of micro-organisms and the susceptibility of such micro-organisms to various antibiotics is given vastly greater resources than is communication of data to physicians. Even in a general hospital situation, laboratory heads care more about generation of data than transmission. As a result, accurate reports arrive too late to influence decisions on antibiotic therapy. Pressure to report partial information to practicing physicians is often resisted as "unscientific". Yet the risks of improper therapy for patients with serious bacterial infections is great enough to warrant a re-ordering of laboratory priorities. Without sacrificing accuracy and details, microbiologists can work with clinicians to improve the flow of information, as well as change its content by revision of methods, susceptibility tests, screening procedures, and reporting.

PRIORITY SYSTEMS

Clinicians and laboratory heads should work together to determine clinical importance of data and how the laboratory generating such data can better transmit answers to physicians. Among others, priorities for generation and transmission of information include:

1. Shared ideas between practicing physicians and laboratory heads. If carried on a regular basis, the laboratory head may learn for example, that a new anti-

biotic has clinical merit and should be added in susceptibility testing, while the practicing physician becomes informed of new uses of antibiotic disc techniques.

2. The clinician must provide information about clinical specimens sent to the laboratory. At the least, this must include the diagnosis under consideration, and the use of antibiotics by the patient at the time the culture was taken. Negative cultures in the face of proven bacterial infections are most commonly a function of concurrent antibiotic therapy, improper handling of specimens, or both. In daily hospital practice, laboratory request slips for tests should be designed to provide "check-off" boxes for presence or absence of antibiotics and a blank space after the box for the name of the drug to be added. In addition, physicians should be called about unclear instructions on clinical specimens. A request for "serologic" tests on a sample of blood transmits no information. If the physician is vague about what he wants, a conversation with the laboratory head or appropriately designated laboratory person can help clarify the matter with regard to the specimen at hand, and help inform the physician.

3. The laboratory should have a flexible policy concerning procedures. This is particularly true for new antibiotics used in susceptibility testing, and new methods such as complement fixation tests to aid in the diagnosis of Mycoplasma pneumonia, rapid pregnancy tests, "direct" antibiotic susceptibility testing, and fluorescent tests for the detection of syphilis (FTA-ABS). In too many instances, new antibiotics are added to the test group after pharmaceutical representatives meet with laboratory heads. Not only does this result in capricious change in methods, but overlap in such testing is the invariable result. In some laboratories recently visited, three kinds of tetracycline discs were used in susceptibility tests on a sample organism, and two kinds of discs containing cephalosporin drugs were used. This

represents needless duplication of efforts.

4. The laboratory should report partial information as soon as possible. The presence of organisms in stained smears of cerebrospinal fluid is a crucial piece of data, to be transmitted at once to the responsible physician. Similiarly, growth of bacteria in samples of blood sent for culture should be reported at once, even if the only information available is that organism stains as gram-negative or gram-positive. In many cases, empiric antibiotic treatment can then be started with later modifications as complete information about the organism is developed. As a corollary to this important priority, a record should be kept of antibiotic susceptibility of various organisms. Thus, a laboratory may find that 90% of E. coli isolated from clinical specimens are sensitive to ampicillin. That information may be included on an initial telephone or written report when an E. coli is cultured from the urine, even while antibiotic susceptibilities of the specific E. coli are still being determined. Similar statements can be made about the sensitivity of Staphylococcus aureus to a variety of antibiotics, based upon the experience of that laboratory and other laboratories.

At the Buffalo General Hospital, this idea has been carried one step further. Since common sputum pathogens are often sensitive to ampicillin or tetracycline, discs containing these antibiotics are put on to the initial plate when a sputum sample is cultured. When growth occurs, after overnight incubation, the organism may be identified as "a gram-negative organism provisionally sensitive to ampicillin". With this information available, the physician may commence therapy before knowing the final identification of the organism, or even the final determination of antibiotic sensitivity. If therapy is underway with another drug, especially one more toxic than ampicillin, a change may be made as more data is awaited.

In patients with urinary tract infections, partial information is crucial. If a single drop of clean urine examined microscopically contains two or more organisms per high power field, one can say with 95% confidence limits that significant bacteriuria is present.[1] This "test" takes less than 5 minutes, requires no staining, and allows for a decision about therapy within a very short time. If small numbers of colonies grow after 24 hours (1,000 colonies or less per ml. of urine), further identification of the organism, a time consuming procedure requiring one or more additional days, need not be carried out unless the physician specifically requests it. Here again, past experience serves as a useful guide to therapeutic decisions. We know, for example, that first episodes of urinary tract infection in women are almost always due to gram-negative organisms such as E. coli or strains of Proteus species and that "first infection" strains are sensitive to nearly all antimicrobial agents (including sulfa drugs) and urinary antiseptics. Thus the information that a patient has a first episode of urinary symptoms associated with significant bacteriuria allows one to state that:

A. Urinary tract infection-defined as significant bacteriuria with symptoms-is present.

B. The organisms are gram-negative rods usually sensitive to certain antimicrobial agents.

Many laboratory heads hesitate to send written information on the basis of such "soft" data. However, this partial information is extremely important in helping a physician make clinical decisions "under uncertainty" and should not be abandoned as unscientific.

5. The laboratory head and practicing physician should determine which sets of tests may be linked, and should attempt to generate linked data as soon as possible. For example, a sputum sample sent on a patient sus-

pected of "viral pneumonia" should lead the laboratory to ask for a sample of serum to determine if cold agglutinins are present, thus helping to make the diagnosis of Mycoplasma pneumonia. In certain laboratories, complement fixing antibody against mycoplasma can also be determined on that serum sample. In similar fashion, a serologic test for syphilis is mandatory in any patient from whom a cervical smear is taken to rule out gonorrhea. In patients with sore throats and throat cultures negative for streptococci, the laboratory should initiate the request for a sample of the serum to determine whether heterophile antibodies are present, helping to make a diagnosis of infectious mononucleosis. In the best possible circumstances, data from another laboratory can be obtained at this point, and if atypical lymphocytes are present in the peripheral blood smear of a patient with heterophile antibodies, the diagnosis of infectious mononucleosis is established.

6. Reassessment of pathogens is a continuing process. Such "non-pathogens" as Staphylococcus albus, species of Candida, and even diphtheroids are increasingly identified as pathogens in the appropriate host.[2] Most laboratories regard S. albus as a contaminant in blood cultures and other clinical samples, yet S. albus is increasingly important as a pathogen in patients with artificial heart valves in place.[3] Conversely, isolation of species of Clostridia often lead to the alarmed consideration of gas gangrene infections. Here it is the physician's responsibility to indicate that wound contamination with clostridia and not true gas gangrene is the likeliest clinical diagnosis.

7. Antibiotic susceptibility testing must be constantly reviewed. Using no more than 10 antibiotics, one can appropriately manage most treatable infectious diseases of man. As the clinician and laboratory head co-operate adjustments can be made in antibiotic susceptibility testing. There is no advantage in testing bacteria

against more than one kind of tetracycline, once cephalosporin drug, and one synthetic penicillin. Other drugs such as dihydrostreptomycin and novobiocin are too toxic for clinical use.

When susceptibility testing for a given antibiotic is deleted, most physicians rapidly lose interest in that antibiotic. This is a negative but sometimes valuable way to aid physicians in their continuing education. In similar fashion, antibiotic susceptibility reports should list the most toxic antibiotics last. In dealing with some bacteria, such as streptococci, very few antibiotics are required in susceptibility testing.

Some clinical situations allow for rapid and confident therapeutic decisions. For example, 90% of adult bacterial meningitis is caused by the meningococcus and pneumococcus, and the treatment of choice for meningitis due to either organism is penicillin. Presumably, the patient is already receiving penicillin by the time the culture report becomes available (after a careful look the stained spinal fluid, in fact), and the sensitivity report merely confirms the therapeutic decision made at an earlier, more uncertain time. In patients allergic to penicillin, data concerning antibiotic susceptibility may be more important, but even here, past experience may be extremely valuable. Since most experts now recommend chloramphenicol as alternative therapy in meningitis due to meningococcus,[4] and chloramphenicol, erythromycin, or cephalothin in bacterial meningitis due to the pneumococcus, decisions on initial therapy in penicillin allergic patients can be made without full data from the microbiology laboratory.

CURRENT RECOMMENDATIONS

As practicing physicians, we often make therapeutic decisions on the basis of relatively little laboratory information. Certain techniques of improving early information have already been mentioned: the importance of gram-stained or direct smears of material from wounds, spinal fluid, skin lesions, or sputum; the knowledge of likely sensitivity patterns for organism known to cause the clinical disease under consideration, and the awareness that in the case of suspected virus infections, antimicrobial agents are of no value.

In the table, current recommendations for initial treatment are listed. This chart is valuable only if the physician remembers that every antibiotic agent is toxic in one or several ways, and that as more information becomes available about the patient's kidney function, circulatory status, and allergic history, modifications can be made. The recommendation can thus be considered as appropriate "starting" therapy until more data is available.

SUMMARY

Successful operation of the microbiology laboratory in a general hospital is a function of close co-operation between clinicians and laboratory heads, ability to report partial information as early as possible in effective ways (telephone rather than mail for example), reassesment of antibiotic sensitivity testing on a regular basis, and the use of linked tests to help make diagnoses more quickly. Although occasions arise where exhaustive and precise identification of a micro-organism is crucial to diagnosis and therapy, hospital microbiology increasingly involves the use of rapid and effective screens. The microbiology laboratory, as others, functions best in the hospital setting when a number of persons with expert training determine both the tactics and strategy for the identification of micro-organisms, their susceptibility to antibiotics, and serologic tests which aid in diagnosis.

References

1. Freedman, L. R. and Epstein, F. H.: Pyelonephritis and other infections of the urinary tract, including prostatitis, in "Harrison's Principles of Internal Medicine," 6th ed., New York, McGraw-Hill Book Company, 1970.
2. Kaplan, K. and Weinstein, L.: "Diphtheroid infections of man.," Ann. Int. Med., 70: 919, 1969.
3. Shafer, R. B. and Hall, W. H.: "Bacterial Endocarditis following open heart surgery," Am. J. Cardiol., 25:602, 1970.
4. DelLove, B. Jr., and Finland, M.: "In vitro susceptibility of meningococci to 11 antibiotics and sulfadiazine," Am. J. Med Sci. 228, 534, 1954.

TABLE I

INITIAL THERAPY FOR BACTERIAL INFECTION BEFORE DATA IS COMPLETE
1971

DIAGNOSIS CONSIDERED	GRAM-STAINED SMEAR RESULTS	ANTIBIOTICS SUGGESTED
MENINGITIS	G+ diplococci, rods, or chains	AMPICILLIN OR PENICILLIN
	G+ clusters only (?Staph)	OXACILLIN OR CEPHALOTHIN
	G-intracellular diplococci	PENICILLIN OR AMPICILLIN
	PATIENT AGE 3-60 months	AMPICILLIN
	G-rod-ADULT	GENTAMICIN
	BURN OR LEUKEMIA PATIENT	GENTAMICIN AND CARBENICLLIN
ALLERGIC TO PENICILLIN	------------	CHLORAMPHENICOL
PNEUMONIA	No bacteria seen	NONE
	No bacteria seen but Mycoplasma clinically likely	ERYTHROMYCIN OR TETRACYCLINE
	G+ organisms only	AMPICILLIN OR OXACILLIN
	G- organisms only	AMPICILLIN OR GENTAMICIN
	Mixed G+ and G-	AMPICILLIN OR GENTAMICIN
WOUND INFECTIONS	G+ rods or chains	PENICILLIN
	G+ clumps (?Staph)	OXACILLIN OR CEPHALOTHIN
	G- organisms	AMPICILLIN OR GENTAMICIN
	Mixed G+ and G-	AMPICILLIN
	None	NONE
PERITONITIS		
No recent surgery	-----------	PENICILLIN AND STREPTOMYCIN
Post-operative; previous antibiotics	-----------	OXACILLIN OR CEPHALOTHIN & KANAMYCIN OR GENTAMICIN
URINARY TRACT INFECTION		
First episode	any	SULPHA OR AMPICILLIN
Second or recurrent	any	AMPICILLIN
On antibiotics	any	NONE (RE-CULTURE)
UNKNOWN SEPSIS		
Age 1-30 days	-------------	OXACILLIN AND GENTAMICIN
Age 30 days-5 years	-------------	AMPICILLIN AND GENTAMICIN
5 years-100 years	-------------	OXACILLIN AND GENTAMICIN

Consult standard texts on doses. DO NOT CONTINUE FULL DOSES OF ANY ANTIBIOTIC IN THE FACE OF RENAL FAILURE.

COMPUTER-ORIENTED THINKING IN HEMATOLOGY

Ralph L. Engle, Jr. M.D. and
Betty J. Flehinger, Ph.D.

The title, Computer-Oriented Thinking in Hematology suggests that the physician should change his pattern of thought to be computer-oriented. The title could just as well have been Physician-Oriented Computer Systems in Hematology. In truth, if we are to take full advantage of the capabilities of computers in medicine it is essential that computers be programmed to maximize the physician's capabilities but at the same time the physician should learn to modify his way of doing things to take full advantage of the computer. There must be a synergistic interface between physician and computer.

For a number of years our group has been evaluating several decision-making models which might be useful to physicians to aid in the differential diagnosis of hematologic diseases. Other members in our group include Dr. Martin Lipkin, Dr. Betty Flehinger (the statistician) Dr. B. J. Davis, Dr. Leo Leveridge, and Dr. Richard Friedman. Dr. Scott Allen of the NIH has done much of the recent programming. Our primary interest has been to get pertinent and useful information into the physicians' hands at the time he is making a decision. At the same time, we have tried to give the information to the physician in the context of an individual patient's illness. We have been going a step beyond presenting textbook type information by programming decision-making into the model. While this may give the impression that we are developing a diagnosis machine, we really believe that the information should be used by a physician to <u>aid in differential</u> diagnosis.

In selecting diagnosis as our decision point, we do not mean to imply that treatment and prognosis are not just as important, if not more important than diagnosis. Indeed, we have plans to include these in the system. Diagnosis is merely the series of first steps in the train of thought of a physician as he approaches the management of a patient.

There has been considerable discussion about the undesireability of automating the present defective system. True enough. However, we must start with something on which there is general agreement and the model to be described is capable of learning as our ideas change. It can also give us information on which to base our new ideas.

Since probability plays such an important part in the physician's thinking as he makes decisions on diagnosis, I want to discuss a modified Bayesian statistical model that we are applying in an experimental way to 35 hematologic diseases. We are, of course, aware of the early work of Ledley and Lusted [1] and of Warner [2] who suggested and used the Bayesian approach to decision making in medical diagnosis. We have used a model similar to that reported by Nugent, Warner, Dunn, and Tyler [3, 4] for Cushing's disease. However, we believe that there are some significant differences in the way in which we use the model. It should be stressed that the model is still relatively crude, using the soft data presently available.

In developing the model, the following steps were taken:

First, we defined the population under consideration to be hematology patients seen as inpatients or outpatients at the New York Hospital.

Second, for each disease we prepared a list of signs, symptoms, and laboratory procedures (hereafter called descriptors) pertinent to the disease utilizing as much information as possible from previous models we have developed. In defining descriptors, a strenuous effort was made to keep them independent because Bayes formula, which we use, makes this assumption. Consider, for example hemoglobin, hematocrit, and red blood cell count. These are obvious highly dependent. We therefore combined them into one descriptor called "red blood cells". We realize, of course, that descriptors are rarely if ever completely independent, even if carefully selected. However, this is a compromise we must make.

Third, for each descriptor, we prepared a list of those findings which, relative to the given disease, were thought to be significantly different. It was required that these findings be mutually exclusive and exhaustive, i.e., for every patient tested, we should be able to select one and only one finding for each descriptor. This was a difficult task. First, Figure 1. After a lenghty discussion about the descriptor, red blood cells, we finally arrived at the set of 10 significantly different findings shown here.

In order to analyze all the diseases from one list of findings, it was important that wereever possible a descriptor relevant to more than one disease be subdivided into the same findings for all the diseases concerned. As the number of diseases analyzed increased, this became an increasingly difficult task, often requiring redefinition of findings in diseases previously analyzed.

On the next slide, is the formula for calculating probabilities. Probability (disease A, given a patient's findings) =

$$\frac{P_A \; \pi \; p_{Aij}}{\text{Patient's findings}}$$

$$P_A \, \pi \; p_{Aij} \; + \; (1-P_A) \, \pi \; q_{Aij}$$

patient's patient's
findings findings

In our model we use a version of Bayes formula which is based on probability concepts originally published in 1763 by Thomas Bayes. (See Appendix I for discussion of formula derivation). The formula is shown here and is read:

The probability that a patient has a particular disease A, given a series of findings, is equal to the probability of someone in the population having the disease A, called capital P_A, times the product, capital π, of the probabilities of someone with disease A having each of the patient's findings, called the p_{Aij}'s or just plain p's; all this divided by the entire numerator plus the probability of someone in the population not having disease A, (1 - capital P_A) times the product of the probabilities of someone without disease A having each of the patient's findings, called the q_{Aij}'s or just q's.

The fourth and fifth steps, then, were to estimate the parameters required for entry into the formula.

For each finding of each descriptor in each disease a group of physicians and the statistician estimated the p's and q's based on judgement and available incidence data:

DOCUMENTATION OF LABORATORY DATA

p is the probability that a patient in the population under consideration who has disease A has a particular finding j for a particular descriptor i

and q is the probability that a patient in the population under consideration who does not have disease A has the same finding for the same descriptor.

The estimates of these probabilities were entered as ratios of two numbers. For any given ratio, the degree of certainty associated with the estimate is represented by the values of the numerator and denominator. For example, if a given finding is thought to occur 50% of the time an entry of 5/10 indicates less certainty than an entry of 50/100 which in turn indicates less certainty than an entry of 500/1000.

The ratio p/q indicates the relevance of a finding to a disease. If p/q is greater than 1, the finding favors the diagnosis of the disease. If the ratio is less than 1, the finding is against the diagnosis of the disease.

The process of estimating the p's and q's was a difficult one. Information about the p's was sometimes available from previous models, sometimes in textbooks, but more often the judgement of the physicians had to be exercised. The q's had to be based almost entirely on judgement. It was always necessary to bear in mind that the p/q ratio had to be consistent with the physician's judgement of the significance of the finding in the diagnosis of the disease. It was necessary that the estimates of q be consistent from one disease to another. This, too, became increasingly difficult as the number of diseases increased.

In the fifth step, physicians estimated the probability of occurrence of each disease in the clinical population, capital P_A, based on hospital experience with relative frequency of various hematologic diseases.

Eventually, the model will be a dynamic one allowing all these probabilities, capital P, p and q's to be automatically and simply modified as data on individual cases accumulate. Each time the diagnosis of a disease is confirmed for a patient, the distributions of p's for that disease and q's for all other diseases will be revised.

For example, for the disease polycythemia vera and the descriptor blood pressure the initial estimates of p and q for three findings are shown below:

Disease: Polycythemia Vera
Descriptor: Blood Pressure
Findings:

	p_{Aij}	q_{Aij}
Hypertension	42/100	10/100
Normal	57/100	88/100
Hypotension	1/100	2/100

If one patient with a confirmed diagnosis of polycythemia vera and two with other diseases all have hypertension, the values are modified as follows:

	p_{Aij}	q_{Aij}
Hypertension	43/101	12/102
Normal	57/101	88/102
Hypotension	1/101	2/102

In this model the values of the less certain ratios are modified more rapidly than the more certain.

A questionnaire relevant to this model was generated by computer from the merged lists of findings relevant to all the diseases in the system. (Next slide, Fig. 2) After this form was checked with information on the findings of a patient, the data in the form of a series of numbers were punched into paper tape and read into the computer. The computer was programmed to print out the following types of information.

DOCUMENTATION OF LABORATORY DATA

First, next slide Fig. 3, an organized summary of the patient's findings.

Second, next slide Fig. 4, a list of most probable diseases in order of probability together with the score. The probability score is the probability of each disease x 100. The estimates of the p's and q's when inserted into the formula sometimes allow a score very close to 100, particularly if the disease in question is of very high probability. In rounding off to two decimal places this may appear as 100 in the printout.

Third , next slide Fig. 5, analysis of the patient's findings in relation to any of the diseases.

This consists of a list of patient's findings which favor the diagnosis where $p/q > 1$ in order of p/q; and second, a list of patient's findings which are against the diagnosis, where $p/q < 1$ in order of p/q.

And, on the last slide Fig. 6, a list of findings to test in order of p/q.

It is also possible to modify any of the findings and retest the system, thereby discovering the practical effects of a new or changed laboratory test or other finding.

When the physician receives information of this type he can compare his own thinking against the programmed "thinking" of the mechanical model. If he feels there is a significant difference in the two he is stimulated to explain it. In a sense, then, this physician-computer interaction can be said to stimulate and aid thought and learning.

The model presently works as an on-line system between my office in New York and the PDP-10 at the National Institutes of Health in Bethesda. Although the model has not been rigorously tested, preliminary experiments indicate that the computer, programmed as described, is capable of providing pertinent and useful information to the physician.

APPENDIX I

The principle of the Bayes' formula we use may be best seen in a scheme modified from Cliffe [5] (Fig. 7). In a population of 400 represented by the large rectangle, 20% have disease A and 80% do not have disease A. They may have other diseases or be normal. Sixty of the 80 people or 75% who have disease A also have a particular finding while 58 of the 320 people or 18.125% who do not have disease A have the same finding. The figures in the blocks are the frequencies that are known or that are capable of being estimated. The probability of disease A given the finding is equal to the number of people with disease A who have the finding divided by the total number of people in the population who have the finding or, in this model,

$$\frac{60}{60+58}$$

We may substitute known or estimated quantities for the 60 and 58. The 60 is 75% of the total population of 400 and the 58 is 18.125% of 80% of the total population. The total population of 400 cancels out. Another way of writing this is

$$\frac{[.20x.75x400]}{[.20x.75x400]+[.80x.18125x400]}$$

If we now generalize these figures we find that the expression is equal to

$$\frac{P_A \times p_{Aij}}{P_A \times p_{Aij} + (1-P_A) \times q_{Aij}}$$

where P_A = probability of occurrence of disease A in the clinical population

P_{Aij} = probability that patient who has disease A has finding j for symptom or descriptor i and

q_{Aij} = probability that a patient in the clinical population who does not have disease A has finding j for descriptor i.

If we now wish to consider multiple findings which are selected to be essentially independent we are able to insert the products of the p's and q's as seen in the formula:

Probability [disease A, given a patient's findings] =

$$\frac{P_A \prod_{\text{patient's findings}} P_{Aij}}{P_A \prod_{\text{patient's findings}} P_{Aij} + (1-P_A) \prod_{\text{patient's findings}} q_{Aij}}$$

Non-mathematicians may need to know that the capital pi stands for product.

References

1. Ledley, R. S., Lusted, L. B., Reasoning foundations of medical diagnosis. Symbolic logic, probability and value theory aid our understanding of how physicians reason. Science 130:9-21, 1959.

2. Warner, J. R., Toronto, A. F., Veasey, G., Stephenson, R., A mathematical approach to medical diagnosis. Application to congenital heart disease. J. A. M. A. 177:177-183, 1961.

3. Nugent, C. A., Warner, H. R., Dunn, J. T., Tyler, F. H., Probability theory in the diagnosis of Cushing's Syndrome, J. Clin. Endocrin. and Metab. 24:621-627, 1964.

4. Nugent, C. A., The diagnosis of Cushing's Syndrome in The Diagnostic Process, ed. Jacquez, J. A., Malloy Lithographing, Inc., Ann Arbor, Michigan, 1964, pp. 185-209.

5. Cliffe, P., Computers in Medicine, in Recent Advances in Medicine, D. N. Baron, N. Compston, and A. M. Dawson, Eds., J. and A. Churchill Ltd., London, 1968, 15th Ed., pp. 1-35.

References to some of our work

1. Lipkin, M., The role of data processing in the diagnostic process, in The Diagnostic Process, Ed. Jacquez, J. A., Malloy Lithographing, Inc., Ann Arbor, Michigan, 1964, pp. 255-280.

2. Engle, R. L., Jr. Computer-aided differential diagnosis of hematologic diseases. Digest of the 7th International Conference on Med. and Biol. Engineering, Stockholm, 1967, Abstract 11-18, page 194.

3. Lipkin,M, Engle, R. L., Jr., Flehinger, B. J., Gerstman, L. J., Atamer, M. A., Computer-aided differential diagnosis of hematologic diseases, Ann. N. Y. Acad. Sci. 161:670-679, 1969.

Descriptor: Red Blood Cells

Findings:
1.	Hgb < 7	MCV > 94	MCH > 30
2.	Hgb < 7	MCV 80-94	MCH > 30
3.	Hgb < 7	MCV < 80	MCH > 30
4.	Hgb < 7	MCV < 80	MCH < 30
5.	Hgb 7-13	MCV > 94	MCH > 30
6.	Hgb 7-13	MCV 80-94	MCH > 30
7.	Hgb 7-13	MCV < 80	MCH > 30
8.	Hgb 7-13	MCV < 80	MCH < 30
9.	Hgb 13-17	RBC 3.5-6	PCV 30-55
10.	Hgb > 17	RBC > 5	PCV > 50

Fig. 1   Findings for descriptor, red blood cells.
Hgb, hemoglobin
RBC, red blood cell count
PCV, packed cell volume
MCV, mean corpuscular volume
MCH, mean corpuscular hemoglobin

```
        282+  LEUKOCYTE COUNT          <   3,000
        283+  LEUKOCYTE COUNT     3,000-   5,000
        284+  LEUKOCYTE COUNT     5,000-  10,000
        285+  LEUKOCYTE COUNT    10,000-  50,000
        286+  LEUKOCYTE COUNT    50,000- 100,000
        287+  LEUKOCYTE COUNT           >100,000
        288+  LYMPHOCYTES    <20%
        289+  LYMPHOCYTES    20-40%
        290+  LYMPHOCYTES    40-60%
        291+  LYMPHOCYTES    60-80%
        292+  LYMPHOCYTES      >80%
        293+  LYMPHOCYTES ATYP IN PB-NONE
        294+  LYMPHOCYTES ATYP IN PB <10% TOTAL LYMPHS
        295+  LYMPHOCYTES ATYP IN PB >10% TOTAL LYMPHS
296- 297+  MONOCYTES > 5%
298- 299+  EOSINOPHIL > 3%
        300+  GRANULOCYTES(NEUT,EOSIN,BASOPHILS)    <2 %
        301+  GRANULOCYTES(NEUT,EOSIN,BASOPHILS)   2-50%
        302+  GRANULOCYTES(NEUT,EOSIN,BASOPHILS)  50-70%
        303+  GRANULOCYTES(NEUT,EOSIN,BASOPHILS)    >70%
304- 305+  NEUTROPHILS HYPERSEGMENTED
306- 307+  GRANULOCYTES IMMATURE IN PB > 4%
```

Fig. 2   Portion of questionnaire for physician
Physician circles or checks proper response
number, either negative or positive. If unknown, no response is made.

```
HIST
    1   AGE <1 WEEK
   12   SEX-MALE
   15   RACE-OTHER
   17   ITALIAN STOCK
   23   SIBLINGS WITH ERYTHROBLASTOSIS FETALIS-YES
   25   MOTHER RH NEGATIVE, FATHER RH POSITIVE-YES
   27   ANTIGLOBULIN TEST-MOTHER(DIR)-POS (INDIR)-NEG
   32   MOTHER-3RD TO 5TH PREGNANCY
PE
  132   SKIN COLOR-JAUNDICE
  133   SKIN COLOR-PALLOR
X-RAY
LAB
  272   LEUKOCYTE COUNT 10-50000
  315   RETICULOCYTE COUNT >10%
  401   BILIRUBIN 5-10 MG%
```

Fig. 3   Printout from computer showing summary of patient's findings.

```
        DIFF DIAGNOSIS IN PERCENT

    # 25   ERYTHROBLASTOSIS FETALIS      100%
    # 24   SPHEROCYTOSIS, HEREDITARY      85%
    # 11   D I HEMOLYTIC ANEMIA           70%
    # 23   FACTOR VIII DEFICIENCY          5%
    # 26   ANEMIA OF INFECTION             4%
    # 19   ANEMIA OF LIVER DISEASE         3%
    # 17   ITP                             3%
```

Fig. 4   Printout from computer showing list of probable diseases with probabilities.

DOCUMENTATION OF LABORATORY DATA

SYMPTOM RATIOS FOR ERYTHROBLASTOSIS FETALIS

P/Q FOR DIAGNOSIS

#315	RETICULOCYTE COUNT >10%	83.000
# 1	AGE <1 WEEK	49.500
# 23	SIBLINGS WITH ERYTHROBLASTOSIS FETALIS-YES	25.000
#401	BILIRUBIN 5-10 MG%	22.500
#132	SKIN COLOR-JAUNDICE	19.000
# 25	MOTHER RH NEGATIVE,FATHER RH POSITIVE-YES	9.900
# 32	MOTHER-3RD TO 5TH PREGNANCY	3.500

P/Q AGAINST DIAGNOSIS

#133	SKIN COLOR-PALLOR	0.167
#191	PERIPHERAL EDEMA-ABSENT	0.204
#193	ABDOMEN-NORMAL	0.235
# 27	ANTIGLOBULIN TEST-MOTHER(DIR)-POS (INDIR)-NEG	0.250

Fig. 5   Printout from computer showing analysis of disease erythroblastosis fetalis in relation to patient's findings. Note p/q ratios for each finding.

QUESTIONNAIRE FOR ERYTHROBLASTOSIS FETALIS

P/Q FOR DIAGNOSIS

#439	ANTIGLOBULIN TEST(DIRECT)-POS. (INDIRECT)-NEG	49.800
#303	NUCLEATED ERYTHROID CELLS IN PB	24.975
#530	VISIBLE EVIDENCE OF CONGENITAL ANOMALY	20.000
# 66	BLEEDING,GEN/LOC.,FR BIRTH/CHILD +/HEMARTH	6.000

P/Q AGAINST DIAGNOSIS

# 65	BLEEDING,GEN/LOC.NOT FR BIR/CHILD,NOT HEMARTH	0.000
#438	ANTIGLOBULIN TEST(DIRECT)-NEG. (INDIRECT)-NEG	0.001
#302	NUCLEATED ERYTHROID CELLS IN PB-ABSENT	0.001

Fig. 6   Printout from computer showing list of additional findings to be tested. Note p/q ratios for each finding.

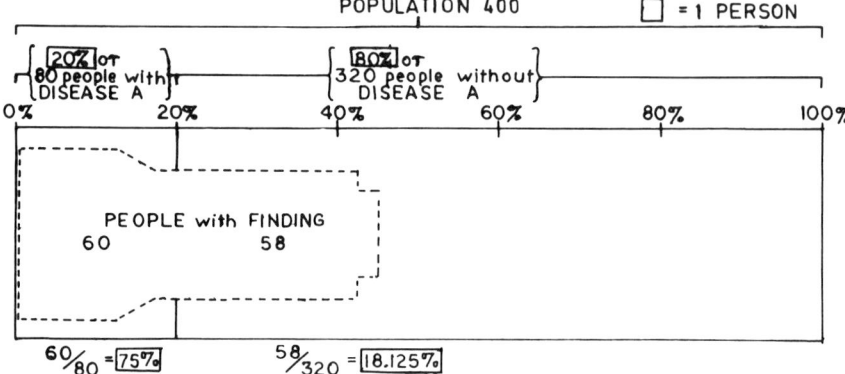

Fig. 7   Scheme to illustrate derivation of Bayes' formula used.

THE HEMATOLOGY CHART

Michael A. Sullivan, M. D.

The purpose of this presentation is to illustrate an attempt at the development of a uniform data base for patients with hematologic disease. Before launching into the specifics, there are several general points to be made which are self-evident but which require frequent restating.

I am sure Doctor Weed, among others here, has emphasized the necessity for an objective elucidation of all of the patient's problems before any one sub-specialty area can be adequately explored. This is, of course, especially true in hematology. Therefore, I am not suggesting that the proposed Hematology chart substitute for the overall medical evaluation forms. However, at the present time these are not available. It must be realized that certain disciplines, for example, some of the surgical sub-specialties, are relatively narrow in scope and well on their way to a standardized form, General Medicine and Psychiatry on the other hand, are extremely wide in scope and it will be a while before uniform standards are developed.

If adopted as an area-wide method, its value is obvious in standardizing the information elicited by physicians of varying backgrounds in different regions and making for easy transmission of this information to a consultant in a distant hospital who will be familiar with the form and contents of the charts.

The slides illustrate a proposed uniform chart for patients who are identified as having a hematologic disorder. The chart is to be used for initial hematology clinic visits and as a supplemental in-patient chart. The accompanying Hematology Consultation Form may be used in conjunction with it, especially the laboratory portions.

The slides are a bit "busy" but they are only meant to illustrate the forms and the data desired and are not necessarily scrutinized by the audience.

I. The first slide is the face sheet of the chart. The Chief Complaints are composed of the 16 most frequently occuring complaints derived from hematologic in-patient charts, in alphabetical order of course, not necessarily the order of frequency.

II. The bottom half of the sheet is occupied by a combination past history symptom review with a total of 99 items which have been extracted from the literature as being of some especial importance in hematologic patients.

The last part of that slide, or page, on the chart is devoted to a brief Dietary History deliberately so because of the extreme difficulty my colleagues, the House Staff, and I have encountered in eliciting a valuable, pertinent dietary history from adults, considering the time and effort involved.

III. The last portion of that dlide, the chart page, is the beginning of an extensive Drug History, based primarily on the work of Alexander and articles by Moser, Meyler, the UNESCO and WHO Symposia and the AMA Registry on blood dyscrasias.

IV. This slide, or page of the chart, is devoted to the Family History, Occupational History, and Geographic History.

The Family History has been modified from the basic

computer compatible charts to include certain hematologic features. A more extensive history might better be developed for a chart devoted to the specialty of Inherited Disease or Genetics.

The Occupational History is left entirely narrative because of the relatively small role occupational disease play in hematologic disorders at present.

The Geographic History is divided into continents with room left for any specific breakdowns regarding particular areas.

Any further pertinent points such as Environmental consideration, habits, etc. not covered in the foregoing can be added at the space left at the end of this sheet.

V. The next slide is an extremely cramped but complete physical exam based on the standard form for the computer compatible charts, but with additions of specific hematologic interest, and designed to eliminate some of the bane of the hematologist's existence, such as the proper measurements of the liver and spleen in centimeters.

VI. The next slide, slide 6, is simply the remainder of that examination. This would complete the Clinic and Inpatient Charts.

VII. The next group of slides, combine a brief Consultation Form which may or may not be used for consultation, but if not can be used as a Summary Sheet for what has gone before. By checking and identifying the number of the pertinent positive information, one can identify a profile of many diseases. There is space left at the right for brief narrative elaboration on the pertinent positive findings. It is deliberately short because most consultants tend to get too verbose. The last part of that slide and the next, VIII, is a rather complete compilation of pertinent laboratory data, with some features that as Doctor Weed would say, teach and tell. Note particularly the use of absolute numbers in the differential for Reticulocyte counts, etc.

The Marrow Report allows room for both an absolute marrow count and a narrative description, hoping to satisfy both factions.

IX. The last slide completes the Laboratory Work and allows for a description of problems and diagnoses arrived at, a space for Additional Information Requested, and then Therapeutic Recommendations.

Now of course, this chart taken out of context could be misconstrued. A pediatric case, for example, could hardly use the extensive Past History-Sympton Review, and could probably use more space for a Dietary History. The usual case of Pernicious Anemia, Sickle Cell Disease, and other straight forward hematologic problems may not require such records, or may pose therapeutic problems rather than diagnostic problems. However, it is just such rather commonplace disorders that are occasionally missed or overdiagnosed and therapeutic problems can probably best be approached from an adequate diagnostic standpoint, complete data base, which often makes the reasons for the therapeutic dilemma evident, and as Doctor Weed has pointed out, oftentimes one might present a relatively untrained individual with all of the patients problems and come up with a more logical line of therapy, rather than presenting a very skilled individual with only part of the problem and oftentimes come up with an illogical or unreasonable line of therapy.

This entire section can be completed by a resident familiar with it in slightly longer time than this paper takes to present. It also lends itself to storage on 3x4 film or 4x5 film.

DOCUMENTATION OF LABORATORY DATA

PHYSICIAN'S ADMISSION FORM

HEMATOLOGY

STANDARD HISTORY
(CROSS OUT QUESTION NUMBER IF ANSWER NOT AVAILABLE)

ADDRESSOGRAPH PLATE

I. IF HISTORY IS NOT RELIABLE CHECK HERE ____

II. CHIEF COMPLAINT(S)
1 ANEMIA ____	5 FEVER ____	9 LEG ULCER ____	13 POLYCYTHEMIA ____
2 ABDOMINAL MASS(ES) ____	6 INFECTIONS ____	10 LYMPH ADENOPATHY ____	14 PRURITIS ____
3 BLEEDING ____	7 JAUNDICE ____	11 PAIN ____	15 WEAKNESS ____
4 BONE PAIN ____	8 JOINT PAIN ____	12 PETECHIAE ____	16 WEIGHT LOSS ____

IF OTHER: SPECIFY 17 _____

III. PRESENT ILLNESS DURATION (FILL IN NUMBER) 1 ____ HOURS 2 ____ DAYS 3 ____ MONTHS 4 ____ YEARS
PATTERN: 5 ____ CONTINUOUS 6 ____ INTERMITTENT 7 ____ PROGRESSIVELY WORSE ____ 8 OTHER

ADDITIONAL PERTINENT DETAILS 9 _____
_____
_____
_____
_____
_____
_____
_____
_____
_____

IV. PAST HISTORY - SYMPTOM REVIEW
1 ADDISONS DISEASE ____	4 ANEMIA ____	7 ARTHRITIS ____
2 ALBUMINURIA ____	5 ANGINA ____	8 ASCITES ____
3 ALLERGIES ____	6 ANTICOAGULANTS ____	9 ASTHMA ____
10 BLEEDING ____	12 BRUCELLOSIS ____	
11 BONE MARROW EXAM ____	13 BURNS ____	
14 CARCINOMA ____	17 COLITIS ____	20 COUMADIN ____
15 CIRRHOSIS ____	18 COOLEYS ANEMIA ____	21 CUSHINGS DISEASE ____
16 CLOTTING DISORDERS ____	19 CORONARY ARTERY DIS ____	
22 ECLAMPSIA ____	24 EPILEPSY ____	26 ERYTHROBLASTOSIS ____
23 EMPHYSEMA ____	25 EPISTAXIS ____	
27 FAVISM ____		
28 FELTYS SYNDROME ____		
29 GALLSTONES ____	31 GLOSSITIS ____	
30 GASTRECTOMY ____	32 GOUT ____	
33 HAIR DYES ____	36 HEMANGIOMA ____	39 HEMOGLOBINOPATHY ____
34 HALOTHANE ____	37 HEMOPHILIA ____	40 HYPERTENSION ____
35 HEART FAILURE ____	38 HEMOCHROMATOSIS ____	41 HYPOTHYROIDISM ____
42 HEMOLYTIC ANEMIA ____	45 HEPATITIS ____	48 HOOKWORM ____
43 HEMORRHAGE ____		
44 HENOCHS PURPURA ____		

Slide I

IV. PAST HISTORY - SYMPTOM REVIEW

49 ILEITIS ____   52 INFLUENZA ____
50 INFECTIONS
51 INFECTIOUS MONONUCLEOSIS ____

53 JAUNDICE ____

54 LEUKEMIA ____   57 LUPUS ERYTHEMATOSUS ____
55 LEUKOPENIA ____   58 LYMPHADENITIS ____
56 LIVER DISEASE ____ 59 LYMPHOMA ____

60 MALARIA ____   64 MELENA ____   67 MULTIPLE MYELOMA ____
61 MALIGNANCY ____   65 MENORRHAGIA ____   68 MYXEDEMA ____
62 MEDITERRANEAN ANEMIA ____ 66 MENINGITIS ____

69 NEPHRITIS ____
70 NOCTURIA ____

70 PANCREATITIS ____   74 POISONING ____
72 PERNICIOUS ANEMIA ____ 75 POLYCYTHEMIA ____
73 PHARYNGITIS RECURRENT ____ 76 PURPURA ____

77 RHEUMATIC FEVER ____

78 SARCOIDOSIS ____   81 SPLEEN - DISEASES ____ 84 SYPHILIS ____
79 SICKLE CELL ANEMIA ____ 82 SPRUE ____
80 SPHEROCYTOSIS ____   83 SURGERY* ____

85 THALASSEMIA ____   88 THROMBOSIS ____   91 TUMORS ____
86 THYROID DISEASE ____ 89 TRANSFUSION ____   92 TWINS ____
87 THROMBOCYTOPENIA ____ 90 TUBERCULOSIS ____

93 ULCERS ____
94 UREMIA ____

95 WORMS ____

96 X-RAYS   97 ISOTOPES
   DIAGNOSTIC   DIAGNOSTIC
   THERAPEUTIC ____   THERAPEUTIC ____

98 List*_____

99 IONIZING RADIATION EXPOSURE ____

V. DIETARY HISTORY
1 ALCOHOL ____   3. FAVA BENAS ____   5 STARCH ____
2 CLAY ____   4 RED MEAT ____

VI DRUG HISTORY
1 ASPIRIN ____   3 ANTIHISTAMINES ____   5 ARSENICALS ____
2 ACETOPHENEDIDIN ____   4 ANTIMALARIALS ____

Slide II

DOCUMENTATION OF LABORATORY DATA

VI. DRUG HISTORY - CONTINUED.

6 BARBITURATES	____	
7 BROMIDES	____	
8 CHEMOTHERAPY	____	11 CORTISONE ____
9 CHLORAMPHENICOL	____	12 CYANOCOBALIN ____
10 CHLORAQUINE	____	
13 DARVON	____	15 DIGITALIS ____
14 DEXTRAN	____	16 DIURETICS ____
17 ESTROGENS	____	
18 FOLATE	____	
19 GOLD	____	
20 HEPARIN	____	22 HYDRANTOINS ____
21 HYDRALAZINE	____	(DILANTIN)
23 INH	____	25 INSULIN ____
24 IODIDES	____	26 IRON ____
27 MEPROBAMATE	____	29 METHMAZOLE ____
28 MERCURIALS	____	
30 NITROFURANTOIN	____	
31 PENICILLIN	____	33 PHENACETIN ____
32 PHENYLBUTAZONE	____	
33 QUININE	____	
34 QUINIDINE	____	
35 RESERPINE	____	
36 SALICYLATES	____	38 STREPTOMYCIN ____
37 SERUMS	____	39 SULFAS ____
40 TESTOSTERONE	____	43 TRIDIONE ____
41 THIOURACIL	____	44 TRIPELANNAMINE ____
42 TOLBUTAMIDE	____	
45 VITAMINS	____	
46 OTHERS	_____	

CODE	SPECIFY DRUG, DOSE, AND DURATION	PAST	PRESENT

Slide III

MICHAEL A. SULLIVAN

VII. FAMILY HISTORY

CODE FOR RELATION	CODE FOR STATUS	CODE FOR ILLNESS
M - MOTHER S - SIBLING	A - ALIVE	1 ALCOHOLISM 4 BLEEDING
F - FATHER C - CHILDREN	D - DEAD	2 ANEMIA 5 CANCER
IF OTHER: SPECIFY	U - UNKNOWN	3 ARTHRITIS 6 CARDIOVASCULAR
7 CONGENITAL ANOMALY	10 DIABETES	13 WELL
8 DEAD OF "OLD AGE"	11 MENTAL ILLNESS	14 OTHER
9 DEAD OF UNKNOWN CAUSE	12 TUBERCULOSIS	

RELATION	STATUS	ILLNESS CODE	SPECIFY - ENCIRCLE CAUSE OF DEATH

VIII OCCUPATIONAL HISTORY _____

IX GEOGRAPHIC HISTORY (PAST 20 YEARS)
   ALASKA   CENTRAL AMERICA   SOUTH AMERICA   NORTH AMERICA
   ASIA   EUROPE
   AFRICA   ITALY
   AUSTRALIA   MALAYSIA

Slide IV

DOCUMENTATION OF LABORATORY DATA

STANDARD PHYSICAL EXAMINATION -- HEMATOLOGY
CROSS OUT QUESTION NUMBER IF ANSWER NOT AVAILABLE

7. GENERAL DESCRIPTION   WELL __ ACUTELY ILL __ CHRONICALLY ILL __   KEMPT? YES __ NO __
                         NUTRITION GOOD __   POOR __   CACHETIC __   OTHER __ _____
8. MENTAL STATUS   ALERT __ CONFUSED __ DISORIENTED __   UNRESPONSIVE __
9 VITAL SIGNS   B.P. _____/_____ MM; PULSE _____/MIN: TEMPERATURE _____ °F
                RESPIRATION RATE _____/MIN;
10 HAIR BALDING __ COARSE __ FINE __
   SKIN NORMAL __ PALE __ JAUNDICE __ ECCHYMOSES __ TALANGECTASIAE __ PETECHIAE __ ULCER __
11

		CHECK		SPECIFY ABNORMAL FINDINGS
---	---	NORMAL	ABNORMAL	---
H	EAR			
E	NOSE			
E	THROAT			
N	ORAL CAVITY			
T	TONGUE			
	NECK			
	EYE: EXTERNAL			
	MUSCLES			
	FUNDUS			
	PUPILS			
	CRANIUM			
	FACE & NECK			

12 CHEST   NORMAL __ ASYMMETRICAL __ INCREASED AP DIAMETER __ SCARS _____
   LUNGS

		NORMAL	DECREASED	INCREASED	RALES	RHONCHI	WHEEZING	RUB
CODE:	BREATH LEFT							
NOT EXAMINED	SOUND RIGHT							
= N.E.	VOICE LEFT							
	SOUNDS RIGHT							
	PERCUSSION LEFT							
	NOTE RIGHT							

OTHER: _____

BREAST   NORMAL YES __ NO __ DISCHARGE NO __ YES __ CHARACTER _____
         MASS: NO __ YES __ SPECIFY SIZE _____ LOCATION: L __ R __

HEART   RHYTHM: REGULAR __ IRREGULAR __ SIZE: NORMAL __ ENLARGED __   LOCATION &
         MURMURS: NONE: __ SYSTOLIC __ DIASTOLIC __ INTENSITY _____ CHARACTER _____
         SPECIFY

13 ABDOMEN   NORMAL __ ASYMMETRICAL __ DISTENDED __ OBESE __ SCAPHOID __
   LIVER   NORMAL __ TENDER __ EDGE _____ CM BELOW COSTAL MARGIN: SURFACE _____
   SPLEEN   PALPABLE? NO __ YES _____ CM BELOW COSTAL MARGIN
   KIDNEY   PALPABLE? NO __ LT __ RT __ TENDERNESS? NO __ ANTERIOR LT __ RT __ POSTERIOR LT __
   BLADDER   NOT PALPABLE? __ ABNORMAL? __ SPECIFY _____ RT __
14 GENITALIA NORMAL __ ABNORMAL __
   PELVIC FINDINGS (A) DEFERRED? CHILD __ MALE __ OTHER REASON SPECIFY _____
                  (B) NORMAL __ ABNORMAL __ SPECIFY: _____
                  (C) PAPANICOLAOU DONE __ NOT DONE __ REASON _____
15 RECTAL NOT EXAMINED __
           NORMAL __ MASS? NO __ DESCRIBE _____ HEMORRHOIDS? NO __ YES __
   STOOL ABSENT __ COLOR (SPECIFY) _____ GROSS BLOOD __ OCCULT BLOOD __ SPHINCTER
           TONE DECREASED NO __ YES __
   PROSTATE   GENERALIZED   DESCRIBE
           NORMAL __   ENLARGED LOCALIZED
16 PULSE

LOCATION	LEFT			RIGHT		
	NORMAL	ABSENT	WEAK	NORMAL	ABSENT	WEAK
FEMORAL	__	__	__	__	__	__
POPLITEAL	__	__	__	__	__	__
ANKLE	__	__	__	__	__	__
RADIAL	__	__	__	__	__	__

Slide V

MICHAEL A. SULLIVAN

STANDARD PHYSICAL EXAMINATION -- HEMATOLOGY --- CONTINUED.

17 EXTREMITIES NO ABNORMALITIES ___ SPECIFY _____
18 EDEMA ABSENT ____ PRESENT ____ SPECIFY _____
19 NEUROLOGICAL STATUS REFLEXES: NORMAL ___ HYPERACTIVE ___ ABSENT ___ UNEQUAL ___ BABINSKI ___
   OTHER (SPECIFY) _____
20 POSITIVE DIAGNOSES AND PROBLEMS

   1 _____ 5 _____

   2 _____ 6 _____

   3 _____ 7 _____

   4 _____ 8 _____

21 CONSULTATION NECESSARY? NO___ STOP (IF YES CONTINUE) SERVICE _____
   PURPOSE (A) EMERGENCY TREATMENT ___ (B) ADVICE ___ (C) CARE BY CONSULTING SERVICE ___
   SPECIFIC INDICATION _____

Slide VI

DOCUMENTATION OF LABORATORY DATA

HEMATOLOGY CONSULTATION

PRIMARY HEMATOLOGIC PROBLEM
   ERYTHROCYTE ___
   LEUKOCYTE ___
   THROMBOCYTE ___
   HEMORRHAGIC ___
   PROTEIN ___
   TUMOR ___
   OTHER: SPECIFY

ADDRESSOGRAPH

NARRATIVE REMARKS
POSITIVE RELATED INFORMATION

  1 INCREASED ___
  2 DECREASED ___
  3 QUALITATIVE ___

RELATED INFORMATION
  1 DISEASE HISTORY POSITIVE ___
  2 DIETARY HISTORY POSITIVE ___
  3 DRUG HISTORY POSITIVE ___
  4 RADIATION HISTORY POSITIVE ___
  5 FAMILY HISTORY POSITIVE ___
  6 OCCUPATIONAL HISTORY POS. ___
  7 GEOGRAPHIC HISTORY POS. ___
  8 ENVIRONMENTAL HISTORY POS. ___
  9 SYMPTOMATIC ___
 10 SYMPTOMS CAUSATIVE ___
 11 SYMPTOMS RESULT ___
 12 PREVIOUS THERAPY ___

EXAMINATION
  1 TEMP ___
  2 HEIGHT ___
  3 WEIGHT ___
  4 HAIR ___
  5 SKIN ___
  6 MUCOUS MEMBRANES ___
  7 TONGUE ___
  8 LYMPH NODES ___
  9 RESPIRATORY SYSTEM ___
 10 LIVER ___
 11 SPLEEN ___
 12 G.I. SYSTEM ___
 13 G.U. SYSTEM ___
 14 NERVOUS SYSTEM ___
 15 BONES, JOINTS ___

LABORATORY
  1 HB ___   5 MCH ___
  2 CRIT ___ 6 MCHC ___
  3 RBC ___   7 WBC ___
  4 MCV ___

Slide VII

MICHAEL A. SULLIVAN

HEMATOLOGY CONSULTATION - CONTINUED

8 DIFF. (ABSOLUTE NUMBERS)
   BLASTS ___   STABS ___   LYMP. ___
   PROMY. ___   SEGS ___   MONO. ___
   MYELO. ___   EOS ___
   JUVEN. ___   BASO. ___

9 PLATELETS _____

10 DIAGNOSTIC MORPHOLOGIC ABNORMALITY ___
11 NON-DIAGNOSTIC MORPHOLOGIC ABNORMALITY ___
12 SPECIFY _____

13 RETICULOCYTES ___   16 B_{12} ___   19 PK ___
14 IRON ___   17 FOLIC ACID ___
15 IRON BINDING ___   18 G-6-PD ___

20 STOOL   23 HAPTOGLOBIN ___
   COOMBS   24 BILIRUBIN ___
   21 DIRECT ___
   22 INDIRECT ___

25 PROTEIN ELECTROPHORESIS ___
26 IMMUNOELECTROPHOESIS ___
27 HEMOGLOBIN ELECTROPHORESIS ___
28 CHEMISTRY _____
               _____
               _____

29 SPECIAL STAIN _____
30 CHROMOSOME ANALYSIS ___

31 MARROW

CELLU LARITY	CELLS COUNTED	MEGA KAR	PLTS	ERYTHRO POIESIS	BLASTS %	MYELOCYTIC PROMY	MYELO	META	% STAB	SEG

LYMPHS %	ERYTHR PRO NORM	% NORM	MONO CYTES %	PLASMA CELLS %	OTHER SPEC. %

REMARKS: _____

Slide VIII

DOCUMENTATION OF LABORATORY DATA

HEMATOLOGY CONSULTATION - CONTINUED.

ISOTOPE STUDIES
    32 RED CELL SURVIVAL ___ NORMAL ___ SHORTENED ___
    SCAN:
        33 BONE   ___
        34 LIVER   ___
        35 LUNG   ___
        36 HEART   ___
        37 SPLEEN ___
        38 SCHILLING NORMAL ___ P.A. ___ MALABS. ___

DIAGNOSES AND PROBLEMS

ADDITIONAL INFORMATION REQUESTED

RECOMMENDATIONS

Slide IX

CONTEXT FREE RESULTS AND THEIR MEANING IN BIOCHEMISTRY

S. Raymond Gambino, M. D.

Specificity, that is the key word. A major reason why laboratory data is difficult to interpret is its lack of specificity. When a physician orders a two hour post prandial blood sugar he is usually asking the laboratory for help in diagnosing diabetes. But the blood sugar test is very unspecific. There is almost no correlation between blood sugars and the clinical disease or diseases called diabetes. Until we develop more specific tests and until we learn the etiologic pathways of complications of diabetes we will continue to have enormous problems handling the millions of blood sugar tests performed each year. It doesn't matter how accurately we make the measurements, how we express the units or how we store the data. The basic measurement has little value.

A similar situation holds for uric acid. Until we know more about the etiology of gout we will not really help our patients when we find an elevated uric acid. In fact, we may harm them. Roger Mills, Jr. has just described severe hypersensitivity reactions associated with allopurinal.$_2$

When a test has chemical specificity we are taking a first step toward easier understanding. For example, it is now possible to measure digoxin. This measurement is highly specific chemically but it is not specific toxicologically. There is a 20% gray area in which it is impossible for the laboratory to say whether or not the patient is dig-toxic. Further improvement of the serum assay will not help. What is needed is a more specific test for dig-toxicity and not just for digoxin. Once we have such a test the problem of interpretation will be quite simple.

The immunologic measurement of heroin is another example of partial success. It is now possible to measure nanogram and even picogram quantities of substances if we have an antibody to that substance and if we can electron-spin label the substance. Then, in a manner similar to radioimmunoassay, we can detect excess free substance through nuclear magnetic resonance. But the process is simpler than radioimmuno-assay, and the electron-spin label is not a giant molecule such as iodine. Soon it will be possible to measure a variety of chemical substances such as heroin by simple, specific and sensitive assays. But this is not enough. All this does is to answer the question, "Is there any drug here?"

There are additional questions that need to be answered. Is the patient addicted to the drug? Through what mechanism or by what biochemical change has the addiction taken place? And even more important--if no drug is found or if the patient is not addicted--is he addictable? Until we can answer these questions in the laboratory we will get minimal problem solving value out of our screening data.

When specific laboratory data is obtained by the physician himself then the problem of meaning may be simplified. For example, when a doctor obtains a Po_2 value from an instrument 30 seconds after he withdrew the sample from the patient then the physician must act on this knowledge. This active response process is an excellent learning experience. The current passive nature of most laboratory data is part of the problem. You know how much more boring it is when you are a passenger rather than the driver. By permitting the physician, and eventually the patient, to obtain his own laboratory data we place the laboratory data in its most appropriate context--right into the hands of the user.

I would like to speak further regarding the need to place laboratory data into the hands of patients. Usually there is no one more interested in the patient than the patient himself. Take pregnancy testing. Why shouldn't any woman be able to self-test herself for pregnancy whenever she wants to? Why does a physician or any other medical person have to intervene? The context of this result should be free of the physician.

I have a young resident on my staff, Dr. Robert Galen, who is getting his Masters in Public Health at the same time he is training in laboratory medicine. Dr. Galen has made a telling point with me regarding laboratory data and laboratory specificity. The blood sugars, the blood gases, the specific drug assays--and most of the rest--are all components of crisis medicine. Even though we improve the reporting, recording and utilization of this crisis data we are still misusing scarce resources. Dr. Galen believes that the laboratory can form an indispensable component of effective public health, but not the laboratory as currently structured by physicians and other clinical scientists.

Dr. Galen would structure laboratory testing to fit the major public health problems of the community in which the patient lived. Everytime a patient made contact with the medical system certain tests would always be performed. For example, a pregnancy test in all women of child bearing age would have higher priority than a blood sugar.

Dr. Gabrieli has shown how impossible it is for any person to remember all that needs to be remembered. The memory of the computer has been offered as a solution. But computer memory is not the only nor necessarily the optimum way to solve the problem. We can also alter what we look at, how we look at it, how we think about it, and how we act on it. Medicine needs its Galileos and its Einsteins. We have too many Cristoforo Colombos adding unexpected discovery upon unexpected discovery.

Our current difficulties may have some similarity to the difficulties the Romans and Greeks had in attempting to improve their science. As Alfred Korzybski said:

"A science of thermodynamics could not have been built on the terms 'cold' and 'warm'. Another language, one of relations and structure, was needed. . . . Could modern mathematics be built on Roman notation for numbers--I, II, III, IV, V.? No, it could not. The simplest and most childlike arithmetic was so difficult as to require an expert; and all progress was very effectively hampered by the symbolism adopted. History has shown that only since the unknown Hindu discovered the most revolutionary and modern principle of positional notation--1, 10, 100, 1000--did modern mathematics become possible. Every child today is more skillful in his arithmetic than the experts of those days."[1]

Our positional notation in arithmetic is a language with strict relationships and structure, whereas the Roman notation had far less structure. This lack of structure required a high degree of skill and memory on the part of the user. There is a lesson here for medicine. One of the reasons physicians require so much skill and memory is that medicine is relatively devoid of language with strict relationships and structure. Our language is more that of a happening and of chaotic events. That is why Lawrence Weed is basically right. His problem oriented chart is more structured than the ordinary medical record. Likewise the ordinary laboratory request and the ordinary laboratory report is founded more on happenstance than on logical circumstance.

Therefore, one of the most important research goals in laboratory medicine is the development of laboratory languages with strict relationships and structure. This conference is a step in that direction.

REFERENCES

1. Korzybski, Alfred. Science and sanity, an introduction to non-aristotelian systems and general semantics. 4th ed. 1958, Colonial Press, Inc., Clinton, Mass. p. 17.
2. Mills, R.M., Jr. Severe hypersensitivity reactions associated with allopurinol. J.A.M.A. 216:799-802, 1971

PROBLEMS OF REGIONAL UNIFORMITY IN BIOCHEMISTRY

By Charles Bishop, Ph. D.
Max E. Chilcote, Ph. D.
Gustavo Reynoso, M. D.

Over the years, the biochemical laboratory has become one of the main focal points in the clinical diagnosis of human disease. Such emphasis places an ever-increasing demand on these laboratories for the rapid and precise dissemination of test results. Such analytical values are used not only for the immediate diagnosis of clinical disorders, but also to detect the presence of underlying, incipient, disease. Such detection, through the advent of mass screening, accentuates the need for some type of universally accepted laboratory output. At a time when rapid data transfer is readily available, it is somewhat alarming to realize that, by and large, clinical laboratories cannot readily utilize test results generated by another similar institution.

If we look at the present system for handling data in the usual hospital, (Figure 1) we find that data whether it be laboratory or clinical data usually come into existence on some sort of document. This document then passes through the hands of some individual who may create from it a punch card. This punch card then enters the computer and the data are transformed to new documents. If perchance the patient enters a second hospital or if the data from the first hospital are for some reason transferred to the second hospital then the process starts all over again. The document is transmuted through the intermediary of a person into some sort of machine readable medium such as a punch card which once again is entered into the computer and further documents are generated. In the COMPARE system, that is Compatible Patient Records System as shown in Fugure 2, the first part of the process in the first hospital may not differ significantly. Data may be picked up on documents. These may be transmitted through people to the computer, but the first thing that is generated is a magnetic tape in defined format. From this this tape then can be generated whatever documentation is required. However, if the data from the first hospital had to flow to the second hospital then no human intermediary is required. The magnetic tape of defined format goes into the computer of the second hospital and generates another up-dated magnetic tape. This tape then may be used to generate documents and again the tape itself is available to travel on to another hospital. These tapes of course will be readily available for transmission over telephone lines or for physical transport to regional agencies such as Blue Cross, or to federal agencies such as the National Institutes of Health. By having defined the format on the tape, it makes no difference how the tape was generated nor how the tape will be used.

Perhaps at this point we should review some features of the COMPARE system. This system was presented by Charles Bishop at a conference held in Buffalo, on October 2-5, 1969, entitled "Use of Computers in Clinical Medicine". The objective of this computer based system is to generate a standard machine readable file for any person's medical record. Any event that occurs in this person's hospital stay, for example may be recorded in this file. Data is entered into the file in flexible strings containing an identifier at the beginning of the string and a delimiter at the end of the string. The identifier consists of 2 letters and indicates what type of information is contained in the string that follows e. g., TM means that time will follow. The data strings may come in from any hospital department and because of standardization of the interfacing, this system can be built in a completely modular fashion. The patient master file is maintained in a prearranged order. New data are merged by periodic up-dating. Interaction of the patient master file with departmental master files allows printout of the patient's medical record as well as billing and statistical analysis. When a patient is discharged, his file is read out onto a storage tape. Because of the standard format and the rigid filing order, data on this patient's hospital stay can be merged with his prior or subsequent medical data whether they come from a hospital, clinic, private physician or social agency. If desired, the patient could carry with him his medical record on a cassette of magnetic computer tape. By using the COMPARE system, a patient's record in one institution becomes compatible with his record in any other institution but without any breach of privacy since each transfer of information would require patient authorization.

In Figure 3 is shown a sample patient record in the COMPARE system. Many strings of data on this particular patient have been assembled and would appear as shown, on magnetic tape. The bottom part of the figure indicates some of the identifiers that have been used in this illustration. These identifiers would obviously need to be rigidly standardized from institution to institution.

Since the authors of this paper were most interested in laboratory data, we began to examine the problems of laboratory interaction or interlaboratory compatibility. Figure 4 shows the request slip used by the Biochemistry Laboratory of the Buffalo General Hospital. Note that CO_2 content of serum has the data processing number 56004, 56 being our department number and 004, the particular test within this department. Since it would be naive to assume that any other hospital anywhere in the world would ever use the designation 56004 to denote serum CO_2 content, it became apparent to us that what we needed was some universal way to designate serum CO_2 content. We were aware that the Canadian government was concerned about this problem of identifying tests, one of their objectives being to assign some sort of work values per test so that laboratories can be intercompared. There is a publication called "Canadian Schedule of Unit Values for Clinical Laboratory Procedures" 1970 edition, published by the Dominion Bureau of Statistics, Health and Welfare Division, Institutions Section, Ottawa, 3 Ontarion, Canada. If one looks at this publication one discovers that bicarbonate on plasma or serum, which is essentially the same as CO_2 content, has been assigned the code number 00437. Presumably now, if one were in Canada, one could use this designation of 00437 and be able to transmit his test designation all across the country.

Even though in Buffalo we are just across the border from Canada, we were reasonably certain that we would not gain great favor by adopting a foreign system, and we were delighted to discover that at about this time the College of American Pathologists had published a long list of laboratory tests. The title of this work is shown in Figure 5, as are some representative numbers. In this system, one can see that the code number 82830 is used for carbon dioxide or bicarbonate and presumably this number could be used more or less universally throughout the U.S. The College of American Pathologists has cleared all its code numbers with the American Medical Association, therefore these numbers would be compatible with the A.M.A.'s Current Medical Terminology. There is also the suspicion that some Blue Cross and some state agencies may also use the same coding system, although the details may vary somewhat from location to location. For example, some systems apparently use a 5 digit code and others use a 6 digit code.

In beginning to experiment with the CAP numbers,

we immediately ran into some difficulties as shown in Figure 6. One of the problems that we ran into was that we couldn't match the test as described the the laboratory with the test described on the CAP list. Sometimes this was because the laboratory designation was unusual and in other cases, the CAP list was ambiguous. Another difficulty that we ran into is that fluids are not necessarily identified. For example, if you look back at Figure 5, you discover that code number 84330 is used for glucose, quantative and does not mention the fluid involved. The code 82310 for calcium, indicates that this might be on blood or urine. It does not indicate whether this could also be on serum, plasma, spinal fluid, chest fluid, feces, or other type of sample. Yet another peculiarity is shown in the final code number on that figure, namely 84160, protein, serum, by refractometry. Here the test is tied to a particular mode of methodology. One wonders whether this list then could be expanded, for example, to include protein by SMA-12 and the like. Yet a third problem was obvious on the CAP list, namely that some tests were not necessarily present on the list. If the CAP were set up to process requests for new test names immediately, then this would be no particular problem. It is not apparent from their literature whether they can in fact do this instantaneously or whether assigning a number will require several committee meetings and coordination with various other groups throughout the country.

Accepting these limitations, we decided to try using the CAP numbers and names to take an inventory of laboratory resources in the Western New York area. To do this we formed a voluntary users group which we called I. D. E. A. L., that is, Information and Data Exchange Among Laboratories. As indicated in Figure 7, our first task was to solicit from all the laboratories that wished to participate, copies of their request slips or lists of those tests which they allegedly performed. The carrot which we used to promote this participation was that we would give each participating laboratory a list of the tests done in all other participating laboratories and a confidential key which they then could use to discover who did a particular test. A fringe benefit which we hadn't anticipated was that any laboratory could now compare its test offerings with the test offerings of the region in general and could find out whether it was doing essentially what everyone else was doing, whether it was not doing certain tests which most other people were doing, or whether it was offering some unique service. In a sense then, we were beginning to get a regional profile of laboratory offerings. Our complacency was shattered however, when we discovered that many laboratories offered to do certain tests but they did not in fact perform these tests on the premises, sending them out instead. We therefore, interrogated all laboratories that were participating, to discover which tests they were actually doing in-house. We were thus able to issue a corrected master list of tests actually performed. The next objective of I.D.E.A.L. was to try to get some information about how the tests were done and what the normal limits were and what units were used for reporting. This phase of the work is in progress now but we run into certain difficulties.

Looking at Figure 8 we discover that we really need more than the test designation. Before we go any further than this, we must make some decision. It is apparent that if we use 5 characters to designate the substance assayed, these characters could be either all numeric or all alphameric or perhaps come combination of the two. A certain number of laboratory report forms are handling glucose, for example, by using the designation GLU. It turns out that in the chemistry laboratory, 3 letters mnemonically selected will give a quick designation of almost all tests performed.

There are obvious advantages in using the mnemonic approach since the laboratory person or the clinician can translate the phrase immediately into meaningful information. Contrawise, there are some definite advantages of using only a numeric designation, namely that this can be rigidly standardized, since it has to be controlled by a code book, and also that the information must be decoded and therefore could be left in an occluded fashion without giving away private information unwittingly. Probably the major disadvantage of using mnemonic letters to designate laboratory tests is the possibility that several laboratories will devise such mnemonic combinations of letters and that they will not rigidly standardize their designations among laboratories. At any rate, we will probably use the 5 numbers of the CAP code for the moment until this whole problem comes into better prespective. After these 5 characters, we believe that we should have a couple of characters for units. If only 2 characters are available, then obviously the units must be carried as coded information since a longer field would be needed to designate actual units. When one starts to code, he has two options: (1) of structuring the code, or creating a matrix; or (2) of assigning codes randomly. The second method is much more economical because it does not force the creation of certain parts of the matrices which will not be used. The hazard of using the random approach to coding however, is that the code may inadvertently link two fundamental or separable attributes together and this will make it very difficult at a later time to separate out these attributes. This was well illustrated in Figure 5 in which the calcium was tied to either blood or urine. This means that if one wanted to have a code for calcium in blood versus a code for calcium in urine, it would be impossible in the present CAP framework. To summarize, we shall probably use a random **two** digit code for units, but we will try to construct this code with extreme care. We believe that we should have one character for origin of the sample. If one uses letters, selected mnemonically insofar as possible, then there are 26 possibilities and this would probably suffice for almost all circumstances. In talking to the clinical chemists in the Toronto area, I discovered that they are using the numeric designation 0-9 for this purpose. This obviously constricts the number of different kinds of fluids that can be coded. Lastly, we would like to add 2 characters for methodology. Again this would probably be by random coding but two avenues present themselves at this point. Once could describe methodology in a very general way. For example, precipitation of calcium as the oxalate and titration with permanganate. Alternatively, one could give a specific literature reference for this particular method. In the former mode of designation, the general principles are readily delineated but the details remain occluded and peculiar to each laboratory using the method. The second approach can give great detail as to the original conditions of the method as first described, but may show little real similarity to the method that has been adapted and readapted for subsequent use in a particular laboratory. We will need some experience along this line before we can solve the problem to our complete satisfaction. If state surveys give some precedence in this area, then we would probably lean toward describing tests in terms of general principles.

There was a time when it appeared that the easiest way to standardize a large group of people was to simply force standardization such as by government decree. In certain situations, this has worked very well. For example, the assignemnt of social security numbers has allowed transfer of data which would be extremely difficult without such numbers. There are still problems in this area including misidentification, duplication, and concern for personal privacy, but the social security numbering system has allowed creation of data bases which would never have been possible without the social security system. In the field of laboratory testing, the random assignment of numbers is not so easy. While one can assign a number to an individual when he is born and have reason to believe that this individual is unique and will remain unique throughout his life time, it is much less easy to identify a particular laboratory test and it is even more difficult to describe this test in detail with all the units and normals that would be associated with it.

One keynote seems to have emerged from this conference, and that is that national problems can often be best solved on a regional basis. When a region has come up with a solution to its particular problems, then not infrequently the same solution can be reapplied in another region. The I. D. E. A. L. group of Western New York Laboratories is an attempt to establish communication among laboratories at a computer-compatible level. If we can achieve this in this area, then we see no reason why similar solutions could not be achieved nationwide or even worldwide.

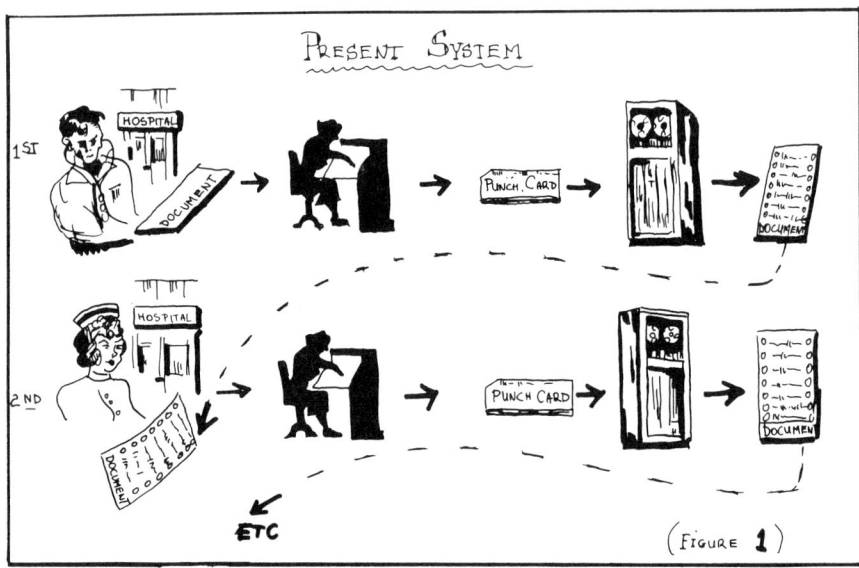
(Figure 1)

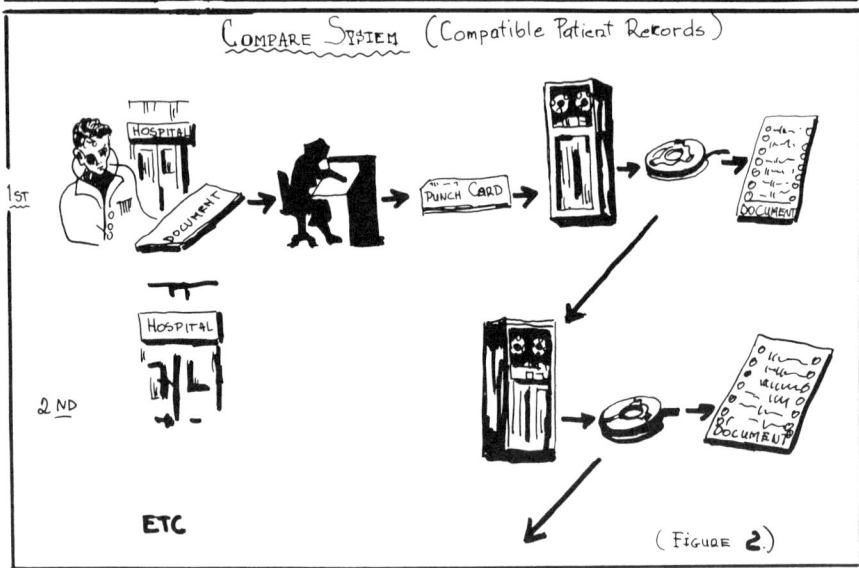
(Figure 2)

Sample Patient Record in COMPARE System

SS123456789WINNER,IMNO:BN8JUN1907:SXM:TM1952:
FN MELENA:TM1941JAUNDICE 1N MIL.SERV.:TM2JAN
70:DX DIVERTICULITIS:TM15JAN70:FN RIGHT ANKLE
EDEMA:RX DIGITALIS:TM2JAN70:FN LEFT ANKLE
SWELLING:RX DIURETICS:TM3FEB70:HA BUFF. GEN.
HOSP.: CC DYSPNEA:PH:24LB.WT. LOSS IN 6 MONTHS /
LOSS OF APPETITE/CHRONIC COUGH: PE ICTERIC
SCLERAE/INCREASED CHEST DULLNESS, DECREASED
BREATH SOUNDS, OCCASIONAL RALES RT. BASE/
IRREG. HEART RATE, 3/6SYSTOLIC EJECTION MURMER
AT APEX/SOFT LIVER EDGE AT UMBILICUS/PETECHIAE,
PRE-TIBIAL, LEFT INGUINAL/4+PITTING EDEMA/
LETHARGIC, SLEEPY: LB GLUCOSE108/UREA14/CO2
24.5/K4.9/NA133/CHLORIDE88L/PO2 64L/PC02 27L/
HC03 21/PH7.511H:EC BLOCK, BIGEM., TRIGEM:XR
INCREASING VASCULARITY WITH INFILTRATES BOTH
COSTOPHRENIC ANGLES:LB HCT39L/WBC7,700,BANDS
37H,FIL.50,LYMPH.7L,MONO.6/URINE SG. 1.022,
PROTEIN 1+, GLUCOSE NEG.:TM4FEB70:BP100/60:UV
260/12HRL:EC BIGEM.,TRIGEM.:....................

BN	Born	PH	Patient history
CC	Chief complaint	RX	Drug therapy
DX	Diagnosis	SS	Social security #
FN	Finding	SX	Sex
HA	Hospital admission	UV	Urine volume
LB	Laboratory test (note L + H flags)	XR	X-ray

Figure 3

DEPT. 56	BIOCHEMISTRY I						
	004	CO₂ Content #					
	017	Sodium #					
	016	Potassium #					
	008	Chloride #					
	011	Glucose #					
	026	Urea N. #					
SERUM	005	Calcium #			018	GOT	
	015	Phosphate			019	GPT	
	009	Creatinine			021	LDH	
	027	Urate		SERUM			
	006	Cholesterol					
	002	Alkaline Phosphatase					
	226	Bilirubin, Total					
	024	Protein, Total #					
	003	Amylase #			012	Glucose Tolerance *	

EMERGENCY OR STAT.   ● * SPECIAL FORM ALSO REQUIRED   PHYSICIAN

THE BUFFALO GENERAL HOSPITAL

Figure 4

A WORKLOAD RECORDING METHOD
FOR CLINICAL LABORATORIES

FIRST EDITION, 1970

COLLEGE OF AMERICAN PATHOLOGISTS
230 NORTH MICHIGAN AVENUE
CHICAGO, ILLINOIS   60610

82830 CARBON DIOXIDE (BICARBONATE)
84330 GLUCOSE, QUANT.
82310 CALCIUM, BLOOD OR URINE
84160 PROTEIN, SERUM, BY REFRACTOMETRY

5 CHAR. FOR SUBSTANCE ASSAYED
2 CHAR. FOR UNITS
1 CHAR. FOR ORIGIN OF SAMPLE, e.g., BLOOD
2 CHAR. FOR METHODOLOGY

Figure 5

PROBLEMS WITH USING CAP LIST

1. COULDN'T IDENTIFY TEST
   1. CONFUSION IN LABORATORY
   2. CONFUSION IN LIST
2. FLUID NOT UNIQUELY IDENTIFIED
3. TEST NOT ON LIST

Figure 6

I.D.E.A.L. INFORMATION & DATA
EXCHANGE AMONG LABORATORIES

1. MASTER LIST OF TESTS
2. DITTO, DONE IN HOUSE
3. DITTO, WITH UNITS, NORMAL
   LIMITS, METHODS

Figure 7

EXPANDING ON TEST NAME

5 CHAR. FOR SUBSTANCE ASSAYED
2 CHAR. FOR UNITS
1 CHAR. FOR ORIGIN OF SAMPLE, e.g., BLOOD
2 CHAR. FOR METHODOLOGY

Figure 8

PROBLEMS IN STANDARDIZATION OF IMMUNOLOGICAL LABORATORY RESULTS

H. Hugh Fudenberg, M.D.

Immunologic standardization represents a difficult problem. As you know, serum sodium, BUN determinations, or white cell counts obtained on the same sample by several different laboratories will give values that are almost identical in each laboratory for any one of these given tests. Modern technology has provided equipment to radpidly and accurately perform these determinations. However, immunological tests have not reached this state of accuracy, thus precluding accurate comparisons between different laboratories.

The reasons for this are several-fold but lie mainly in the fact that each given antiserum to a given antigen, even in the same laboratory, differs. First, each animal responds differently to a given antigen. Second, an antiserum obtained at one time from a given animal may differ in titer and specificity from that obtained at another time. All antisera vary in potency and may also vary in specificity, since thay are usually made against proteins that contain many different antigenic determinants. Thus, for example, standard values for gamma globulin concentrations of normal serum vary from one research laboratory to another when measured by immunologic methods, even when each laboratory uses its own reagents. Antisera supplied by varying commercial laboratories were tested by a group convened by the NIH myeloma task force, and none were found to be consistently satisfactory for accurate quantitation.[1] The antisera proved adequate for clinical screening of hypergammaglobulinemia and marked hypogammaglobulinemia but were not precise enough to permit sufficient accuracy to warrant computer analysis of the data obtained.

However, even with these limitations, measurement of immunoglobulins (Ig's) by immunologic techniques is useful. For example, hypergammaglobulinemia can confirm a suspected diagnosis of chronic liver disease or may help confirm the diagnosis of one or the other of many diseases associated with hypergammaglobulinemia. In this context, it is important to note that the normal values supplied by commercial firms are based on those in normal Caucasian adults, (usually, technicians, medical students, or house staff, aged twenty to thirty five and usually Caucasian). However, Ig values in Negroes and Orientals are considerably higher (20 - 30% greater) than in Caucasians [2]. Hence, a laboratory result stating that hypergammablobulinemia is present in someone of non-Caucasian ethnic origin has little validity. Secondly, Ig levels vary with age [3]. The data illustrated in Figure 1 (a, b, and c) show that IgG, IgA, and IgM levels rise from birth at different rates to eventually obtain their adult levels. The rate of rise varies for the three Ig's but it is apparent that the value 400 mg% for IgG, for example which would be more than two standard deviations below the normal level for an adult, is normal for a six-month old infant. IgA levels take even longer to rise; therefore, it is important to evaluate levels obtained against a norm for the population of the given age, rather than using norms supplied by the manufacturer. A composite is shown in Figure 1 (d).

I IMMUNE DEFICIENCY

Another important point is that simple electrophoresis is no longer sufficient to exclude immune deficiency. For example, marked diminution of one or two of the three major Ig's, i.e., IgG, A or M may be associated with marked elevation in a third; for example, low normal electrophoretic values may be obtained for "gamma globulin" in the hereditary disorder known as infantile dysgammaglobulinemia with hyper IgM [4]. In this condition, the IgG and IgA are greatly reduced, but IgM levels are sufficiently increased so that on electrophoresis, the gamma globulin area looks normal. Such patients are predisposed to recurrent infection (as are patients with isolated absence of IgM). In fact, in someone with recurrent infection, it is important to measure each of the three Ig's simultaneously. Screening is usually done by immunoelectrophoresis (IEP), using both antiserum to total immunoglobins and mono-specific serum to IgG, A, and M. Antisera to the three major immunoglobulins can define isolated Ig deficiency; e.g., IgA deficiency which is associated with increased incidence of infections (especially gastrointestinal infections and bronchial tract infections [5] but occurs in approximately one in five hundred apparently healthy individuals [6]. Figure 2 shows a normal IEP, using antisera to whole sera. In contrast, is the IEP obtained in a patient with deficiency of all three major Ig's, using anti-sera to pooled Ig's. In classic agammablobulinemia, all three IgG bands are markedly diminished (Figure 3a). Figure 3b shows isolated IgM deficiency [7] which is rare. Isolated absence of IgG also occurs. Figure 3c shows serum from a child with markedly elevated IgA and markedly decreased IgG and IgM [8]. Figure 3d shows serum from a patient with normal IgG but absence of IgA and IgM [9].

If diminution in one or another of the Ig's is shown by IEP, quantative values should then be obtained before therapy is started. The method most commonly used at present is the Mancini radial-diffusion technique*[10] in

*Radial diffusion procedures are capable of great precision and high sensitivity when proper care is taken. Mancini and colleagues demonstrated a co-efficient of variation of 2% at high antigen concentration (9mg. of albumin per milliliter) and a limiting detection sensitivity of 1.2 µg per milliliter.

which the antigen is placed in a well and allowed to diffuse into, antibody containing agar. Isolated proteins or serum containing known quantities of the antigen are also run as controls. After standard periods of time, the rate of diffusion of antigens into the antibody containing agar stops and a precipitin band forms (Figure 4). The area of the circle formed by the diffusion of the antigen is directly proportional to the antigen concentration in the serum or other test solution. A newer method, "rocket electrophoresis"[11] appears to provide the same results in a quicker and less laborious fashion. In this case, the antigen is inserted in wells in an antibody containing agar but is electrophoresed into the antibody containing agar, rather than merely passively diffusing into it. The distance of migration is directly proportional to the antigen concentration (Figure 5).

IEP is also useful for the diagnosis of multiple myeloma and macroglobulinemia. Demonstration of a serum spike on electrophoresis does not discriminate between myeloma and macroglobulinemia. The natural history and preferred mode of therapy for these two disorders is quite dissimilar; the latter is a relatively benign disease that can often be treated solely by plasmaphoresis, which reduces the hyper viscosity symptoms[12], often without the necessity for using protoplasmic poisons, such as cytoxan, chlorambucil or similar agents. Bone marrow morphology is often helpful in differentiating between the two, but 10-15% of cases with macroglobulinemia have marrows that are indistinguishable from those with myeloma[12]. IEP using monospecific antiserum to IgG, A, and M will then disclose whether the serum spike in question is due to macroglobulinemia or to IgG A, D, or E myeloma. (IgD and IgE myelomas are rare; the concentration of IgD and IgE in normal serum is too low to be detectable with antiserum to normal human serum.) It is also essential that sera of patients with spikes be tested by IEP with antisera to the μ-and κ light chains. Normal individuals have immunoglobulin molecules of

two light chain types in their serum, one type containing
μ chains and the other type containing ƛ chains (Table 1).
The paraproteins of each patient with macroglobulinemia
or myeloma contain only one of the two light chain types.
Commercial antisera for light chains vary from one
company to another, and from batch to batch from the
same company. Further, some react only when the light
chains are attached to heavy chains[13]. Another problem
is that some IgA and some IgM proteins cannot be typed
unless the light and heavy chains are separated by reduction[14]. A group of related disorders of the so-called
heavy chain diseases[15] are characterized by the presence of three heavy chains, either γ, α, or μ, which are
devoid of light chains. The use of light chain antisera in
the lymphoplasmacytic dyscrasias will occasionally turn
up "heavy chain disease." This identification is not
possible without the use of anti-light chain sera.

II. Other tests for immunologic deficiency. Earlier
we discussed humoral immune deficiency which, as you
know, is due to diminution in serum antibodies; these
may be decreased, either in agammaglobulinemia of the
typical variety (deficiency of all three major Ig's) or in
the atypical variety (only one or two of three major Ig's
are missing) or in macroglobulinemia and myeloma, in
which so much paraprotein is present that the residual
normal antibody concentration is greatly reduced.

Genetic defects of cellular immunity in the presence
of normal Ig also predispose to infection. There are
many test methods for measuring cellular immunity.
Table 2 lists criteria for evaluation of cellular and
humoral immune mechanisms. Initially, skin tests were
used and absence of reactivity to six common skin test
antigens were accepted as evidence for deficiency in cellular immunity. Space limitations preclude the listing of
the antigens recommended for tests, but our recommendation for skin tests and for the manner in which they
should be applied is published in "Pediatrics"[16a] and

in the "Bulletin of the World Health Organization" (16b). (This was a report of a WHO expert committee on primary immunodeficiencies.)

In vitro methods for assaying cellular immunity also exist. Cellular immunity is due to thymic dependent cells, (in contrast to humoral immunity, which is due to "B-cells" (B for bone marrow in mammals and for bursa in chickens) [16]. Incorporation of tritiated thymidine into DNA during a standard period is one in vitro assay of cellular immunity. A better assay is the inhibition of macrophage migration in capillary tubes, by supernatants obtained after incubation of a sensitized donor's lymphocytes with the antigen in question (Figure 6a). Figure 6b shows typical MIF response, i.e., inhibition of migration of the macrophages out of the glass tube by the lymphocyte supernatants of two subjects, one tuberculin (PPD) positive, the other, tuberculin negative, along with the appropriate controls. We have found that the MIF test is a better index of cellular immunity than blast transformation and is also better than skin tests. This has been demonstrated by our group both in experimental animals [17] and in patients with genetic disorders associated with defective cellular immunity (e.g., Wiscott-Aldrich Syndrome),[18] in which therapy with transfer factor converted MIF production to normal before skin tests became positive. Lymphocyte responses to antigen in vitro culture remined impaired, even though the patients had dramatic clinical remissions.

With gross absence of cellular immunity, merely looking at the lymphocytes after phytohemagglutinin (PHA) simulation, will demonstrate the failure of the transformation from the small round cell to the large pyroninophilic blast cell, which is seen in a normal individual or in an individual who has only mildly impaired cellular immunity. Milder T-cell impairment is often demonstrable by the response of lymphocytes in culture, in terms of DNA or RNA synthesis, to specific stimuli antigens or mitogens). These systems must be rigorously controlled. For example, the lymphocytes are incubated (usually in a multiple of 10 to 6 per ml) in fetal calf sera or autologous serum of normal serum. Since autologous serum contain inhibitors and simulators of DNA synthesis, results obtained with it are often meaningless. The fetal calf serum (preferably agammaglobulinemic fetal calf serum should be from the same batch. However, some patients have antibodies to constitutents in cow sera, and thus give a high baseline. It is preferable to use AB plasma from a non-secretor of ABO substance for the incubation mixture, using the same donor throughout. Counts are usually expressed as counts incorporated per 10^6 cells, divided by counts in control cells, i.e., cells to which PHA are not added (experiment/control ratios). However, some patients show high and diverse rates of DNA synthesis in the absence of stimulation. We prefer to subtract baseline counts from counts obtained upon stimulation. Dose-response curves are important if the control cells are not from an age-matched control, as the optimal dose of PHA is different in infants than in adults[19].

Another disease that causes recurrent infection and is associated with still another genetic defect is "chronic granulomatous disease"* This is, in reality, a group of diseases. As first shown by our own group, at least three forms exist and probably, more[20]. This disease is characterized by the inability of the patient's neutrophils to kill ingested bacteria. Ingestion is normal but killing is impaired. Standard techniques involve exposure of a given number of granulocytes to a given number of bacteria, incubation for a standard time period (this must be standardized for each laboratory), subsequent addition of antibiotics to the media to kill organisms not ingested further incubation, then lysis of the white cells and plating of their contents. Normal granulocytes will kill

*We prefer the term "phagocyte dysfunction syndrome."

the bacteria so that colonies do not grow and there is at least a two-log kill. (Figure 7a).

The same defect is present in the monocytes as is in the granulocytes [21]. The most common form of the phagocyte dysfunction syndrome is an autosomal recessive form, in which the mothers often show intermediate killing curves (Figure 7b). It is essential to use at least two organisms in these tests, as some patients may show a selective defect to one organism alone [22] as shown by our own laboratory, some years ago, and as recently confirmed by Hobbs [23]. The two organisms most commonly used are staph 502A and serratia. In our own laboratory, we test with five organisms and, if at all possible, we use the organism with which the patient is infected. Screening tests for this syndrome, based on reduction of the dye, nitro-blue tetrazolium, have been described, but these will fail to detect the isolated defects for one organism [24].

III. Protease inhibitors. Another genetic syndrome associated with recurrent infection, especially bronchitis and pneumonia, is a genetic defect for $_1$-antitrypsin ($_1$AT), one of the serum protease inhibitors. Patients who are homozygous for the abnormal gene causing $_1$-AT deficiency develop emphysema at an early age [25]. Emphysema subsequently results in repeated bronchitis and pulmonary infection. The diagnosis can be made by a biochemical means, i.e., measurement of the amount of $_1$-AT by methods which measure the inhibitory capacity of the serum during trypsin digestion of the synthetic subtrates, such as T.A.M.E. Quantitative methods are not fully adequate unless adequate controls are used. Lipemic sera, sera that have been hemolyzed, or sera that have been repeatedly frozen and thawed, can give spurious results:

Furthermore, about 10% of the $_1$-AT capacity of normal sera resides in the intra α-globulin area, which is under different genetic control than the α_1-AT. Immunologic assay of α_1-AT can also provide needed information (Figure 8)[126] but the commercial standards now available must be diluted 1:10 for use. Several thawings of this diluted material render it antigenically unreliable and may be responsible for the conflicting data regarding the possible increased incidence of emphysema in heterozygotes for α_1 AT deficiency. Further, acute infection[27], contraceptive pills, or pregnancy, can raise the level of this protease inhibitor (Pi).

Further complications arise in that the crystalline trypsin (from Worthington Biochemicals) used by most investigators varies in activity from one batch to another from as much as 40-70%. There is never 100% activity. In view of this huge variation, it is mandatory to include sera of known α_1-AT concentration in all assays. As noted earlier, storage conditions of the sera may influence the results.

New genetic typing systems, based on differences in antigen antibody crossed electrophoresis[28a] and on differences in mobility in acid starch gel electrophoresis[28b] detect the various phenotypes of α_1-AT (called Pi phenotypes, since α_1-AT is a protease inhibitor) and appear capable of resolving this problem; these will, undoubtedly, become widely useful in the near future. The normal gene, producing normal levels, is called Pi^M; the abnormal gene, associated with low levels, is called Pi^Z. (At least seven other genetic variants have been described.) The vast discrepancies in the literature can probably be accounted for by methodological errors, as many investigators are unaware of these various pitfalls[29].

IV. Immunohematologic tests. The most common immunohematologic test is the Coombs' test. There are two main types of antibodies to red cells; "complete" antibodies binding the cells to form a lattice and causing agglutination (Figure 9 top) and "incomplete" antibodies binding the cells but not causing agglutination (Figure 9 bottom, left.) Subsequent washing of the cells, coated by incomplete antibodies, several times with saline, removes serum proteins from the cell suspension solution. Subsequent addition of a rabbit antisera containing antibodies to human immunoglobulin cause lattice formation and clumping of the cells. One common laboratory error is failure to run a control tube through the washing procedure and to add saline, rather than Coombs' antiglobulin sera, to the tube. To reiterate, a saline control should be added to a separate tube each time cells are tested for positive Coombs' test. Without this precaution, false-positive Coombs' test may occur, since high-titer cold agglutinins or cold agglutins of moderate titer of a high thermal amplitude will cause spontaneous agglutination of the cells, even without addition of the Coombs' serum. This might, otherwise, be missed. This is important, since high-titer cold agglutinins and hemolytic anemia almost never respond to steroids, whereas warm antibody hemolytic anemia of the IgG type usually responds to steroids, [30,31].

Further, it should be emphasized that the presence of IgG on red cells does not necessarily prove that the IgG is auto-antibody-directed against red cells. For example, penicillin and insulin given in large doses may bind red cells in vivo: if serum antibody to these compounds develops, the antibody may bind to the antigen absorbed to the cells to give a positive Coombs' test and result in a hemolytic anemia, where the red cell is not the antigen but only an innocent bystander [32,33] (Figure 10).

In some warm antibody hemolytic anemias and in some patients without anemia, complement is present on the red cells and is detectable by conventional serologic techniques, using antisera to complement components. Recent studies of commercial antisera show that their titer of anti-complement is extremely low [34]. Table 3 indicate that commercial antisera, which are standardized against Rh positive red cells coated with anti-Rh, performed well against cells coated with IgG auto-antibody when compared with antisera made in our own laboratory. However, most gave only a very weak agglutination against complement-coated cells, when compared to the specific anti-complement reagents that we use. This proved to be true whether the complement-coated cells were obtained from patients with hemolytic anemia, in which the cells were coated by complement in vivo, or by cells sensitized by complement-fixing blood group antibodies in vitro. Thus commercial Coombs' sera cannot be relied upon for the detection of complement unless the cells are strongly coated.

Quantitative complement assays are useful in the diagnosis and management of the renal diseases associated with lupus. Serum levels of total complement, especially C3, are usually depressed, and on therapy they rise toward normal before overt clinical improvement occurs and before improvement of renal functions tests occurs [35]. Recent data by our group indicates that neurologic or psychiatric symptoms in lupus, due to involvement of the central sacral nervous system by the disease process, can be differentiated from corticoid-induced CNS symptoms by measurement of spinal fluid C4 and IgG levels; both are invariably depressed in CNS lupus [36,37].

While on the subject of lupus, it should be mentioned that the antinuclear antibody test, which is often positive in other diseases, perhaps because of the neutrophil receptors for IgG [38] and the lack of appropriate controls, is being replaced by specific assays of lupus sera for antibodies to DNA, RNA, and for another antigen called extractable nuclear antigen [39-41]. One or more of these antibodies are usually present in the sera of lupus patients, and on their kidneys when lupus renal disease is

present. It should also be mentioned that more and more
is being learned about the nine different complement components and their interrelation to other systems, such as
the Kinin system, the clotting system, etc. Specific
assay of certain of these components have already uncovered genetic disorders resulting in defects in phagocytosis ^{42,42} and will probably reveal defects in other
biological functions when measurements of other complement components (e.g., C7, C8, and C9) become
feasible.

V. Rheumatoid Factor. Most commercial firms
selling diagnostic reagents provide latex particles coated
with human IgG as a test reagent for rheumatoid factor.
The vast majority of sera from patients with rheumatoid
arthritis do, indeed, react to such particles. However,
50% of sera from patients with chronic liver disease
(sacroidosis), pulmonary fibrosis, and a host of other
conditions give positive reactions with the reagents $^{44,45)}$. In rheumatoid arthritis, the rheumatoid factors
react preferentially with rabbit IgG. It is difficult to put
rabbit IgG in antigenically reactive form on latex particles. It can, however, be placed on human or sheep
red cells. We use a rabbit antibody to human red cells
in subagglutinating doses. About 70% of the sera from
patients with rheumatoid arthritis give positive agglutination reactions in this system, whereas only a small percentage of patients with liver disease, etc. do. Further,
there are antiglobulins of other types than the rheumatoid
factor, for example, anti-antibodies, which react with
human IgG on latex particles in red cells. Thus, if a
positive reaction occurs, we attempt to inhibit the reaction with normal IgG . Rheumatoid factor is inhibited,
anti-antibodies are not ^{45}.

VI. Immunoflourescence. Any immunoflouresence
test is only as good as the specificity of the antisera
used. Most commercial antisera are goat or rabbit antihuman IgG. Thus, sera containing IgA anti-antibody,

for example, to gastric mucosa, adrenal cortex, or to cell nuclei (i.e., antinuclear antibody) may give false negative results when commercial antisera are used. The potency of the antisera is also important, as is the specificity. Most commercial firms test specificity by IEP or simple diffusion in agar. This is not sensitive enough for immunoflourescence, which is at least 100 times as sensitive. Thus, an antisera thought to be monospecific against IgM, for example, might by immunoflourescence also react with IgG. Differentiation between IgG and IgM antinuclear antibodies is considered by some immunologists to be very helpful in the differential diagnosis between lupus and rheumatoid arthritis. Thus, adequate information concerning the reagents used for immunoflourescence is mandatory. Titration scores mean little between one laboratory and another, unless the same antisera are used in the indirect immunoflouresence technique. Most research laboratories prefer to make their own antiserum and properly absorb it.

In closing, it is obvious that attempts to standardize immunologic techniques are resulting in the opening of Pandora's box. However, the International Union of Immunologic Societies and the World Health Organization are now attempting to bring some order from this chaos. Provision of standard reagents and the testing of these is now underway by both of these organizations, as well as by the Committee on Standardization of the International Society of Blood Transfusion. As a member of all three organizations, I can only plead that you allow us time to compare and contrast the results of different laboratories using reagents obtained from other laboratories and to compare these results with those in which each laboratory's own reagents are used. From this beginning, perhaps an adequate panel of standards can emerge from which commercial firms can take their clue. If so, the day when results are reproduceable between different laboratories may soon be coming. Then, and only then, will immunological results be ready for computer analysis.

REFERENCES

1. Claman, H., Fudenberg, H.H., Rosen, F., Tomasi T.B. et al: Unpublished observations.
2. Fudenberg, H.H.: Gamma globulin levels in several populations. Vox Sang. 8:249-254, 1963.
3. Stiehm, E.R., and Fudenberg, H.H.: Serum levels of immune globulins in health and disease: A survey. Pediatrics 37: 715-727, 1966.
4. Stiehm, E.R., and Fudenberg, H.H. Clinical and immunologic features of dysgammaglobulinemia type I. Report of a case diagnosed in the first year of life. Amer. J. Med. 40: 805-815, 1966.
5. Tomasi, T.B., Jr., and Bienenstock, J.: Secretory immunoglobulins. In Advances in Immunology, edited by F.J. Dixon, Jr. and H.G. Kunkel. New York, Academic Press, 1968.
6. Bachmann, R.: Studies on the serum γA-Globulin level. III The frequency of a-γA-globulinemia. Scandinav. J. Clin. & Lab. Invest. 17: 316, 1965.
7. Faulk, W.P., Kiyasu, W.S., Cooper, M. and Fudenberg, H.H.: Deficiency of IgM. Pediatrics 47: 399-404, 1971.
8. Stites, D.P., Levin, A.S., Costom, B.H., and Fudenberg, H.H.: Selective "dysgammaglobulinemia" with elevated Serum IgA and Chronic Salmonellosis. Am. J. Med. (In press).
9. Fudenberg, H.H., Heremans, J.F., and Franklin, E.C.: A hypothesis for the genetic control of synthesis of the gamma-glodulins. Ann. Inst. Pasteur (par) 104: 155:168, 1963.
10. Mancini, G., Carbonara, A.O., and J.F. Heremans Immunochemical quantitation of antigens by single radial immunodiffusion, Int. J. Immunochem. 2: 235-254, 1965.
11. Laurell, C.B.: Quantitative estimation of proteins

by electrophoresis in agarose gel containing antibodies. Analyt. Biochem. 15: 45, 1966.
12. Fudenberg, H. H.: Waldenstrom's Macroglobulinemia. In Cancer chemotherapy, edited by I. Brodsky and S. Kahn, New York; Academic Press (In press).
13. Korngold, L., Madalinski, K.: Sub-groups of G-myeloma globulins of type K and type L. Immunochemistry 4: 353-362, 1967.
14. Osterland, C. K., Chaplin, Jr., H.: Atypical antigenic properties of an IgA myeloma protein. J. Immunol. 96: 842-848, 1966.
15. Franklin, E. C.: Heavy Chain diseases. New Eng. J. Med. 282: 1098, 1970.
16. a) Fudenberg, H. H., Good, R. A., Hitzig, W. H., et al.: Primary immune deficiencies: Report of a WHO committee. Pediatrics 47:927-945, 1971.
b) Fudenberg, H. H., Good, R. A., Hitzig, W. H. et al. Primary immune deficiencies: Report of a WHO committee. Bulletin, World Health Organization (In press.)
17. Spitler, L. E., Benjamini, E., Young, J. D., Kaplan, H., and Fudenberg, H. H.: Studies on immune response to a characterized antigenic determinant of the tobacco mosaic virus protein (TMVP). J. Exp. Med. 131: 133-148, 1970.
18. Levin, A. S., Spitler, L. E., Stites, D. P., and Fudenberg, H. H.: Wiskott-Aldrich syndrome, a genetically determined cellular immunologic deficiency: Clinical and laboratory responses to therapy with "transfer factor." Proc. Nat. Acad. Sci. (USA) 67: 821-828,
19. Stites, D., Carr, M., and Fudenberg, H. H. In preparation.
20. Douglas, S. D., Davis, W. C. and Fudenberg, H. H. Granulocytopathies: Pleomorphism of neutrophil dysfunction. Am. J. Med. 46: 901-909, 1969.
21. Davis, W. C., Huber, H., Douglas, S. D., and Fudenberg, H. H.: A defect in circulating mononuclear phagocytes in chronic granulomatous disease of childhood. J. Immun. (Brief reports) 101:1093-1095, 1968.

22. Davis, W. C., Douglas, S. D., and Fudenberg, H. H., A selective neutrophil dysfunction syndrome: Impaired killing of staphylocci. An. Int. Med. 69: 1237-1243, 1968.
23. Hobbs, J.: Personal communication, 1970.
24. Fudenberg, H. H., and Douglas, S. D.: Unpublished observations.
25. Eriksson, S.: Pulmonary emphysema and α_1-antitrypsin deficiency. Acta Med. Scand. 175: 197-205, 1964.
26. Laurell, C. B., and Eriksson, S.: The serum α_1-antitrypsin in families with Hypo-α_1-antitrypsinemia. Clinica Chimica Acta 2: 395-398, 1965.
27. Laurell, C. B., Kullander, S., and J. Thorell: Effect of administration of a combined estrogen-progestin contraceptive on the level of individual plasma proteins. Scand. J. Clin. Lab. Invest. 21: 337-343, 1968.
28. a) Laurell, C. B., and Eriksson, S.: Antigen-antibody crossed electrophoresis. Anal. Biochem. 10: 358-361, 1965.

b) Fagerhol, M. K., and Laurell, C.: The Pi system-inherited variants of serum α_1-antitrypsin. In Progress in Medical Genetics, edited by A. G. Steinberg and A. G. Bearn. New York: Grune & Stratton, pp. 96-111, 1970.
29. Adamson, J., Baker, A. L., Fagerhol, M. K., Falk G. A., Freier, E. F., and Fudenberg, H. H.: International Smyposium on Proteolysis and Pulmonary Emphysema, Pasadena, California, January 1971.
30. Dacie, J. V.: The Haemolytic Anaemias, Congenital and Acquired, Part IV, 2nd ed. New York: Grune & Stratton, 1967.
31. Fudenberg, H. H., and Petz, L. D.: Unpublished observations.
32. Petz, L. D., and Fudenberg, H. H.: Coombs-positive hemolytic anemia caused by penicillin administration. New Engl. J. Med. 274; 171-178, 1966.
33. Faulk, W. P., Tomsovic, E. J., and Fudenberg, H. H.: Insulin-resistance in juvenile diabetes mellitus; immunologic studies. Am. J. Med. 49: 133-139, 1970.
34. Garratty, G., and Petz, L. D.: An evaluation of commercial antiglobulin sera with particular reference to

their anticomplement properties. Transfusion 2: 79, 1971.

35. Gotoff, S. P., Isaacs, E. W., Muehrcke, R. C., and Smith, Roger D.: Serum Beta$_{1c}$ Globulin in Glomerulonephritis and Systemic Lupus Erythematosus. Annals of Internal Med. 71: 327-333, 1969.

36. Petz, L. D., Sharp, G. C., Cooper, N. R., and Irvin, W. S.: Serum and cerebio spinal fluid complement and serum autoantibodies in systemic lupus erythematosis. Medicine (in press).

37. Levin, A. S., Fudenberg, H. H., Petz, L. D., and Sharp, G. C.: IgG levels in cerebrospinal fluid of patients with central nervous system lupus. (In preparation).

38. Messner, R. P., and Jelinek, J.: Receptors for human γ G Globulin on human neutrophils. J. Clin. Invest. 49: 2165-2171, 1970.

39. a) Barbu, E., Seligmann, M., and Joly, M.: Reactions between anti-DNA antibodies from serum of patients with disseminated lupus erythematosus and denatured or degraded DNA. Annales de l'Institut Pasteur 99: 695, 1960.

b. Stollar, D., and Levine, L.: Antibodies to denatured desoxyribonucleic acid in a lupus erythematous serum. J. of Immunology 87: 477-484, 1961.

40. Schur, P. H., and Monroe, N.: Antibodies to ribonucleic acid in systemic lupus erythematosus. Proc. Nat. Acad. Sci. 63: 1108-1112, 1969.

41. Holman, H. R.: Partial purification and characterization of an extractible nuclear antigen which reacts with SLE sera. Ann. N. Y. Acad. Sci. 124: 800-806, 1965.

42. Miller, M. E., and Nilsson, U. R.: A familial deficiency of the phagocytosis-enhancing activity of serum related to a dysfunction of the fifth component and complement. New Eng. J. Med. 282: 354, 1970.

43. Alper, C. A., Abramson, N., Johnston, R. B., Jandl, J. H., and Rosen, F. S.: Studies in vivo and in vitro on an abnormality in the metabolism of C3 in a patient with increased susceptibility to infection. J. Clin. Invest. 19: 1975, 1970.

44. Kunkel, H. G., Simon, H. J., and Fudenberg, H. H.: Observations concerning positive serologic reactions for rheumatoid factor in certain patients with sacroidosis and other hyperglobulinemic states. Arthritis Rheum. 1: 289-296, 1958.
45. Fudenberg, H. H.: Complete immunology: Science or septophrenia? Clin. Exp. Immun. 2: 1-18, 1967.

Table 1. **Human immunoglobulins and their structural units.** The newest immunoglobulin described, (IgE), present in only trace amounts in normal human serum, is not listed. Its heavy chain is termed Epsilon ( ). Thus, normal human serum contains immunoglobulin molecules of at least 10 kinds (i.e., 5 kinds of heavy chains X 2 kinds of light chains). In myeloma or macroglobulinemia, 1 of the 10 kinds is increased markedly in concentration, with the others being considerably reduced.

IMMUNOGLOBULIN CLASS		GLOBULIN STRUCTURAL SUBUNITS		
New Terms	Old Terms & Synonyms	Heavy Chains		Light Chains
IgG (γ G)	γ_2, 7sγ, γss	Gamma (γ)	K (I)	Kappa
			L (II)	Lambda
IgA (γ A)	γ_{1A} β_{2A}	Alpha (α)	K (I)	Kappa
IgM (γ M)	γ_{1M}, β_{2M}, 19Sγ		L (II)	Lambda
IgD (γ D)		Mu (μ)	K (I)	Kappa
			L (II)	Lambda
		Delta (δ)	K (I)	Kappa
			L (II)	Lambda
γ_u	γ_L Microglobulins, Micro-molecular urinary proteins		K (I)- Kappa L (II)-Lambda	

Preferred terminology of the immunoglobulins.

Table 2. Criteria for evaluation of cellular and humoral immunity.

Cellular Immunity
Circulating lymphocytes (absolute number !)
Anatomy of the lymphoid organs
Antigenic stimulation of lymphocytes :
  in vitro (homologous cells, pure antigens, PHA)
  in vivo (skin transplants, allergens)

Humoral Immunity
Circulating immunoglobulins
Circulating antibodies
Anatomy of lymphoid organs and bone marrow
Antigenic stimulation with various antigens
→ antibody titers
→ anatomical changes

Table 3. Direct antiglobulin tests on cells sensitized in vivo with complement components, using various antisera.*

Antiglobulin Sera	Cold Agglutinin Disease				S.L.E.		"Warm" A.I.H.A.	
	F.M.	S.F.	M.C.	B.L.	E.T.	G.Y.	C.R.	M.W.
Authors' reagents								
Anti-W.H.S.	3	3	4	1½	1½	1½	1½	1½
Anti-IgG	0	0	0	0	0	0	0	0
Neutralized anti-W.H.S.	3	3	4	2	1½	1½	1½	1½
Anti-C3	3	3	4	2	2	1	1½	1½
Anti-C4	1	1	1½	0	0	1½	½	0
Commercial reagents								
A	2½	2	3	1	0	0	½	0
B	0	0	0	0	0	0	½	0
C	0	0	0	0	0	0	½	0
D	0	0	0	0	0	0	0	0
E	0	0	½	0	0	0	0	0
F	0	0	1½	0	0	0	0	0
G	0	1	1½	0	0	0	0	0
H	1½	0	½	½	0	0	½	0
I	0	0	½	0	0	0	0	0
J	½	0	½	0	0	0	0	0

*Anti-WHS means rabbit anti whole normal human serum. "Neutralized" antiglobulin serum is anti-WHS absorbed with IgG.

*Reproduced from Garratty, G., and Petz, L.D., Transfusion 2: 79, 1971.

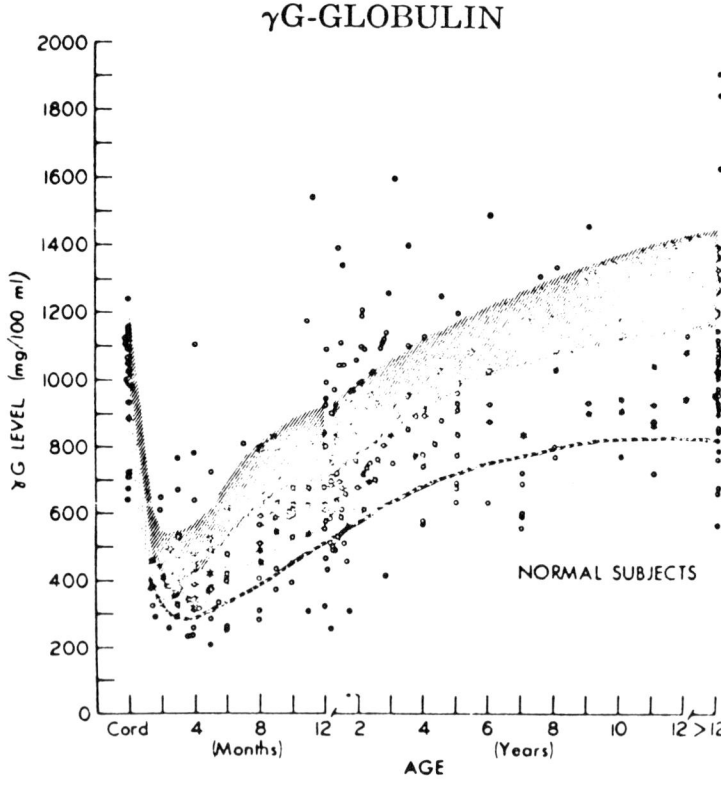

Fig. 1(a)

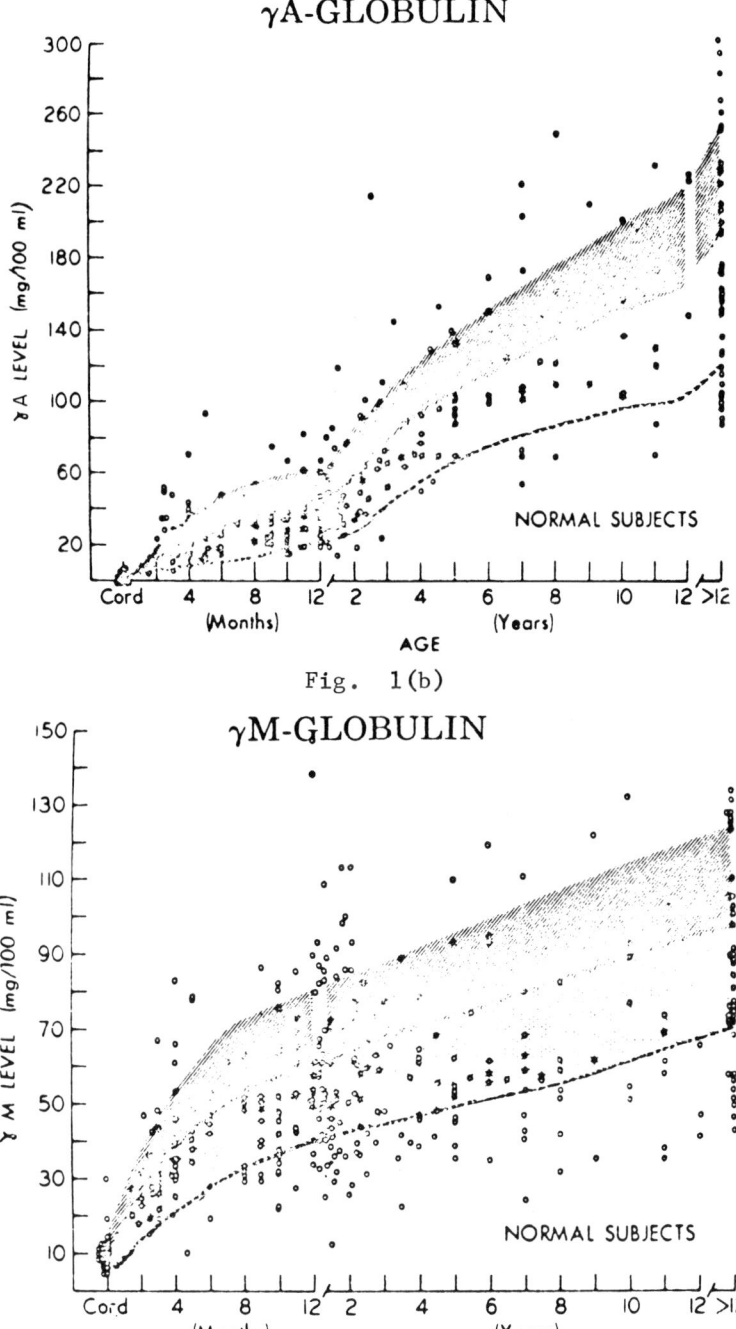

Fig. 1(b)

Fig. 1(c)

SERUM IMMUNOGLOBULINS AT DIFFERENT AGES

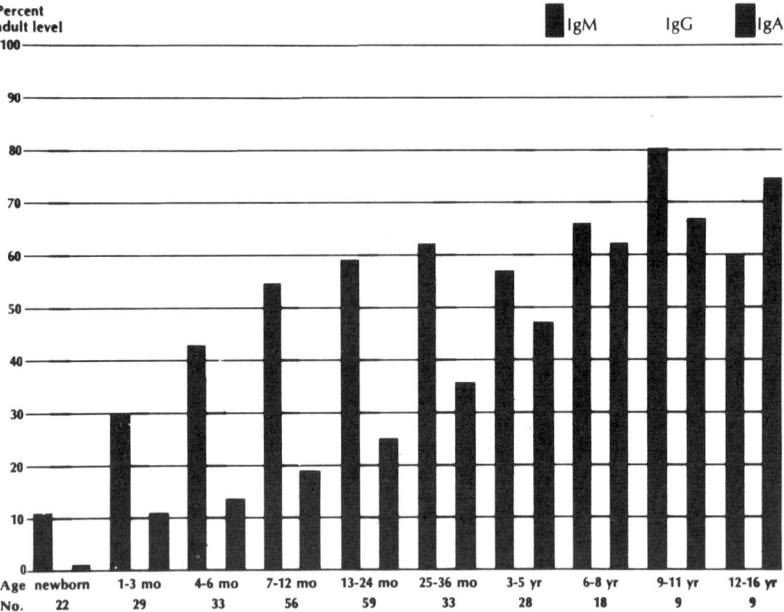

In 296 normal children of different ages, mean levels of serum immunoglobulins are compared with those in 30 normal adults. The transmission of IgG across the placenta is reflected in the high IgG levels in the newborn. IgM is synthesized rapidly in the neonatal period, while IgA increases slowly during infancy and childhood. Adult levels for IgG and IgM are reached earlier than for IgA, which continues to rise during early adulthood.

Figs. 1(a) -(d). Immunoglobulin (Ig) levels at different ages. (a) IgG (b) IgA (c) IgM (d) Composite. (Reproduced from Stiehm, E. R., and Fudenberg, H. H., Pediatrics 37, 715-727 (1966) with the permission of the journal.)

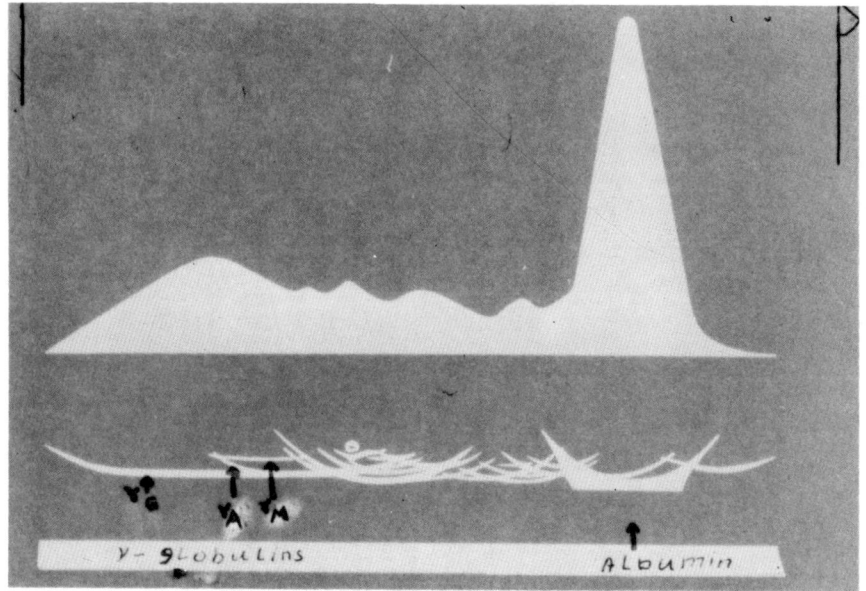

Fig. 2. Electrophoretic patterns of normal human serum. Moving boundary electrophoresis (top) and immunoelectrophoresis (IEP) (bottom). Note the 3 precipitin bands in the region electrophoretically designated as -globulin characteristic of IgG, IgA, and IgM.

IEP with Rabbit anti-Normal Human Serum

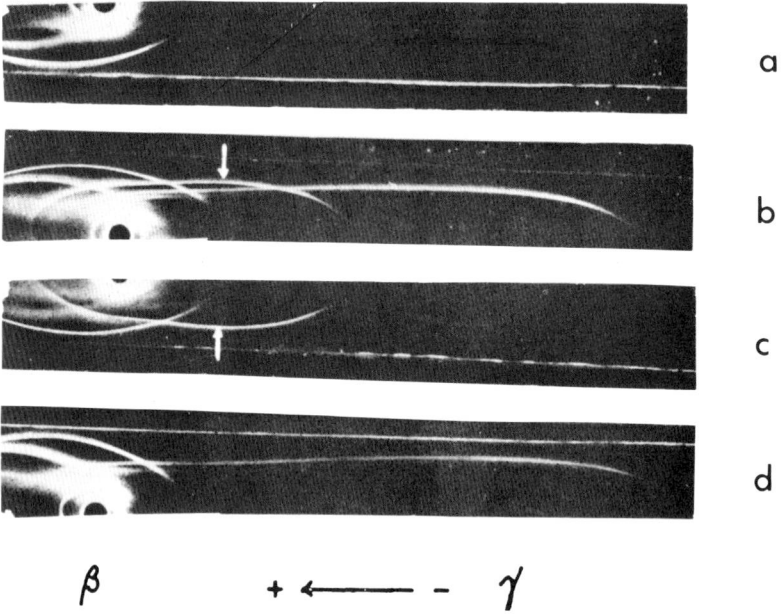

Fig. 3. Immunoelectrophoretic (IEP) patterns in immunoglobulin deficiency syndromes. (a) Classical aggammaglobulinemia: diminution of all 3 major immunoglobulins (b) Selective deficiency of IgM; arrow points to normal IgA band (c). Marked diminution in IgG and IgM; arrow points to IgA band, which was increased markedly for this infant's age (d) Marked diminution in IgA and IgM with normal IgG.

DOCUMENTATION OF LABORATORY DATA

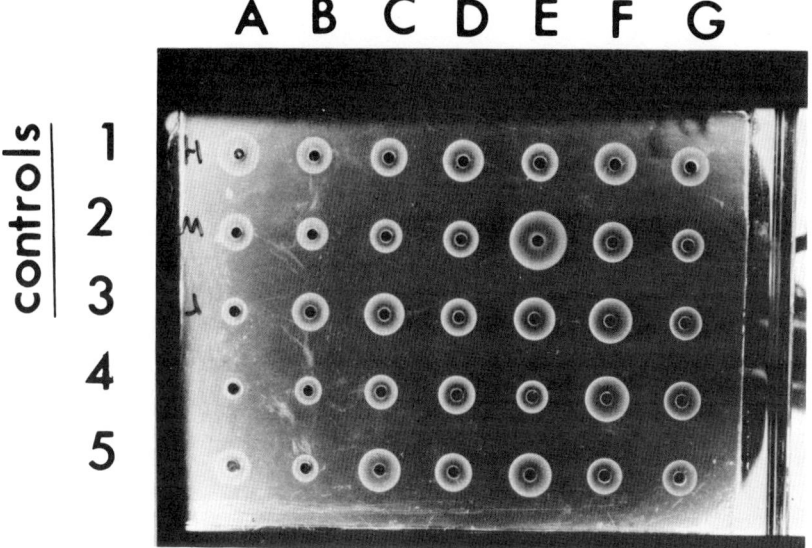

Fig. 4. Radial immunodiffusion measurements of IgA in serum. 1-A, 1-B, and 1-C represent standard sera of high, medium, and low concentration. 2E represents a serum with marked increase in IgA and 4-A a serum with very low IgA. The area of migration produced by each serum is directly proportional to the IgA concentration in the serum.

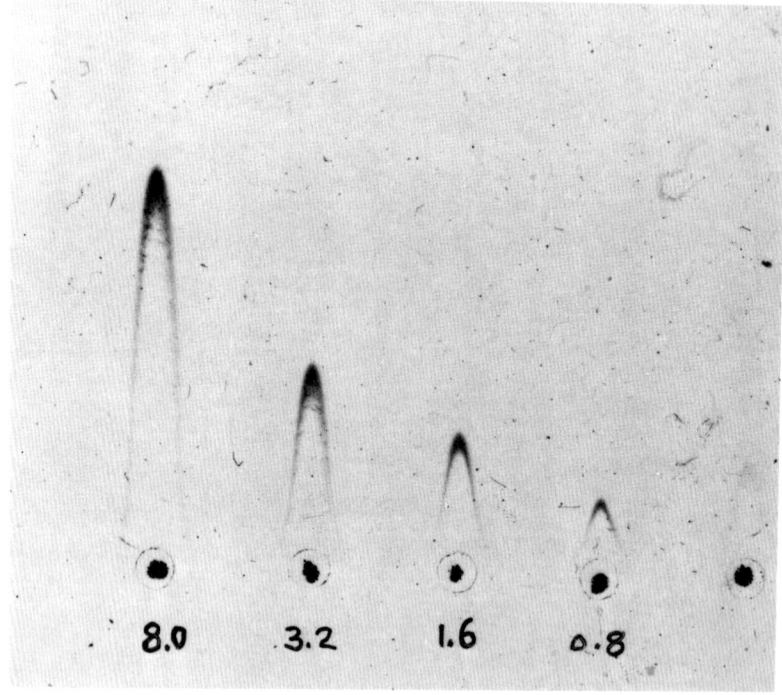

Fig. 5. "Rocket electrophoresis" measurements of IgA. Distance of migration of the antigen from the insertion site is directly proportional to the IgA concentration, noted below each serum in mg/ml.

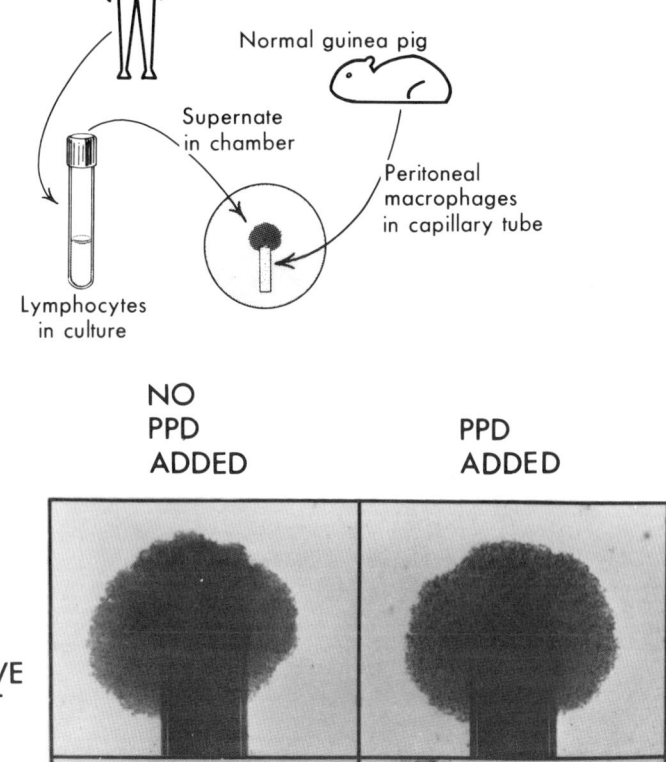

Fig. 6(a) & (b). Macrophage inhibition factor (MIF) test. (a) Method and (b) results in 2 patients, one PPD negative, the other not.

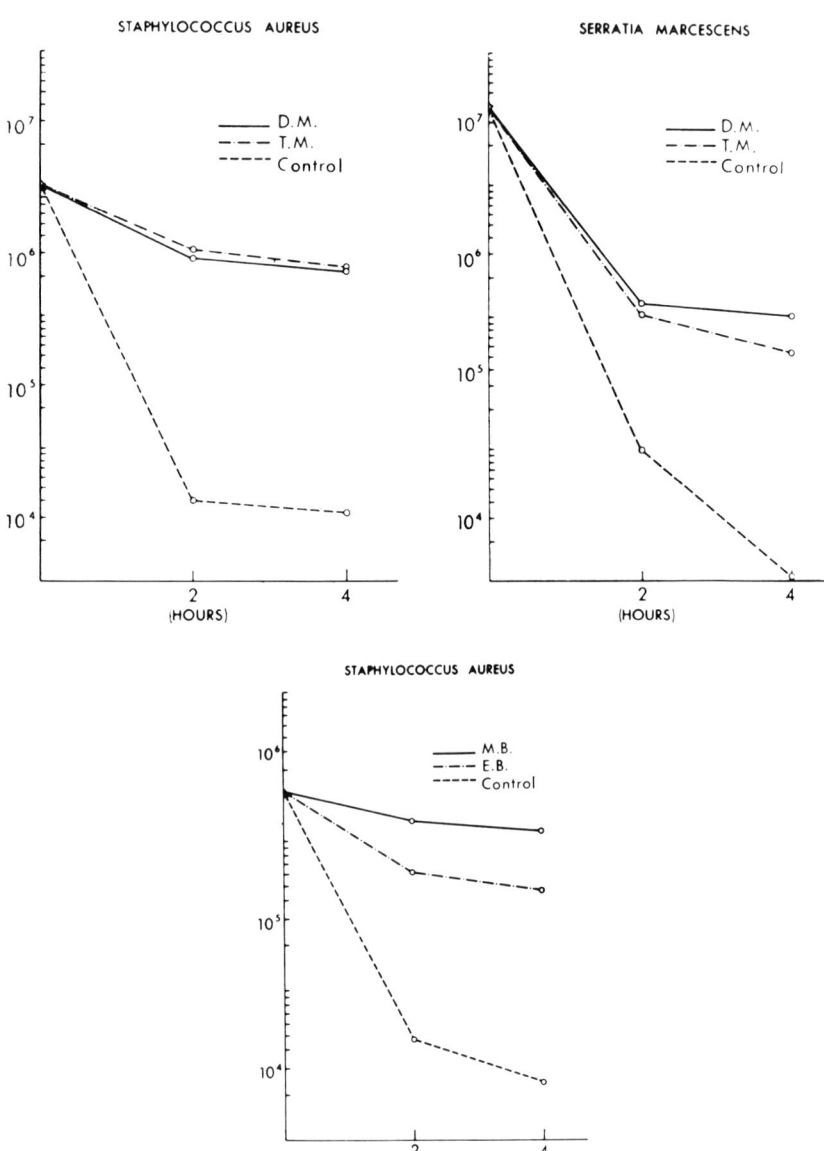

Fig. 7(a) & (b). In vivo killing of opsonized bacteria by leucocytes in (a) 2 patients with the phagocyte dysfunction syndrome, (D.M and T.M.) and normal control; (b) similar curves in another patient and his mother (M. B. and E. B.) and normal control. (note that mother has a partial defect.) Numbers indicate viable bacteria.

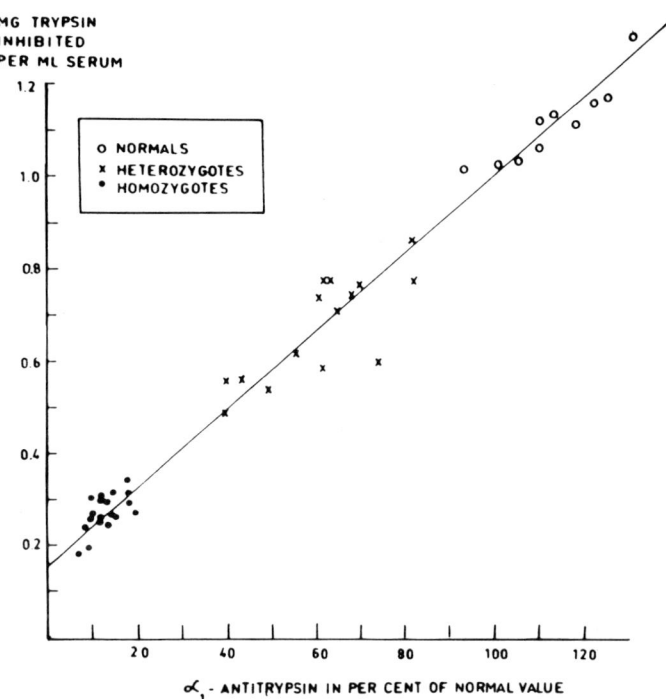

Fig. 8. Correlation of immunologic assay of α_1-antitrypsin with trypsin inhibitory papacity, measured by biochemical test. (Reproduced from Laurell, C.B., and Eriksson, S., Clinica Chimica Acta 2, 395-398 (1965) with permission of the authors and Elsevier Publishing Company, Inc.)

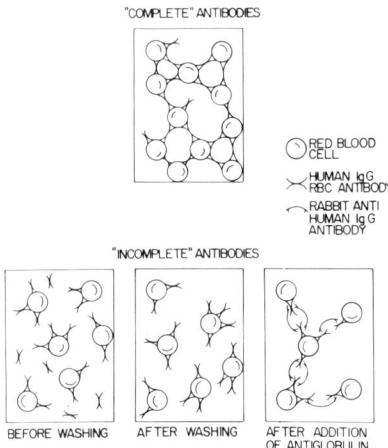

Fig. 9. Red cell antibodies. "Complete" antibodies (top) and "incomplete" antibodies (bottom): (left) coated red cells in suspension, before washing (middle) Coated red cells, after washing 3X with 20-fold volumes of saline (right) agglutination of washed coated red cells, after addition of antiglobulin (Coombs') serum.

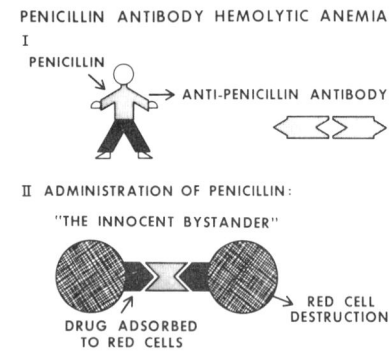

Fig. 10. Mechanism of penicillin antibody hemolytic anemia.

EXPLICIT DOCUMENTATION OF LABORATORY DATA

A. INTRODUCTION - Dr. Gerald R. Cooper

Communication of laboratory data is worthwile only if the produced data is documented. Production of valid data demands that certain precautions and requirements must be met with respect to basic analytical performance. In addition, explicit documentation insists that data be valid for the purposes it will be used. The session today will be concerned with the inherent difficulties and basic essentials for explicit documentation of the analytical operation of the clinical laboratory. First, presentations will be given by the four panelists; after this, a question and answer period will be held; and last, a summary and a list of recommendations will close the session.

B. PRINCIPLES OF USEFULLY REPORTING LABORATORY DATA - Dr. Edward L. Burns

C. PANEL PRESENTATIONS
  1. THE PROBLEM AND PROGRESS OF EXPLICIT DOCUMENTATION OF LABORATORY DATA FOR COMMUNICATION
       Dr. Gerald R. Cooper

  2. DOCUMENTATION AS A CONCERN OF PROFESSIONAL SOCIETIES AND INDIVIDUAL LABORATORY DIRECTORS
       Dr. Roy N. Barnett

3. DOCUMENTATION CONCERNS OF STATE AND COMMUNITY FOR COMMUNICATION OF LABORATORY RESULTS

Dr. William Kaufmann

4. DOCUMENTATION INTERESTS OF NATIONAL BUREAU OF STANDARDS AND COLLABORATING GROUPS FOR COMMUNICATION OF LABORATORY RESULTS

Dr. Robert Schaffer

PRINCIPLES OF USEFULLY REPORTING LABORATORY DATA*

Edward L. Burns, M. D.

Accurate and useful communication of data from the laboratory to the clinician is difficult and no ideal method has as yet been found. In speaking on this subject one must avoid being specific since laboratories operate in too many individual manners to permit designation of one best way. We believe, however, that communication can be improved if we delineate certain principles of laboratory reporting, from which individual laboratories may design the methods most suitable to their own particular operation.

In general, a laboratory report should be compact, of consistent format and terminology, clearly understandable and when combined with a larger medical record, logically located and accessible. It should carry the date and time of collection and, where pertinent, a gross description of the specimen. Whatever method of reporting is used the results should be displayed so that the normal and abnormal values are sharply differentiated, and when multiple results on a single substance are shown they should be placed in a logical sequential order. Since the report is generated by a request or order from a physician, the physician, his patient and the patient location should be clearly identified and assurance should be given that the requests are accu-

*Prepared from data collected by The Standards Committee, College of American Pathologists Subcommittee on Medical Usefulness Criteria, Roy N. Barnett, M. D. Chairman

rately transmitted to the laboratory. If possible, the original request should be sent directly to the laboratory; if copying is necessary some verification should be performed to insure that the transcription was done accurately. Finally, for the sake of economy, the communication should be easily prepared and have administrative and record keeping value. These desirable general qualities may be listed as follows:

1. Compactness
2. Consistency of terminology and format
3. Clear understandability
4. Logical location in medical chart
5. Statement of date and time of collection
6. Gross description and source of specimen when pertinent
7. Sharp differentiation of normal and abnormal values
8. Sequential order of multiple results on a single specimen
9. Identification of patient, patient location and physician
10. Assurance of accuracy of transcription of request
11. Ease of preparation
12. Administrative and record keeping value

THE PROBLEM AND PROGRESS OF EXPLICIT DOCUMENTATION OF LABORATORY DATA FOR COMMUNICATIONS

Gerald R. Cooper, M.D., Ph.D.

The problems of communication among clinical laboratories have increased appreciably with the tremendous growth of results produced in the laboratories. Rapid computer systems and high volume analytical equipment produce and handle large quantities of data. Many laboratory programs, previously impossible, are now possible. A great concern is that the clinical laboratory, pressed to install large volume analytical and computer systems, may produce massive but incorrect and insignificant data. We should remember that, regardless of the quantity, worthless data lead to worthless conclusions and are worse than no data. Data production and collection techniques must be suited to the functions of the clinical laboratory, and the data collected will be useful only if it is documented and has a determinable relationship to reference data. This paper will be primarily concerned with the general problems of documentation in the clinical laboratory and recent progress made toward documentation. The assumption is made that documentation should be defined as any information about observed data that makes the data useful to a user.

PROBLEM OF EXPLICIT DOCUMENTATION IN THE CLINICAL LABORATORY

General Nature. The development of the clinical laboratory in the United States has been influenced by the independent courses of some laboratories, regional communication among laboratories, and varying economic support. The independence of laboratory directors and the influence of regional communication have led to the introduction of different methods, different automation, different standards, and different nomenclature. Economic support in different places has varied so much that many different types of laboratories, with all levels of competency, have developed. In some places, the value of laboratory data has been undermined by improper planning; poor facilities; unsatisfactory equipment; non-specific methods; insufficiently trained, impatient, or lowly motivated personnel; and lack of effective quality control. Systematic bias exists in the laboratory determinations of all disciplines. New uses of the clinical laboratory have highlighted disadvantages that arise from lack of data documentation. Admission laboratory profiles in the hospitals, automated multiphasic health testing and services, collaborative clinical investigations, and cooperative epidemiologic studies have been limited in usefulness by apparent lack of documentation in some clinical laboratories.

Documentation is needed among laboratories. Each of several laboratories may attain high precision, but the results from these same laboratories cannot be validly compared. This problem arises mainly because relatively nonspecific rapid procedures that are susceptible to various types of interferences and to changes in conditions are necessarily used with many types of automation and diagnostic kits. The problem of systematic bias is illustrated vividly by the experience of ten hospital laboratories that decided to determine the comparability of results of the determination of cholestrol. Two samples of different concentration were distributed to all of the hospitals. The performance within each hospital revealed an acceptable standard deviation, but comparison of mean values among the hospitals revealed unacceptable differences, some as large as 100 mg/dl. Happily, many of these problems can be solved by rigidly following directions, checking on stability of reagents and equipment, and using effective internal and external quality control.

Many clinicians are limited in the opportunity to learn and keep informed on the reliability and interpretation of clinical laboratory data. Changes in procedures, automation, or personnel can cause continuing alteration in normal values for a determination. Choice of limits of permissible error can influence the number of false positive tests in a battery of tests performed upon the same individual. In interpreting laboratory tests, one must recognize that one test out of 12 in a battery will be abnormal in about 50 percent of the reported batteries if 95 percent confidence limits are used for each determination. Thus, if follow-ups are done on only 5 percent instead of 50 percent of the patients, tighter limits must be used for each test in the battery. Interpretation is also complicated by certain tests, such as determinations of enzymes, which give highly variable results and abnormal values more often than the other tests used in the battery. Guidelines on documentation of data will prove of immediate benefit to clinicians.

Hospital records, journals, textbooks, and monographs contain an immense amount of useful laboratory data, if it is documented. The data may have been collected without considering many essential factors, such as sampling, repetitive determinations, or variability of disease. Retrospective studies in hospitals are currently in high disfavor because of apparent lack of documentation. The usefulness of clinical laboratory data retrieval systems in hospitals depends greatly on the validity of the laboratory data placed in the hospital records. Editors tend to check documentation of data presented in journals, monographs, and textbooks with respect to proof of statements, but they usually do not check the comparability of data with that of other articles. Documentation of laboratory data could eventually permit investigators to gain confidence in retrospective as well as prospective studies.

Standardization Problems. Obstacles to standardization which are intimately related to documentation exist in all disciplines in the clinical laboratory. In fact, each determination in a discipline may or may not have suitable methods, satisfactory standards or reference materials, or widespread accepted units. Explicit documentation cannot be gained in clinical laboratories until the tools necessary for calibration, quality control, and standardization are readily available to all clinical laboratories.

In clinical chemistry, major obstacles to explicit documentation exist even for the tests that have been widely used for years. For the determinations of glucose, urea, and uric acid, there is indecision about the best reference method, lack of confidence in serum and blood reference materials, recognition that collection, handling, and preservation techniques may cause deterioration in the sample or add interferences to the sample, and recognition that results from various methods differ. Contamination of the specimen particularly influences the determination of glucose, but it has some effect on essentially all determinations in clinical chemistry. With the determination of urea, questions have been raised about the specificity of certain methods, interferences of amino groups and atmospheric constituents, increased breakdown of urea by variable analytical factors, such as pH and heat, and uncontrolled errors in automation from deterioration by reactive recipient streams, settling of sediment into the flow cell, consistency of enzymatic reactions, and lack of similar reaction on standard solutions, reference materials, and unknown samples. Concern has been expressed repeatedly about the purity and stability of preparations of uric acid, the specificity of colorimetric methods, and the suitability of the available serum pools of uric acid for use as reference materials.

Many practical standardization problems still exist with the determinations of calcium, electrolytes, bilirubin, and serum proteins. To explicitly standardize the determination of calcium, the precision and accuracy required for clinical usefulness must be attained, an acceptable reference method must be available, differences in levels with different methods must be eliminated, and contamination and changes in the pH of samples must be controlled. The so-called simple battery of tests for electrolytes of Na, K, Cl, and CO_2 still have the problems of misuse of standards; improper collection, handling, and storage of samples; and error by careless analysts. Methodology has improved for the determination of bilirubin, but progress in the development of suitable standards and reference materials is slow. The determination of total protein and distribution of proteins suffers mainly from lack of a widely accepted standard. In determining total protein, different clinical laboratories use different nitrogen to protein conversion factors, various methods based on essentially different physical and chemical properties, and, often, unstable reagents. A decision is needed about whether to base the calculation of results upon calibration with a pure compound such as ammonium sulfate, or a highly purified animal albumin or human albumin, or a human serum of defined "normal" characteristics. Serum protein electrophoretic analysis still lacks a widely accepted reference material, reference analytical technique, and guidelines for calculating results.

During recent years, the clinical laboratory has extended its services to the determination of diagnostic enzymes and lipids. Tests for diagnostic enzymes do not have pure standards because enzyme preparations are not absolutely pure. Points of reference, therefore, are based on functional activity, which is variable and highly sensitive to conditions. Multiple types of procedures, confused nomenclature, and different units of measurement cause variation in values and interfere with comparison of results.

The determinations of cholesterol, triglyceride, and lipoproteins are increasingly requested of the clinical laboratory, and each of these lipid determinations has unique problems in documentation(3). The widespread use of multiple methods relatively nonspecific for cholesterol but each sensitive to different interferences, lack of proper referencing to available cholesterol standards, and use of a single reference serum instead of multiple reference serums covering the "normal" and abnormal ranges limit the documentation of the determination of cholesterol. A major effort must be made to increase the specificity of methods used in the clinical laboratories and to gain widespread use of external quality control before explicit documentation can be accomplished for the determination of cholesterol. The triglyceride determination suffers from lack of one accepted standard and use of multiple units. The results of the determination of triglyceride in the clinical laboratories are currently quite variable because the procedure involves steps which are difficult to reproduce. Prospects appear good for improving the precision and comparability of results of the basic colorimetric, fluorometric, and enzymatic methods. Documenting the lipoprotein determination in the clinical laboratory will mainly require selection of appropriate methods, choice of techniques, and development of accepted guidelines for interpreting results.

In hematology, documentation problems exist for each clinical laboratory test. For all hematological tests, errors can result from improper preparation of the patient, careless technique in collecting and handling specimens, and delayed testing of improperly preserved samples. Continuing surveillance is needed for reagents, equipment, and techniques to produce valid data.

DOCUMENTATION OF LABORATORY DATA

The determination of hemoglobin presents a remarkable example of the tremendous advance that can be made in quality performance by documentation. Since 1960, the determination of hemoglobin changed from among the worst analyses to among the best analyses in the clinical laboratory because effective internal and external standardization procedures were instituted. This determination now almost has explicit documentation, yet an entire symposium was held recently on the problems of standardization that must be controlled if explicit documentation is to be achieved (4). Determinations of red and white cells and platelet counts need reference points, preparations applicable to calibration by instruments, and specimens controlled as to source, diurnal variations, emotional stress, anticoagulants, and any condition that changes the relation of cells to plasma. Clarification of nomenclature, recognition of cells of defined characteristics, and guidelines for preparing, staining, and examining smears are needed for documentation of the blood cell differential test. The determination of prothrombin time needs documentation of thromboplastin, the analytic technique employed, the temperature of the reaction, and the measurement of endpoint. The use of reference plasmas and reference thromboplastins are essential for documentation. To be fully useful, reference plasmas for the determination of prothrombin must be characterized for content of other coagulation and lytic factors.

The hematology discipline in the clinical laboratory is being extended to unique chemical and enzymatic tests on constitutents of cells, procedures for individual coagulation and lytic factors, host resistance, and toxic factors. Documentation must plan for control and standardization of such tests.

In immunohematology, explicit documentation of the laboratory techniques necessary to guide and safely operate a blood bank and to obtain information about blood type prevalence requires highly specific methods, the development of reliable equipment, use of sensitive reagents, and strict standardization of tests. Reference methods, stable reference materials, and available reference laboratories appear to be essential.

In microbiology, documentation is difficult because of the wide field of specialized interests, such as bacteriology, parasitology, mycology, and virology. Quality control applicable to each discipline must be developed for documentation of the respective procedures. Documentation demands control of specimen collection, handling, shipping and storage, maintenance of the quality of reagents and media, sensitivity and specificity of the technical procedures, and reliability of chemical and immunological reactions used in detection and identification. Reference specimens, reference methods, and guidelines for interpreting results are essential for documentation of microbiological procedures.

In urinalysis, documentation of bacteriuria, cellular constituents, casts, screening tests, and collection techniques requires methodology guidelines, reference materials, and rules for interpretation. Such so-called simple qualitative and quantitative tests have been woefully neglected so far as quality control and standardization are concerned. This situation must be corrected before explicit documentation can be achieved.

A review of the essentials of documentation for the different disciplines in the clinical laboratory clearly shows that the requirements generally demand availability and proper use of specific methods, reliable equipment, standards, reference materials, guidelines for interpreting data, and the presence of motivated and well-trained personnel. Documentation cannot be accomplished within or among clinical laboratories unless internal and external quality control systems are effective within each laboratory and performance meets allowable limits of error compatible with documentation.

Progress Made Toward Documentation in the Clinical Laboratories

There are groups who are interested in documentation.

Professional Groups. Committees of national professional societies in the various disciplines have provided leadership and encouragement in the development and maintenance of quality performance in the clinical laboratory. These committees have introduced measures aimed at gaining comparability of results, which is so essential to documentation. Committees on standards, reference methods, automation, nomenclature, and special topics such as enzymes, true values, and normal values have outlined problems, studied approaches for correction, and, whenever possible, instituted measures for documentation. Proficiency testing programs, on-site visits to laboratories, consultation and assistance by reference laboratories, and guidelines on what is expected of members of certain professional organizations are available in selected disciplines and in certain regions. In addition, professional organizations have offered educational programs, manuals, and opportunities for all types of training. These efforts have tended to improve documentation in the clinical laboratory during recent years.

National Committee for Clinical Laboratory Standards (NCCLS). The NCCLS has been formed in the United States from representatives of various professional societies, industrial organizations, and governmental agencies to develop and help establish standards and provide a forum for promoting improvements in the clinical laboratory. Attempts are being made to develop standard specifications for biological and chemical reagents or reference materials, reference methods or reference procedures, systems of nomenclature, classifications of operating methods, and controls for equipment. Committees on microbiology, clinical chemistry, instrumentation, hematology, immunohematology, and blood banking are now at work. In 1970, five written specifications in microbiology and one in instrumentation were announced as tentative standards. These standards are now being distributed, tested, and evaluated. Comments are being collected from the laboratory community. After a one year period, the NCCLS will vote whether to make these standards NCCLS standards. All accepted NCCLS standards are subject to three year review.

International Committees. The Commission on World Standards of the World Association of Anatomic and Clinical Pathology Societies has encouraged and assisted in developing specifications for standards, reference materials, and reference methods. International surveys, investigation of normal values and medical usefulness, and encouragement of national quality control and standardization programs have been a part of the Commission's program. Symposia have been arranged on critical standardization topics. Special international projects have been initiated on antibiotic sensitivity testing, immunofluorescence reagents and methods, the one-stage prothrombin test, and international surveys in clinical chemistry in selected countries.

The Committee on Standards of the International Federation of Clinical Chemistry has sponsored publications on standardization of quantities and units in clinical chemistry and has reviewed the development of standards and reference materials. The Committee is now attempting to clarify and delineate the nomenclature and principles of quality control.

The International Committee for Standardization in Hematology (ICSH) is working hard to achieve reliable and reproducible results in diagnostic hematologic laboratory analysis. It deliberates on standardizing possibilities, stimulates and coordinates research on standardization, and attempts international comparability trials. This Committee has already sponsored outstanding symposia on the standardization of hematologic procedures in the clinical laboratory.

The Commission on Quantities and Units of the Section of Clinical Chemistry of the International Union of Pure and Applied Chemistry (IUPAC) has prepared a pamphlet entitled "List of Quantities, Draft Recommendations, 1971." Nomenclature on quantities and units is discussed thoroughly.

National Conferences. A Conference on Automated Multiphasic Health Testing and Services (AMHTS), sponsored by the National Center for Health Services Research and Development, was held in 1970 to examine, evaluate, and prepare guidelines for comprehensive health screening services and other preventive services designed to contribute to the early detection and prevention of disease in old age (5). Provisional guidelines were proposed for selecting tests and procedures and for establishing technical personnel requirements, instrumentation requirements, quality control, data processing, and follow-up procedures for designing and operating an AMHTS system.

In 1970, the National Research Council (NRC) sponsored a conference on "Documentation of Procedures and Results in Laboratory Medicine" (6). It recommended that (a) the NRC set up pilot projects to solve specific documentation problems on a regional level before attempting to set up a national project; (b) the NRC subcommittee continue as an on-going agency and coordinating group for documentation; and (c) that regional quality control pool reference samples be used for translating laboratory values from one laboratory to another because they are more reliable than "normal" values. This conference proposed that documentation be defined as any information about observed data that makes the data useful to a user. It pointed out that documentation information may vary according to how the data is used. Generally, however, it includes such information as condition of specimen collection, quality control of analytical procedure, usual population values, method of analysis, instrument used, and standards. The need for documentation was identified with the mobility of the present U. S. population, the increase in number of medical data banks, the difference in methodology and equipment used by small-volume and large-volume production laboratories, and the potential saving of millions of dollars by making repeated tests unnecessary. Investigations were recommended on (a) the exchange of documentation data by 100 to 200 large laboratories; (b) the common use of a single manual and a single automated procedure in a group of small and large laboratories; (c) collaborative planning with medical data banks; (d) identification of repeated tests that could be avoided if documentation was available; (e) evaluation of regional quality control programs; (f) publication of experiences on what and how tests and changes in methodology should be documented and how to educate physicians in the use of documented data; and (g) the usefulness of documenting medical data within the Government Armed Forces.

National and International Agencies. The National Bureau of Standards (NBS), the National Institutes of Health (NIH), the Center for Disease Control (CDC), and many other governmental groups are contributing to documentation. NBS, NIH, and CDC are collaborating in developing and furthering the proper use of quality control and standardization in documenting clinical and epidemiological investigations.

At the CDC, a primary interest is to develop the tools needed for documentation in all disciplines of the clinical laboratory. Investigators in each discipline are attempting to (a) develop or improve the available primary standards and reference materials; (b) find out how to collect, store, and ship biological samples; (c) develop reference methods for labeling reference materials as points of reference; (d) investigate and compare commonly used methodology; and (e) evaluate automation, develop appropriate use of automation, and establish standards and reference materials for automation. Experimental proficiency testing concerned with the best ways to carry out proficiency testing and the problems, limitations, and economical disadvantages of such testing provides useful information for CDC's proficiency testing for interstate licensed laboratories and for other national proficiency testing programs.

Research projects for instance, in clinical chemistry have been directed at seeking practical criteria for purity of standards and "true" values of reference materials for such procedures as the determinations of cholesterol, triglyceride, glucose, urea, uric acid, and creatinine. Investigators are seeking the best reference compound or material for interpreting analysis of cholesterol, triglyceride, and lipoproteins; ways to produce stable reference materials of different concentrations of lipids and other constituents in combination with the lipids; and reference points and suitable diagnostic procedures for selected hormone and genetic abnormalities. Reference analyses for about 14 different clinical chemistry determinations are performed to further documentation of results of investigative groups seeking standardization among themselves, proficiency testing operations, and laboratories serving collaborative clinical and epidemiological investigations. Two laboratories were recently established: (a) reference and standardization laboratory in nutritional biochemistry to provide collaborative analytical services to the National Health Nutritional Surveys and to render documentation assistance to nutritional epidemiological and clinical investigatons across the country, and (b) a reference and standardization laboratory in clinical laboratory toxicology to develop a self-evaluation assistance program for clinical laboratories. Experience in the practical problems of automation, such as sample identification, control of operation of instruments and analysts, use of a computer, and special checks needed for maintaining the accuracy of massive amounts of data is gained by operating a high-volume automated central laboratory serving 55 clinics across the country. This central laboratory processes the results of 12 clinical chemistry procedures used to study the effect of drugs on coronary heart disease. In addition, manuals, movies, mimeographed material, and microphotographs are prepared for training and consultation. Cooperative standardization programs for the determinations of cholesterol, triglyceride, glucose, and urea have been in progress in collaboration with approximately 300 to 400 laboratories on a national and international basis.

The CDC continues to strengthen its resources for developing and offering documentation services in microbiology by establishing specialty research groups, reference diagnostic laboratories, and training and consultation services. Groups in these areas are working closely with different professional organizations and with industry, especially in attempting to improve applications of automation, specific diagnostic procedures, reliability of reagents and reference materials, and clinical laboratory procedures. In addition, during the past five years, more attention has been given to the problems of documentation in hematology, histopathology, and clinical immunology. In hematology, activities are concentrated on developing reference materials and reference methods for usual clinical laboratory hematologic procedures and for coagulation and lytic tests. In histopathology, documentation activities are directly concerned with developing a repository of highly positive tissue specimens for use as a reference material and with evaluating cytologic and cytogenetic diagnostic procedures.

National agencies in other countries such as Canada and many Pacific area and European countries are contributing greatly to documentation in the clinical laboratory. Most of these efforts are now coordinated to some extent by international societies in the various disciplines.

The World Health Organization (WHO) in Geneva has always been concerned with documentation in the world's clinical laboratories. In the past, WHO has exerted most of its efforts in the field of communicable diseases, but during the past five years it has gradually increased its activities in non-communicable disease areas of the clinical laboratory. The WHO Cardiovascular Disease Section, the Health Laboratory Services Section, and the Epidemiology of Non-Communicable Diseases Section, as well as the immunology, nutrition, and pesticide groups have held conferences and worked with various laboratories over the world in attempting to further documentation of laboratory services. The WHO has intensely attempted to document the results of laboratories serving WHO epidemiological studies, but in many cases it has been limited in success because of circumstances and wide differences in conditions. The Cardiovascular Disease Section has established an International Reference Center for Lipid Determination in Cardiovascular Research at the CDC to offer documentation services to international laboratories. The Health Laboratory Services Section is establishing a documentation service in glucose and urea determinations for international laboratories. This section hopes to be able to coordinate documentation activities for the clinical laboratories on an international basis.

In conclusion, worldwide concern about documentation in the clinical laboratory is growing. Conferences and planning are timely. A concerted action toward documentation by interested laboratorians, professional societies, industry, and national and international agencies can be successful on both a national and international scale.

References

1. Cooper, Gerald R.: "Quality Performance in Clinical Pathology." Progress in Clinical Pathology, Vol. III; M. Stefanini, Ed., Grune & Stratton, Inc., N. Y. (1969). Pages 1-71.
2. Cooper, Gerald R.: "Standardization and Control of Quantitative Analyses." Z. Anal. Chem. 243, 816-824 (1968).
3. Cooper, Gerald R.: "The Importance of Valid Chemical Laboratory Services for Studies of Cardiovascular Diseases." Ann. N. Y. Acad. Sci. 126, 841-850 (1965) August.
4. Standardization in Hematology. G. Astaldi, C. Sirtori, and G. Vanzetti, Editors. Franco Angeli Editore, Viale Monza 106, Milano, Italy (1970).
5. Report of Conference on "Provisional Guidelines for Automated Multiphasic Health Testing and Services." National Center for Health Services Research and Development, Washington, D. C., January 21-23, 1970. Volume I. U. S. Government Printing Office 0-407-381 (1970).
6. Informal Summary Report of Conference on "Documentation of Procedures and Results in Laboratory Medicine. Bradley E. Copeland, M. D., Chairman. Division of Medical Sciences, National Research Council, Washington, D. C. May 7-8, 1970. Am. J. Clin. Pathol. 55, #3, 380-383 (1971) March.

DOCUMENTATION AS A CONCERN OF PROFESSIONAL SOCIETIES AND INDIVIDUAL LABORATORY DIRECTORS

Roy N. Barnett, M.D.

At an earlier conference held in May 1970 in Washington, D. C. the following definition was accepted (3). "Documentation was defined as any information with respect to observed data that makes the data more useful to the user". This definition is excessively broad for our present purposes. Perhaps we might do better to divide this into three questions from the clinician to the laboratory.
1. How does this result fit in your laboratory data?
2. How does this result fit in my patient's case?
3. How does this result compare with those from other laboratories?

The first question refers to the general problems of precision and quality control. Although it would be scientifically valid to report a blood sugar as 70mg/dl with a 95% chance that it is truly between 60 and 80mg, it is unrealistic to believe that we could routinely generate laboratory reports of this type without overwhelming both the laboratory and the clinician. Nevertheless this information should be known in the laboratory and available to the clinician on request.

The second question concerns normal limits under the defined conditions of collection and processing, and for the specific age, sex and other variables represented by the patient. Such data must be generated locally for individual installations, and actually is generally lacking. It should also include limits for specific diseases, and this is rarely available.

The third question can be answered with proficiency survey data properly used - but it rarely is made known to the clinician. Even when the facts are made known concerning performance on specific samples, the question of sample collection and handling is left open. For example, Laboratory A may be 5mg/dl lower than the mean glucose value, but because Laboratory A ordinarily examines plasma rather than whole blood the values available to the local clinicians may be 5mg higher than the mean values for whole blood generally reported in the community.

Having indicated some problems in documentation I would like to proceed to some contributions to solving these problems, specifically the role of the College of American Pathologists and of the American Society of Clinical Pathologists. The CAP Proficiency Surveys in which specimens are sent periodically to participating laboratories are now by far the largest in the world with over 5000 participants. This provides a huge data base permitting analysis of data by time periods, types of tests, methods, single laboratories, various groupings of laboratories and in some instances by instruments and reagent manufacturer. Additional tests are being constantly added to widen the data base. Although extensive use has been made of this information by the CAP Standards Committee much more can be done. One practical result is the identification of clearly outlying values so that laboratories and regulatory agencies can take prompt action to remedy gross errors. However, there still remains a wide range of values considered acceptable, and this identifies one limitation on clinical interpretation of results (2).

The ASCP through its Commission on Continuing Education programs, such as Check Samples, Workshops and Summary Reports, makes available tools for improving performance in the many fields of Clinical and Anatomic Pathology. Used in conjunction with survey results these

DOCUMENTATION OF LABORATORY DATA

provide an opportunity to change inadequate procedures and to identify causes of discrepant results.

Going now to the problems of narrowing interlaboratory variation I would like to consider the possible effects of adopting standard methods, instrumentation, reagents, etc. This solution has often been proposed with the idea that we would thereby eliminate many variables and develop a desirable nationwide uniformity. One example of the effect of such a system in the clinical field is Hemoglobinometry: since general adoption of the Cyanmethemoglobin method and the use of Certified standards there has been a substantial improvement in the field nationally.

Here are some results from a month's quality control program in which a group of laboratories use a single pool of material.

Test	Method	Mean Value**	CV (%)
Sodium	SMA	136.2-140.0	0.7-1.8
Sodium	Manual	137.0-144.6	0.6-3.2
Chloride	Cotlove	93.2- 99.4	1.0-2.8
BUN	AA	15.3-17.4	2.9-9.0
Glucose	SMA	71.7-90.4	1.5-8.4

I believe this indicates clearly the substantial difference in laboratory accuracy and precision between different installations. Furthermore the use of common machinery methods and reference material as illustrated by SMA values does not seem to solve the problem at all.

Another thought has been to document differences

* Outlying values and laboratories excluded.
  N about 20 for each figure.
** In usual units.

between different installations and then "correct" the values to eliminate these differences. For example if Laboratory A were 10mg./dl lower than the mean for its peers, we would merely add 10mg. to all its results and file the corrected answers in our national data bank.

Dr. Irwin Weisbrot of the Norwalk Hospital did a study of this proposal as follows. He compared the results for the normal and abnormal pools of lyophilized material which we analyze for glucose daily. He used the following format:
    1. Find mean value for normal pool.
    2. Find difference from this value for each day, actual analysis. This is correction factor and is signed.
    3. Find mean value for abnormal pool.
    4. Find difference from this value for each day, actual analysis. This he called error score and is unsigned.
    5. Use correction factor from normal pool and apply this to the day's actual analysis for the abnormal pool arithmetically. Calculate error score against the abnormal mean value.
    6. Use correction factor from normal pool and apply this to the day's actual analysis for the abnormal pool proportionally: for example if the normal pool were 5% high, make the abnormal result 5% higher than observed. Calculate error score against the abnormal mean value. He added the error scores for 15 consecutive days.

Here is what he found.

Table 2

Error score, abnormal glucose: 15 days

Not corrected	Arithmatic Correction	Proportional Correction
157	198	291

Note that these corrections increased rather than decreased the discrepancies from the mean. This experiment tends to emphasize random error rather than systematic bias, but does point out that any attempt to make daily corrections in observed values is unlikely to succeed.

Suppose, instead, we made an arithmetic correction of all the data for a certain laboratory based on its average difference from the mean for its peers. Would this necessarily diminish systematic bias between laboratories?

In examining this proposal I have taken some figures from a Magruder Fertilizer Survey which Mr. Ed Glocker of W. R. Grace Company gave Dr. Roger Gilbert of Waterbury Hospital. The values are taken from 13 analyses done at 3 month intervals over a 3 year period.

Table 3

Magruder Fertilizer Survey

	Laboratory*			
	A	B	F	H
Av. bias	+0.05	-0.13	+0.67	+0.10
bias S_b	0.39	0.35	1.11	1.34
random S_r	0.43	0.45	1.20	1.38
data S_d	0.58	0.58	1.76	1.92

*All figures in normalized units

Note that the poorer laboratories F and H exhibit such marked imprecision that no realistic use of their bias figures for individual surveys is possible, whereas the better laboratories A and B do not present this obstacle to use of their data.

We conclude then that correction for bias in a peer group can be made only for laboratories which provide adequate precision of analysis. This is true even though systematic bias is by far the major reason for interlaboratory variation (5), an observation recently confirmed in the clinical laboratory field by Dr. Gilbert . (4).

My final area of discussion concerns the clinical usefulness of laboratory data at present, and how it may be improved in the future.

Dr. Joseph Amenta (1) recently wrote a fine paper on discriminant functions in laboratory medicine and explained the statistical analysis necessary to find which laboratory tests helped and which did not help in diagnosing disease. I quote from this paper. "One could easily visualize---a proposed new test which improved discriminant power while at the same time reducing to insignificance an older established test. ---For example new tests of thyroid function are being proposed constantly. To our knowledge this statistical technique has not been applied in determining which combination of tests best differentiates between the hyperthroid and the euthyroid or the hypothyroid and the euthyroid patient." Unfortunately there is a real weakness in this proposal. It involves the circular reasoning illustrated in the following dialogue:

    Doctor: You have thosis.
    Patient: How do you know?
    Doctor: Your thosis test is positive.
    Patient: Why is that?
    Doctor: Because you have thosis.
    Patient: Oh !

Actually in discriminating between diseases by laboratory tests we can draw up the following chart:

Table 4

Test	DISEASE		
	Yes	Maybe	No
Yes	Yes*	?	No
Maybe	?	?	?
No	No	?	No**

For the one-starred results, a positive test when the disease is present, and the two-starred result, the negative test when the disease is absent, we have excellent correlations. For all the other results which are inconclusive or false the correlation is poor.

Dr. Gabrieli speaks of hard data, namely laboratory data which is quantitative and whose reproducibility is known, as contrasted to soft data, namely clinical data which is generally qualitative and of unknown precision. There is, I believe, a substantial danger that because of this distinction we will permit the "good", or hard data, to replace the "bad" or soft data as the index of clinical diagnosis. Although I applaud the idea of documenting laboratory data in the many ways discussed at this conference, I feel that a much more important step, though a more difficult one will be to document clinical data.

In discussing screening laboratory procedures with clinicians I find that my ability to document laboratory data already far outweighs their ability to tell me reliable facts about their patients. Furthermore although they are not too busy to order and presumably examine masses of laboratory values, they are invariably too busy to develop even simple records of what benefits the patient derived from these studies. This is why the question "what is the clinical usefulness of the data?" cannot be satisfactorily answered except for a very few tests and for very few patients. I urge that all of us support such long-term clinically oriented studies as the Framingham study and the UGDP Diabetes study so that we may learn what is useful. I suspect that our ability to generate adequate laboratory data is already considerably greater than the clinicians ability to use it.

Finally I doubt that we can presently develop a workable scheme for a nationwide documented laboratory data bank in which all values are corrected for known analytic variation. I believe a number of regional studies using a variety of statistical approaches should be carried out first, the best format selected and then an attempt made for a wider application. I would also suggest that partial documentation adjusted to our present state of knowledge might be a feasible interim step.

References

1. Amenta, J. S. and Harkins, M. L. The use of discriminant functions in laboratory medicine: evaluation of phosphate clearance studies in the diagnosis of hyperparathyroidism. Amer. J. Clin. Path. 55, 330 - 341, 1971.
2. Barnett, R. N. Medical significance of laboratory results: Amer. J. Clin. Path. 50, 671 - 676, 1968.
3. Copeland, B. E. Informal summary report of conference on documentation of procedures and results in laboratory medicine: Amer. J. Clin. Path. 55, 380 -383, 1971.
4. Gilbert, R. K. Systematic bias revealed by surveys. Meeting of Conn. Society of Pathologists, Mar. 17, 1971.
5. Youden, W. J. The sample, the procedure and the laboratory. Anal. Chem. 32, 23A - 37A, 1960.

DOCUMENTATION INTEREST OF THE NATIONAL
BUREAU OF STANDARDS AND COLLABORATING
GROUPS FOR COMMUNICATION OF LABORATORY
RESULTS IN CLINICAL ANALYSIS

Robert Schaffer, Ph.D.

Dr. Vannevar Bush wrote "If men are to accomplish together anything useful whatever, they must, above all, be able to understand one another. That is the basic reason for a National Bureau of Standards."[1] By these words, Dr. Bush was denoting the goals of the National Bureau of Standards: strengthening and advancing the Nation's science and technology, and facilitating the effective application of science and technology to the public benefit. To achieve these purposes, the Bureau's activities include programs that range from providing the experimental basis for establishing the highest attainable accuracy in the definition of our basic physical standards: the meter, the kilogram, the second, the degree Kelvin, the ampere, and the candela, to seeking to ensure that this national measurement capability is transferable to all who need assurance that their work is (a) sufficiently accurate, and (b) compatible with that of others.

Thus, the meter and the second are at present defined on the basis of fundamental atomic properties to nine and ten significant figures, respectively, but current work at NBS shows promise of increasing these in accuracy by

[1]See Foreword by Vannevar Bush to "Measure for Progress. A History of the National Bureau of Standards" by R. C. Cochrane, U.S. Government Printing Office, Washington, D. C., 1966.

419

several factors of ten, and of improving the other standards as well. To be sure, only certain segments of our Nation's science and technology are directly strengthened by such discriminating advances. NBS recognizes this, and recognizes as well that other scientific fields have needs for standards of far less exactness--and that these are urgently needed. Certainly, work in clinical chemical analysis is in this latter category. I particularize only because clinical chemistry is a subject of this conference.

Until recently, NBS gave little direct attention to the clinical chemical field, primarily because the field of health appeared to be outside the purview of an Agency of the Department of Commerce. However, such a differentiation has been discarded at NBS in the present framework of concern for seeking to aid all areas of science and technology where the Bureau's measurement capability can facilitate problem-solving, especially where the problems are subjects of national importance. Hence, when Dr. Bradley E. Copeland, Chairman of the Standards Committee of the College of American Pathologists, addressed us with the need for a purified, highly characterized cholesterol standard, and Dr. George N. Bowers, Jr. Chairman of the Standards Committee of American Association of Clinical Chemists, sought our help with a number of other clinical standards, Dr. W. Wayne Meinke, Chief of the NBS Chemistry Division (and then also Chief of the Office of Standard Reference Materials), responded by directing part of his program to the development of standard materials for the clinical laboratory. Cholesterol, uric acid, urea, and creatinine were the first of the Standard Reference Materials to be issued for use in clinical chemical analysis.

The National Institute of General Medical Sciences (through Dr. Robert S. Melville's committee, Automation in the Medical Laboratory Sciences) subsequently recognized the importance of NBS standard materials for automated clinical analysis, and established a cooperative agreement with us to promote development of these clinical standards.

The May 1971 issue of "Analytical Chemistry"[2] contains W. W. Meinke's thorough review of the SRMs produced for the clinical laboratory.

Standard Reference Materials (SRMs) issued through the Bureau's Office of Standard Reference Materials, are materials of certified composition that are made widely available to interested users who require a homogeneous material having well characterized properties for calibrating a measurement system so that meaningful scientific data can be produced. Much effort is given to the analysis of candidate preparations so that a most satisfactory material can be put through the Bureau's certification process --- which stresses the homogeneity of the macro and trace constituents to afford NBS and the user a maximum of assurance as to the composition of the standard material. NBS's concern for an SRM continues, with frequent reexaminations of the SRM after it is issued, to ensure that no change of composition has occurred (the finding of evidence of decomposition would signal notification to all purchasers), and with tests of the applicability of newer techniques for studying the SRM. To ensure uninterrupted availability to users, the recertification of new supplies of an SRM is begun before a supply of it is exhausted.

Table 1 lists SRMs for clinical analysis that have already been issued. Table 2 lists other SRMs that also have been recently issued, and should be of interest to clinical chemist. In addition, we now have in process of certification: cortisol, D-mannitol (as standard for the glycerol obtained by saponification of triglycerides), and

---

[2] W. Wayne Meinke, "Standard Reference Materials for Clinical Measurement", Anal. Chem., 43, 28A (1971).

4 hydroxy-3methoxy-DL-mandelic acid (VMA). Completion of these SRMs is expected in the next few months. Also, liquids for use as spectrophotometric standards are nearing completion of certification.

Only for one of the SRMs thus far issued, bilirubin, has it been considered necessary to seek a more satisfactory method than is currently available to prepare standard solutions from crystalline preparations; in particular, we wished to provide secure directions for the use of the bilirubin SRM. Our work on standard solutions is now near completion, and we expect soon to be able to offer our suggestions to purchasers of the SRM and to others by the usual publication procedure.

Finally, in seeking to make clinical measurements more meaningful, the Bureau and a group of interested clinical chemists and pathologists are beginning a joint effort to develop referee methods, that is, methods of known accuracy. Mr. J. Paul Cali, at present Chief of the Office of Standards Reference Materials, has organized this program. The objective is to develop, and define the accuracy of, a method for each serum constituent. The referee method must be capable of being run in some clinical laboratories, but because it may be too cumbersome to be used routinely, only relatively few laboratories would have the means by which routine clinical methods for that constituent might be evaluated and as required, have their systematic biases corrected.

The initial effort is centered on developing a referee method for serum calcium. For its part of the work, NBS is using its highly accurate, isotope-dilution, mass-spectrometry method to determine the calcium content of serum samples, and these samples will be tested in the cooperating clinical laboratories by a carefully described, atomic-absorption method. Statistical evaluations of the clinical lab data by NBS experts, coupled as needed, to modification of the atomic-absorption procedure, will ultimately afford the referee method. At all stages in this development, cooperating laboratories will be in quality control through use of the Bureau's SRM calcium carbonate, and the SRM will also serve to tie together the referee method with other routine methods used for serum calcium.

Thus, the steps taken at NBS to transfer to the clinical laboratory an accuracy base for measurement are (a) the issuance of SRMs and (b) the initiation of an interaction program with a select cluster of clinical laboratories dedicated to the development of referee methods for clinical analysis.

Table I. SRMs issued by NBS for clinical chemical Analysis

SRM NO.	Name
911	Cholestrol
912	Uric acid
913	Urea
914	Calcium carbonate
915	Bilirubin
917	$\underline{\underline{D}}$-Glucose
918	Potassium chloride
922	Tris(hydroxymethyl) aminomethane
923	Tris(hydroxymethyl) aminomethane hydrochloride
930	Glass filters for spectrophotometry
2201	Sodium chloride for pNa and pCl
2202	Potassium chloride for pK and pCl

Table 2. SRMs issued by NBS and used in clinical analysis

SRM NO.	Name
40h	Sodium oxalate
83C	Arsenic trioxide
84H	Acid potassium phthalate
136C	Potassium dichromate
350	Benzoic acid
1591	Orchard leaves
1861C	Potassium dihydrogen phosphate

DOCUMENTATION CONCERNS OF STATE AND COMMUNITY FOR COMMUNICATION OF LABORATORY RESULTS*

William Kaufmann, M. D.

In discussing the State's proficiency testing program as it relates to the accumulation of clinical laboratory data, it was suggested that I explain the difference between the State's proficiency testing program and a quality control system. The suggested outline I was given contained the statement that "a laboratory may satisfy State requirements without adequately supporting clinical medicine." I am not sure that I fully understand this statement but if I do then I think that it is incorrect. In fact, I submit that as part of such requirements a properly operated State proficiency testing program cannot but support or better still prove to be the foundation upon which clinical medicine is built.

I shall try to illustrate this as well as the inevitable pitfalls of this concept on the basis of experience gained with the proficiency testing program of New York State. Evidence will be presented to show how laboratory data gathered by accurate, precise and reproducible means allow for standardization of laboratory testing and consequently for the issuance or revocation of licenses, thus

---

*Data for this presentation were supplied by:
Drs. Hassan A. Gaafar, James H. Kelly, Walter Stahl and Raymone E. Vanderlinde, of the Clinical Laboratory Center of the Division of Laboratories and Research.

aiding and supporting the practice of clinical medicine. Admittedly the process is an on-going effort and the end result is not yet in sight. Experience is still recent, in our case only 5 years, and much more experience, research and trial are needed until we find and can present the standard model.

I do not question that there is a difference between a State operated proficiency testing program and one operated by a voluntary agency. This difference does not necessarily lie in the program itself, but more likely in the consequences resulting from its application by either organization. Of all the quality control programs described so far, a proficiency testing program is the most readily identifiable one by which proficiency, efficiency and reliability of a laboratory can be identified and documented. It is by no means the best method for evaluating a laboratory's capability to perform, nor does it reflect achievement of every day excellence, which must be relegated to internal quality control, but it is the only way which allows for the accumulation of retrievable data on which the State can often base far-reaching decisions. It is one thing to inform a laboratory that its performance in the proficiency testing program is not satisfactory and then exhort it to "strive for better performance", but it is another when on the basis of poor performance a license may be revoked and the laboratory is instructed to "cease and desist" from doing laboratory tests. Thus, for the State it is essential that its program have total validity so that its decisions can be firmly and unequivocably established and upheld.

Two questions immediately arise: Is this really necessary and is the profession as a whole not in a position or willing to police itself and so to ascertain that the patient is assured of the best possible diagnostic care? The answer to the last question may well be in the affirmative in most hospitals where traditionally self control by professional organizations has been responsible for continuous improvement in the delivery of medical care, including that emanating from the laboratory. However, since laboratory practice is definitely a growth industry in which the profit motive plays an important role with a view to investment opportunities, the answer to the first question must also be in the affirmative and uniform application of regulations is inevitable.

I should like to demonstrate now with the help of observations made in several categories of laboratory practice over a period of years how the State evaluates performance and arrives at decisions. Only certain specific areas will be discussed since they represent prototypes of the broad field of laboratory medicine. They will suffice, hopefully, to illustrate the point I wish to make.

Let us look at the field of parasitology. We began operating this program only recently and for the test year 1970-71 prepared two sets of specimens which after being checked by reference laboratories were submitted to participating laboratories. The organisms contained in the sets are outlined in table 1. As can readily be seen the percentage of accuracy ranges in the first set of specimens in October 1970, showed that achievement was far from what should be expected to be of clinical value. Following an intensive educational effort by the State, attended by 767 laboratorians the March 1971 testing revealed remarkable improvement in performance. There are two deductions possible: one, that a deficiency actually existed and, two, that it was correctible. We like to interpret this achievable correction as the direct result of our efforts, of course!

If we now turn to the category of bacteriology, conditions were almost identical to the above in the assembly of material, but identification of organisms required a broader range of methodology. Again reference laboratories, as in all proficiency testing programs determined the feasibillty, the targets and the ranges of allowable deviations and the organisms to be identified are outlined in table 2. As can be seen in the slide, accuracy of performance seemed to be directly related to the intricacy and difficulty with which certain organisms can be identified. Nevertheless there is considerable improvement in the performance in bacteriology in 1970-71 as compared to that observed before 1969 and illustrated in table 3. Table 4 shows the arbitrary grading of the total performance which again illustrates the greater reliability in 1970-71 as compared to that prior to 1969. This is of important clinical significance.

Prothrombin time determinations offer another opportunity to demonstrate our point. Table 5 shows the performance in about 450 laboratories in the normal prothrombin time range with Warner Chilcote, Dade and a combination thromboplastin. There is good evidence of accuracy, precision and reproducibility in this performance regardless of the material used and so there is no reason to believe that laboratories have difficulty in performing in this area. However, this assurance is shattered promptly as we turn to the next observation in table 6 where we notice an unusually wide range of figures in the abnormal prothrombin time range. Again thromboplastin identical to that used in the normal range was used. In fact we actually observe two peaks, one in the 20 to 26 second range, and one in the 28 to 36 second range. We must therefore conclude that when the same laboratories test prothrombin time in the abnormal range, there is considerably less accuracy while precision may still be acceptable.

The discrepancies in the two ranges obviously require an explanation which I shall attempt to offer. First, let me compare the results presented with those observed in 1968. In table 7 the normal range is demonstrated and in table 8, the abnormal. Comparison of these two observations with those of 1970 at least illustrates that the curves have narrowed somewhat with time and that things are not quite as bad as they used to be. But this is not much comfort. The real shocker is most likely seen in table 9, when on voluntarily offered information we are told that 38% of all laboratories never calibrated their hemoglobinometers. One wonders what the fate of the tools for prothrombin time determination was. It is hoped that the use of controls was and is more widespread than appears from the next table (10) in hemoglobinometry. That there is a definite relationship of accuracy and reproducibility of one method to the other in prothrombin time determinations is evident by a look at table 11, where the standard deviation of the automated method is demonstrably narrower than that observed with the manual method.

Recent experience with a drug abuse toxicology proficiency testing program is also of interest. There are a number of laboratories claiming that they are capable of detecting abusive drugs in the urine of suspected individuals. There is no need to emphasize the absolute necessity of being accurate and dependable in this identification because of the dire consequences which errors may produce. Therefore, to test the proficiency of laboratories in this area reasonable combinations of drugs subject to abuse were added to pooled urine collected from individuals known to be free of medication. The concentration of drugs added were high but in keeping with levels that might be expected from an individual who has quite recently undergone a drug abuse experience. In addition, pooled positive specimens were obtained from individuals attending methadone clinics.

While 12 coded specimens were submitted, 4 of the specimens were duplicates. The combination of drugs as well as their concentration in the various specimens are presented in table 12. The scoring system was designed to penalize more heavily false-positive than false-negative reports. In addition, penalties were weighed in terms of the relative importance of the particular drug in a drug abuse screening program. To obtain a permit to perform tests in drug abuse toxicology the Department of Health of the State and City of New York agreed that the laboratory tested must demonstrate proficiency in the testing of barbiturates, amphetamines, morphine, methadone, codeine, quinine and glutethimide. Consequently, laboratories were penalized when they failed to report these drugs, if they were present. Phenothiazine errors were not scored. This drug was added to some urines to determine the possibility of incorrectly reporting the phenothiazine as some other drug.

Tables 13, 14, and 15 are illustrative of the detailed achievement of our participating laboratories and identify the methods used for the discovery of the abused drugs. A minimum of 90% was set as the acceptable rate of identification.

In most instances, false positive findings are probably due to cross contamination during the handling of the specimens in the laboratory. In some instances, normally present ninhydrin reacting material was incorrectly identified as amphetamine. The reported false positive quinines were probably due to the failure of the analyst to separate the urine from the chloroform extract completely. False negative findings for the various drugs were due to incomplete transfer of the extracted residue to the thin layer chromatographic plate. Some laboratories experienced difficulties with the identification of methadone because they were not able to distinguish the methadone from other material which moved with the solvent front. In one case the laboratory's poor performance was obviously related to a mix-up in the identification of the specimens.

Aside from the points discussed above, no particular problems were encountered. The number of drugs not detected or falsely reported as being positive appear to be randomly distributed. From this, we conclude that the errors that did occur were due to the failure of the laboratory to perform the test properly.

The results of the testing in this really new field are illustrated in the next tables.

This table (16) shows the results with the urine specimens tested this past November and March. Of the 22 laboratories participating in both series of tests, seven false positives were found in blank urines submitted in duplicate by six laboratories in November and six false positives by three laboratories in March. Incorrect identification in the form of false positives occured as follows: 21 by fourteen laboratories in November and 34 by seven laboratories in March. In addition, in the first series, 17 laboratories failed to identify 58 drugs; in the second series 13 laboratories failed to identify 38 drugs. In summary, in the November series, 18 laboratories made a total of 96 errors and in the March series 14 laboratories a total of 79 errors. Obviously, four laboratories obtained 100% in the November series and eight laboratories in the March series.

The next table (17) repeats the results for March for the 22 laboratories but it also includes data on six laboratories which had not previously participated. Only one of these laboratories correctly identified all of the drugs present. The other results are as follows: two false positives in the blanks by one laboratory; 22 false positives or incorrect identifications by five laboratories; and a failure to detect 27 drugs by these five laboratories. The errors totaled 51 for the five laboratories or approximately 10 errors per laboratory. It should be realized that this is the qualitative detection of the presence of drugs in the urine when sufficient quantities of the drug are present to represent an overdose. Experience is a definite factor of performing well in this particular area of specialization. Because of the implications and label that one is placing on an individual if a major addictive drug is found in the urine, we are very much concerned about having laboratories pass proficiency testing at a level of 90% or greater before they begin work on patient specimens in this very vital area.

Finally I should like to demonstrate some observations made in the field of Clinical Chemistry. Acid phosphatase determinations, an important clinical diagnostic enzyme test, will illustrate the point.

In this next table (18), seventeen laboratories using the Bodansky procedure reported coefficients of variations of 38.5% and 30.7% on the grossly and slightly elevated specimens, respectively. Thirteen laboratories using the almost identical Shinowara-Jones-Reinhart procedure showed coefficients of variation of 29.3% and 25.0%, respectively. We have no explanation for the better results by the Shinowara-Jones-Reinhart modification. The 12 laboratories using the Gutman and Gutman procedure reported 14.7% and 22.9% variation, and 19 laboratories using the practically identical King-Armstrong method showed 40.0% and 28.3% respectively. The 65 laboratories using the Babson-Read and Babson-Phillips procedure reported coefficients of variations of 15.5% and 21.5% respectively on these two specimens. The largest number of laboratories - 111 - employed the Bessey-Lowry-Brock procedure. They showed a variation of 21.0% and 15.1%, respectively. On the grossly elevated specimen this is the lowest coefficient of variation by any of the methods and for the slightly abnormal specimen there is considerable difference in the precision of results by the various methods.

The next table (19) summarizes the overall results. On the grossly elevated specimen, five laboratories out of 286 or 1.8% would have reported this grossly abnormal specimen as being within the normal range of their method. On the slightly elevated specimen an additional

28 participated voluntarily. These were mostly mental hygiene units, to which these specimens were sent only as duplicates. Of the 314 laboratories 22 or 7% would have reported this slightly elevated specimen to be within normal limits by their procedure. In addition, the reports showed that 14 laboratories, or almost 5% of those reporting interchanged the results on these two specimens. We therefore believe data handling may represent a significant source of error.

That errors of this nature can have serious effect on management of disease needs no reiteration. Inherent problems in methodology interfere with reproducibility and equally interfere with decision-making on the State level. Thus continuous investigative efforts are essential to pinpoint inherent problems and to detect their causes. One example of this is demonstrated in the next table. (20).

Table 20 shows the effects of a proper standard and an interfering constituent on cholesterol results. A large pool of serum with a target value of 236 mg/100 ml was split and 30 mg% bilirubin added to 1/2 of the material. Both specimens were submitted to laboratories. Laboratories using standards, A, B, and C showed excellent agreement between the mean results obtained and the target (reference laboratory mean). Fair agreement is shown when standard D was used and poor agreement with standards E, F, and G. Due to the fact that many laboratories do not use extraction procedures to remove bilirubin, column three shows all laboratories to have obtained a higher mean value on the specimen containing bilirubin. Thus, failure to remove an interfering substance can result in inaccuracy even though a proper standard has been used to calibrate the method.

In summary therefore, as the State has assumed the responsibility to establish achievable standards in laboratory practice for the purpose of providing its citizens with the best obtainable support in medical practice, it also charged its department of Health to devise ways and means to do so. Evaluation of laboratory practice was specifically introduced in the law by the designation of a proficiency testing program (Laboratory Reference System). While not the only and not necessarily the best means to evaluate continuous quality performance, it is at present the only recognized one for documentation of any performance. Since the State must depend on such retrievable documentation as a prime requisite for decision making, such as issuing and revoking licenses, proficiency testing is assured a primary and determining role in the total State Program of Laboratory Evaluation. Research should be directed towards the development of quality control programs capable of surveying daily and routine unbaised performance with automatic monitoring and retrievable data collection. When properly developed and proven reliable, they should replace external quality control programs (proficiency testing) and the latter should be used as educational tools only.

DOCUMENTATION OF LABORATORY DATA

TABLE 1

Parasitology 1970-1971

Specimens submitted on:	TOTAL Sent	TOTAL Ret'd	Hospital #	Hospital % Sat	Independent #	Independent % Sat	County #	County % Sat	State #	State % Sat	City #	City % Sat
Oct. 26, 1970	247	240	137	56.2	68	44.1	19	52.6	13	69.2	3	33.3
March 15, 1971	136	126	66	86.4	44	81.8	5	80	9	66.6	2	50
Results based on the two shipments		259	145	92.4	76	86.8	19	73.6	16	62.5	3	66.6

Organisms Submitted

Entamoeba histolytica trophs   Ascaris lumbricoides eggs
Entamoeba coli cysts & trophs   Hookworm eggs
Giardia lamblia cysts & trophs   Strongyloides stercoralis larvae

TABLE 2

Bacteriology 1970-1971
Performance as related to organisms submitted

	Number examined	Per cent correct
Streptococcus (Diplococcus) pneumoniae	335	85%
Streptococcus pyogenes	325	94.7%
Streptococcus agalactiae	215	74.8%
Staphylococcus aureus	49	93.8%
Staphylococcus epidermidis	49	75.5%
Hemophilus influenzae	49	38.7%
Alpha hemolytic streptococcus	287	72.8%
Neisseria lactamicus	287	74.2%
Citrobacter freundii	245	89.2%
Listeria monocytogenes	245	91.8%
Salmonella enteritidis	245	87.0%
Enteropathogenic Escherichia coli	245	96.3%
Clostridium perfringens	245	78.8%

TABLE 3

Bacteriology. Performance results per organism

	Total Number Sent	Per Cent 75 Per Cent +
Coagulase positive Staphylococcus	123	86.9
Klebsiella pneumoniae	123	73.1
Salmonella typhimurium	143	72.7
Citrobacter	129	69.7
Salmonella typhi	144	69.4
Pseudomonas aeruginosa	207	69.0
Klebsiella, Enterobacteriaceae	70	68.5
Enteropathogenic Escherichia coli	121	66.9
Beta hemolytic Streptococcus, group A	151	66.8
Diplococcus pneumoniae	185	64.3
Beta hemolytic Streptococcus, group C	180	60.0
Corynebacterium xerose	146	57.5
Listeria monocytogenes	127	57.4
Hemophilus influenzae	175	56.5
Shigella sonnei	148	55.4
Alpha hemolytic Streptococcus, group D	111	54.9
Enterococcus	87	54.0
Herellea vaginicola	154	53.2
Clostridium perfringens	87	52.8
Mima polymorpha	175	50.2
Neisseria meningitidis	66	48.4
Alcaligenes faecalis	88	47.7
Pasteurella multocida	135	46.6
Proteus morganii	49	38.7
Proteus vulgaris	72	30.5
Clostridium bifermentans	156	22.4

TABLE 4

Bacteriology 1970-1971
Summary of performance

	Number of Reports	Percentage of Laboratories
Excellent (90-100%)	328	56.9%
Very good (80-89%)	95	16.5%
Good (75-79%)	53	9.1%
Unsatisfactory (60-74%)	56	9.7%
Poor (below 60%)	45	7.8%

TABLE 5

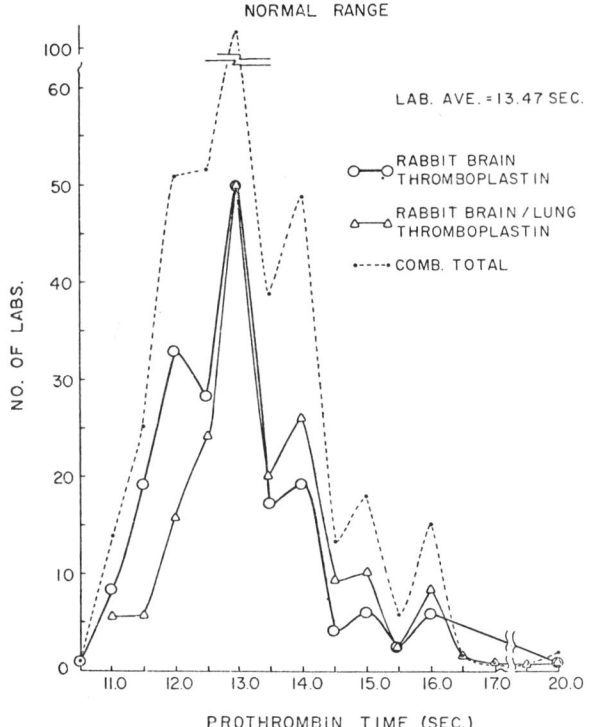

TABLE 6
N.Y. STATE LABORATORY IMPROVEMENT PROGRAM
PROTHROMBIN ESTIMATION – 1971
THERAPEUTIC RANGE

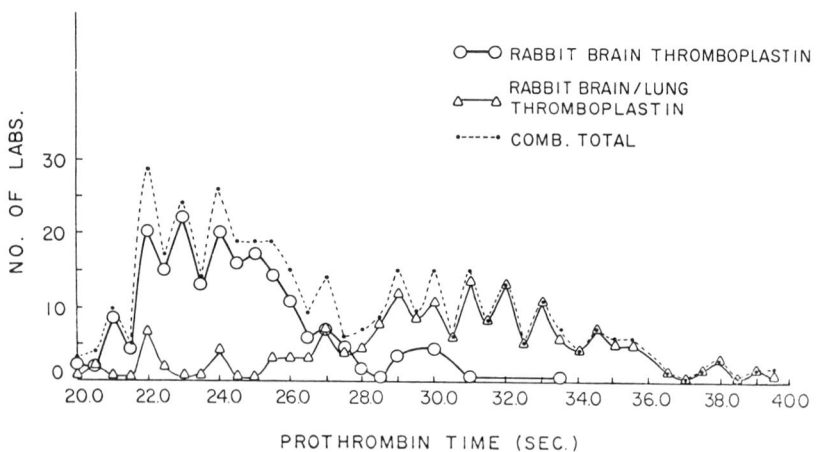

TABLE 7
LABORATORY RANGE OF NORMAL PLASMA PROTHROMBIN TIME DETERMINATIONS

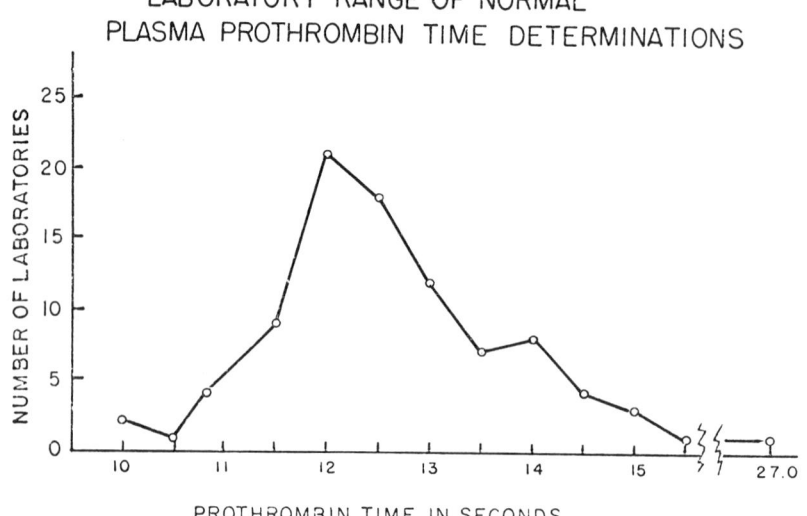

DOCUMENTATION OF LABORATORY DATA

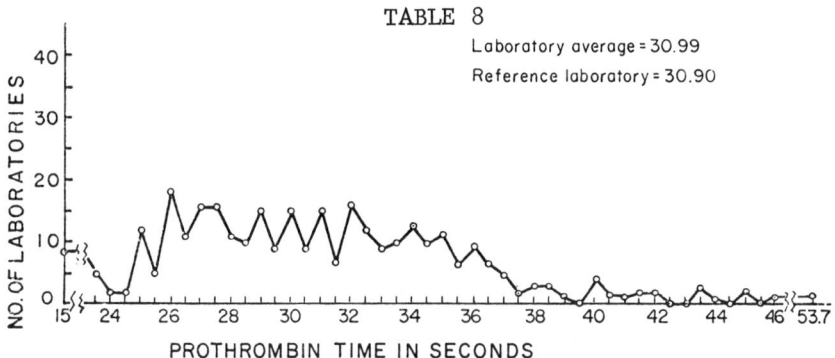

TABLE 8
Laboratory average = 30.99
Reference laboratory = 30.90

TABLE 9
New York State
Laboratory Improvement Program
Hematology 1967

Calibration of Hemoglobinometer

Once a day	(58)	17.5%
Once a week	(60)	18.1%
Occasionally	(47)	14.0%
Never	(126)	38.0%
Other	(41)	12.4%
Laboratories	332	100%

TABLE 10
New York State
Laboratory Improvement Program
Comparison of Hemoglobin Results

	Within 3 S.D.	Over 3 S.D.
Controls Used	91%	9%
Controls Not Used	88%	12%

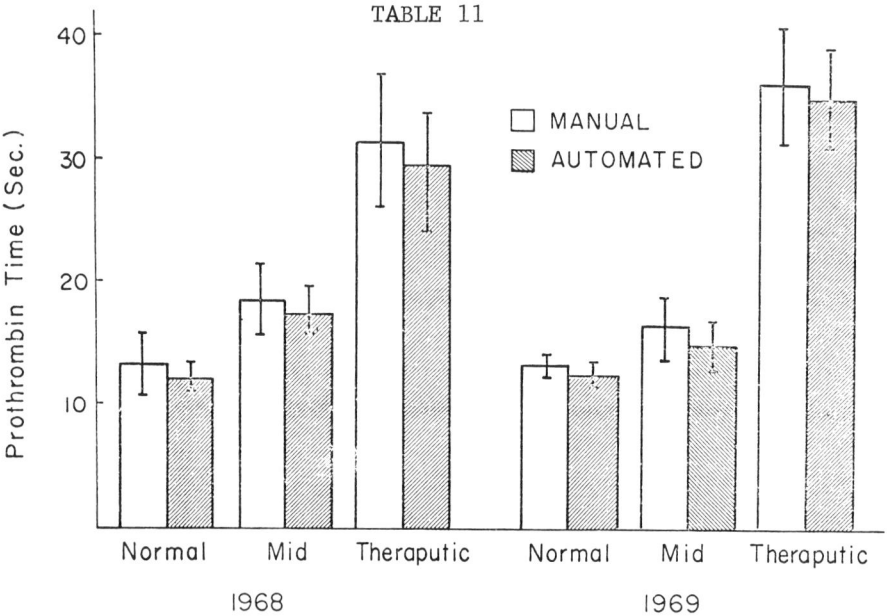

TABLE 11

TABLE 12

NUMBER OF SPECIMENS	DRUGS	CONCENTRATION µg/ml URINE
2	none	0
2	amphetamine quinine	8 0.3
2	pentobarbital chlorpromazine	5 3
2	morphine methadone	1.5 8
1	quinine methadone morphine	0.3 8 1.5
1	morphine	1.5
1	amphetamine morphine quinine methadone	8 1.5 0.3 8
1	phenobarbital glutethimide	5 8

DOCUMENTATION OF LABORATORY DATA

NEW YORK STATE
DEPARTMENT OF HEALTH
Division of Laboratories and Research
Albany, New York 12201

Drugs in Urine Testing
March - 1971

YOUR LABORATORY NUMBER IS _____

TABLE 13

Laboratory	A & B BLANK	C & D Barbiturates	C & D Phenothiazines	C & D False +	E & F Amphetamines	E & F Quinine	E & F False +	G & H Morphine	G & H Methadone	G & H False +	I Barbiturates	I Glutethimide	I False +	J Amphetamine	J Quinine	J Morphine	J Methadone	J False +	K Quinine	K Morphine	K Methadone	K False +	L Morphine	L False +	Point Score	METHOD
	A B	C,D	C,D		E,F	E,F		G,H	G,H			I			J					K				L		
1	0/0	+/+	+/+		+/+	+/+		+/+	+/+		+	+		+	+	+	+		+	+	+		+		100	Dole; Stain
2	0/0	+/+	+/+		+/+	+/+		+/+	+/+		+	+		+	+	+	+		+	+	+		+		100	Dole
3	0/0	+/+	+/+		+/+	+/+		+/+	+/+		+	+		+	+	+	+		+	+	+		+		63	Davidow
4	0/0	?/+	+/+		0/0	+/+		+/?	+/+		+	+	Me	+	+	+	o	P.	+	+	o	P.?	+		76	Broich et al
5	0/0	?/+	+/+		+/+	+/+		+/?	+/+		+	+		+	+	+	+	B	+	+	+	A B	+		94	Mule modification
6	0/0	+/+	+/+		+/+	+/+		+/+	+/+		+	+		+	+	+	+		+	+	+		+		100	Davidow
7	0/0	+/+	+/+		+/+	+/+		+/+	+/+		+	+		+	+	+	+		+	+	+		+		100	Davidow
8	0/0	+/+	+/+		+/+	+/+		+/+	+/+		+	+		+	+	+	+		+	+	+		+		100	Davidow
9	0/0	+/+	+/+		+/+	+/+		+/+	+/+		+	+	A	+	+	+	o		+	+	+		+		85	Davidow
10	0/0	+/+	+/+		+/+	+/+		+/+	+/+		+	+		+	+	+	+		+	+	+		+		100	Modified TLC

TABLE 14

NEW YORK STATE
DEPARTMENT OF HEALTH
Division of Laboratories and Research
Albany, New York 12201

Drugs in Urine Testing
March - 1971

YOUR LABORATORY NUMBER IS ____

DOCUMENTATION OF LABORATORY DATA

TABLE 15

NEW YORK STATE
DEPARTMENT OF HEALTH
Division of Laboratories and Research
Albany, New York 12201

Drugs in Urine Testing
March - 1971

YOUR LABORATORY NUMBER IS ___

	A & B	C & D			E & F			G & H			I			J				K				L		Point Score	METHOD
SPECIMENS	Blank	Barbiturates	Phenothiazines	False +	Amphetamines	Quinine	False +	Morphine	Methadone	False +	Barbiturates	Glutethimide	False +	Amphetamine	Quinine	Morphine	Methadone	False +	Quinine	Morphine	Methadone	False +	Morphine	False +		
	B	C, D	C, D	D	E, F, E, F	E, F, E, F	B	G, H	G, H	P P	I		me	N	J	J		C G B		K		C	L	Me	49	Dole
22	0	+ +	+ +		? ?	+ +		+ +	+ +		+ +	+ ?		+ +	+ +	+ +	+ +		+ +	+ +	+ +		+		98	TLC
23	0	+ +	+ +	+	? ?	+ +		+ +	+ +		+ 0	+ 0		+ ?	+ +	+ +	+ +		+ +	+ +	+ +		+		0	Davidow
24	B na me	0 +	+ +	me	+ +	+ +		+ +	+ +		0	0	me	0	+ +	0	+ +	B G	+ +	0	+ +		0		69	Davidow
25	0	+ +	+ +		? ?	+ +	?me	+ +	+ +		+ +	+ +		0	+ +	+ +	+ +		+ +	+ +	+ +		+		93	Del Cortivo
26	0	+ +	+ +		? ?	+ +	?me	+ +	+ +		+ +	+ +		0	+ +	+ +	+ +		+ +	+ +	+ +		+		93	Del Cortivo
27	0	+ +	+ +		+ +	+ +		+ +	+ +		+ +	+ +		0	+ +	+ +	+ +		+ +	+ +	+ +	Co	+		52	Davidow
28	0 ?G	+ +	+ +	?G ?G	+ +	0 0		+ +	+ +		0 +	0 +		0	+ +	?	+ +		+ +	+ +	+ +		?			
	4 false+	3 1 false -	2 false -	15 false+	5 2 4 3 false- fal+		12 fal+	2 2 false	3 3 false	3 fal+	3 3 false-fal+		4 false-fal+	7 false	1 4 false -	3 false -	3 false	8 fal+	1 false	1 2 false	2 false	12 Co	3 ?	3 fal+fal-fal+		

TABLE 16
Upstate Labs - Drug Testing

	Nov. - 70 22 labs	Mar. - 71 22 labs
False + in blanks	7(6 labs)	6 (3 labs)
Other False +	31(14 labs)	34 (7 labs)
False -	58(17 labs)	38 (13 labs)
Total Errors	96(18 labs)	79 (14 labs)

TABLE 17
Upstate Labs - Drug Testing

March - 1971

	22 labs	6 new labs
False + in blanks	6 (3 labs)	2 (1 lab)
Other False +	35 (7 labs)	22 (5 labs)
False -	38 (13 labs)	27 (5 labs)
Total Errors	79 (14 labs)	51 (5 labs)

TABLE 18
June 1969

Method	Labs (Nos.)	Low Samp. (C.V.)	High Samp. (C.V.)
BOD	17	38.5	30.7
SJR	13	29.3	25.0
G&G	12	14.7	22.9
K.A.	19	40.0	28.3
B.R.	65	15.5	21.5
B.L.B.	111	21.0	15.1

TABLE 19
TOTALS

	No. of Labs	Reported Normal
P1-4	286	5 (1.8%)
P5-8	314	22 (7%)

Sample Mix-up 14 labs. 4.9%

TABLE 20
N.Y.S. - Cholesterol (mg/100ml)

June - 1970

Std.	Unknown	Ict. Unknown
A	236	293
B	237	329
C	234	275
D	229	305
E	221	290
F	255	318
G	218	250
Target	236	236

PRACTICAL PLANS SUGGESTED BY PANEL FOR
EXPLICIT DOCUMENTATION OF CLINICAL LABORA-
TORY DATA IN COMMUNICATIONS

Practical plans should suggest sensible ways to start planning, to initiate what can be done now, and to outline long-term goals. The following are suggestions that seem appropriate at this time:

General Plans:
1. To define and select a single standardized language for laboratory medicine. Efforts should be continued, in collaboration with the AMA, to select a common language such as SNOP. Inter-laboratory regional and national communication of data can only be effective if there is national agreement on a common language for laboratory data.
2. To develop guidelines for documentation of each analytical method used in the clinical laboratory to cover manual or automated procedures. These guidelines should include all disciplines in the clinical laboratory.
3. To establish points of reference suitable for documentation of each test performed in the clinical laboratory. "True" values shall serve as reference points and for labeling whenever possible.
4. To encourage research on development of information and tools needed for documentation of each test in each discipline where these are not available. The documentation of each test in each discipline where these are not available. The documentations should be satisfactory for both internal and external uses.
5. To find an acceptable way to relate the laboratory data in context of the patient. Laboratorians and clinicians must develop a meaningful report to meet needs of patient. This is necessary to ensure all med-

ical groups are interested in documentation of data. Laboratory data should be closely coordinated with the rest of the data of the patient.

6. To initiate the evaluation of internal and external documentation procedures in small groups of clinical laboratories in close communication with each other.

Specific Plans: (For all disciplines in the clinical laboratory).

1. To establish an information center on documentation to help in education and training on documentation procedures, and to point out deficiencies in documentation in methods, techniques, and automation.

2. To encourage committees on documentation of different professional organizations to establish communication channels and work together toward goals.

3. To establish mimimum quality control requirements necessary for documentation of each test used in the clinical laboratory.

4. To encourage methodology research on how to "clean up" chemical, hematological, or microbiological basis used in automation.

5. To devise guidelines for sampling, handling, and preservation of specimens for each test in the clinical laboratory. This includes directions to accompany sample.

6. To review and develop concensus on nomenclature, units, and basis of calculations for each test used in the clinical laboratory.

7. To develop guidelines for changing reference materials, analytical techniques, personnel, or other factors influencing analytical results.

8. To tabulate physiologic and environmental effects that influence the results of each test for development of appropriate reference values for the patient.

9. To list and examine potential uses of each test in the clinical laboratory and establish limits of permissible error for each function.

10. To develop guidelines for interpretation of each test or group of tests that lead to further clinical class-

ification.

11. To consider the need for percentiles, or another mechanism, for common laboratory language.

12. To continue development of ways to express probability of significance of a result for interpretation of laboratory values.

13. To outline documentation procedures specifically applicable to the determination of diagnostic enzymatic reactions.

14. To accumulate experiences of how to control operations of a large-volume clinical laboratory. Information should be collected on control needs for clinical laboratories of different sizes.

15. To continue modifying and testing of Canadian and U.S. workload recording method for clinical laboratories.

16. To initiate workshops, or sessions, at national professional meetings on documentation procedures.

17. To recommend that funding agencies demand laboratories prove ability to do the work and proper documentation has been installed in the laboratory before initiation of analyses.

18. To suggest that accreditation, license, or offer to participate in a national documentation program not be extended unless a laboratory meets guidelines for documentation.

SUMMARY OF PANEL - Dr. Gerald R. Cooper

The presentations of the panelists and discussions with the audience crystallized certain statements or concepts. Dr. Barnett emphasized the need to relate laboratory data in the context of the patient, and the absolute necessity that acceptable and similar precision exist within laboratories for comparison of data among laboratories. Dr. Schaffer stated that laboratories must establish a sound analytical base for documentation and analysts must follow directions for use of standards and reference materials. Dr. Kaufmann pointed out that quality performance in the individual laboratory must be acquired before documentation can be acquired on a national basis. Dr. Burns has suggested that while reports of laboratory data must contain certain essentials, they must be flexible to fit various functions and contribute rapidly to patient care.

In the discussion period, the use of the reference laboratories was described as a means to play fair with peers and at the same time to demonstrate what should be the goals. A concerted effort is now being made to help clinical laboratories to truly become reference laboratories. Setting of limits of permissible error so far has been largely arbitrary, but was considered from the point of view of performance of peer and reference laboratories and clinical significance of results.

Inconsistencies will occur in results returned to participants by different proficiency testing programs. The positive outlook is not to criticize the proficiency testing, but to look for possible errors within the laboratory that could have caused a poor result on a single sample, or a mixup of reported results. This can happen to any laboratory in the range of borderline performance. Methodology differences, though, can cause such inconsistencies when one proficiency testing corrects for methodology and the other does not.

Daily calibration can consist of either checking validity of expected standard curve or actually using a new standard curve. The nature of the determination and effect of run-to-run factors, as seen by extent of variation of standard curve from day to day, indicate whether new standard curves need to be run within each run. Stable standard curves may be checked satisfactorily by single point determinations within each run. Lastly, suggestions were outlined about how explicit documentation could be stimulated and implemented progressively by professional and economic actions.

PLANNING THE FUTURE

R. S. Melville, Ph. D.

If you think our problems are unique to today's problems in communication you are mistaken. As an example of this I would refer to the Holy Bible for documentation!:

GENESIS 11:7, 9

"Let us go down, and there confound their language, that they may not understand one anothers speech."

"Therefore is the name of the city called Babel because the Lord did there confound the language of all the earth, and from thence did the Lord scatter them abroad upon the face of the earth."

During the past two days you have all had the opportunity to listen and learn about the exciting developments going on in the clinical laboratory with regard to computer applications.

This morning Gerry Cooper's panel presented a discussion of specific recommendations evolved during the conference.

My job is to see how some of these recommendations can be implemented. First, I would like to talk in a more general vein for a few minutes. It has been said that "all the materials needed by the clinical laboratory to achieve its complete automation are already in existence - if only we knew where to find them."

The "digital revolution" in industrial process control has been a little over 10 years in developing and has now finally arrived in full bloom. This is exemplified by the following lead paragraph from the editorial in the January 1971 issue of "Instrumentation Technology," the journal of the Instrument Society of America.

I quote, "As our lead article in this issue summarizes--the time is now in sight when digital computers will execute process control almost universally. Given a few more technical improvements that are even now on the way, the digital computer will become an easily justified and routine implement of control throughout the process industries."

Recent major developments which have helped gain this acceptance are:

1. The integrated mini-computer with its high reliability and low cost.
2. Small, inexpensive data collection and distribution devices such as A to D and D to A converters and multiplexers which can be used remotely from the computer thus reducing wiring and installation costs.
3. The appearance and promotion of efforts to achieve a standardization of computer programming languages to obtain:
    a. The emulation of programming of small machines onto large central machines reduces the memory requirements of the small machines since compilers and other programming aids need not be carried in them at all times.
    b. Transportability of a given program, written in a higher level language, from one computer to another.
4. An economic need to achieve a much more exact control of the process and a much better coordination of its various operating units in order to achieve higher productivity, better quality, and lower operating costs.

This growth is now at a point where a major effort can be expended towards developing an overall hospital operating system. Using the knowledge already acquired from the industrial process, control effort looks promising.

Our point of contact with the overall hospital operating system is the patient. In our own Institute, NIGMS, a fool-proof positive laboratory sample identification system is still top priority. One of the reasons for this is that sample identification represents a limiting factor in the further development of mechanized and automated analytical instrumentation, especially in such instruments as the GeMSAEC.

Despite its intrinsic importance for the laboratory, sample identification is a relatively minor problem in the total complex mechanism for the delivery of health services to the individual.

Viewed in this broad context, several general considerations should be evident for the building of a satisfactory identification system.

1. It must fit smoothly into present procedures and yet must clearly make provisions for future changes.
2.a The laboratory system whatever it may be must be capable of direct communication by computer with all other systems in the hospital.
2.b. Even a casual familiarity with the extraordinary interlocking inter-dependence of hospital operations brings the realization that seemingly minor changes in procedure at one point can result in vigorous and unanticipated vibrations elsewhere in the web of patient services. Thus, it is not too soon to consider in our newer hospitals a total automation system at least in so far as information is concerned.
3. Only a minimal burden of alteration of ongoing staff routines can be tolerated in such a system.

4.a Even more significant than the convenience of the staff is the comfort of the patient which should be our first consideration.

4.b Any method which increases patient discomfort would be unacceptable since in the final analysis it would decrease the effectiveness of medical care.

In addition to these general considerations, the "ideal" sample identification system should meet some specific goals:

1. The sample must be unambiguously linked to the individual from whom it was derived.
2. The identification must carry through the entire chain of analytical and data processing to the final report of results.
3. For the purposes of the laboratory, the sample requires correlation with the circumstances of its origin. These include time and location at which it was obtained, the anticoagulent used and the tests to be completed.
4. The system must have a greater reliability and freedom from error than the procedure it would replace.
5. The initial cost must be justified by the savings demonstrable through increased operating efficiency and enhanced productivity.
6. Beyond this, the information needed relates to good housekeeping procedures of any reputable lab such as quality control information etc. and I will not discuss them further.

As for other future planning I would like to mention the patient's chart, or record, as it relates to the laboratory.

First, we should constantly be aware that if it were not for the patient there would be no need for the clinical laboratory, and that our interface between the clinical laboratory and the patient is the patient's physician. Our reports must be so constructed that this busy man can read and understand the messages generated in the clinical laboratory. I recently spent two days at a conference where formatting was the principal subject discussed. No decisions were made and a committee was formed to look into the matter. I realize that different physicians look for different things in a report but why can't we compromise on perhaps one format as a working pattern and then work out the differences.

Actually the documentation of the patients' data and the validity of test results is part of the routine houskeeping of any laboratory, and in my opinion have no business cluttering up the chart. As Dr. Weed said--the physician wants to know what the "serum rhubarb" level is and if you can guarantee him reliable results. Of course, the basic data necessary to back up your claims of reliability should always be available in the laboratory for your own in-house statistical message. In fact, in order to comply with Federal requirements, this statistical material must be maintained and available for inspection.

Normal Values

Unless and until we can reduce the analytical errors involved in the composite result of any given test at least to within the physiological range of the same parameter I feel that it is useless to attempt the definition of normal values. Dr. George Z. Williams is now working on this aspect of the clinical laboratory sciences and we hope before long to have considerable insight into this problem. However, whenever anyone begins to sit down and determine (arbitratily) normal values for the clinical parameters with which the laboratory is involved, we must be assured that pathologists, and clinical chemists will be at the negotiating table.

Language

This applies in two ways: We should develop a language common to all computers or translatable from one computer to another, and we must develop a language comprised of standard terms for our own lexicon. Logically, this could be an extension of SNOP (systematized nomenclature of pathology) to include enzymes, and hormones for example.

In summary--as Dr. Gabrieli said day before yesterday, we have a task--to develop and maintain communications with the physician, and unless we do establish this we will lose all contact between science and medicine.

Planning the Future - A Panel Discussion

Roy N. Barnett, M.D.
E. R. Gabrieli, M.D.
Robert S. Melville, Ph.D.
Wellington B. Stewart, M.D.

Dr. Wellington B. Stewart: Dr. E. K. Jennings, the President of the American Society of Clinical Pathologists has appointed me as official representative. This Society has a longstanding interest in the types of problems we have discussed during this Conference and has had various educational programs along the lines of this Conference. We are aware of the task of communicating with our clinical colleagues, and as Dr. Gambino suggested in his presentation, frequent participation in clinical problem solving is also our duty. In areas of standardization, such as standardization of reagents, methods, terms, codes, we support the efforts of the College of American Pathologists. Dr. Barnett represents the College in this panel discussion. I only want to encourage any suggestions or comments about these problems which the American Society of Clinical Pathologists will welcome and will give careful consideration.

This Conference stressed computer-oriented communication. I want to emphasize, computers aside, that extensive standardization of our language, our numbers, our form of reporting is needed, just for the sake of better communication. We need to keep this principle in proper context and this Conference succeeded in focusing on this problem.

We physicians have developed our own language. Information scientists have also developed a language of their own. A large effort is being made now, particularly by physicians interested in computers, and interestingly enough, largely by pathologists, to translate our rather basic English into standard codeable terminology. Dr. Arnold Pratt at the N.I.H. has developed a linguistic computer capability. His program is able to handle 90-95 per cent of the diagnostic terms submitted in natural language by pathologists. The output is in SNOP code. Dr. Lamson of UCLA approached the problem differently and he was also successful translating undisciplined English into an internal code.

Computers can put in storage vast amounts of data. It is, however, a large task to retrieve these data on demand. Information technologists successful in business or industry have not successfully solved the seemingly similar tasks when they attempt to automate the hospital. The operational hierarchy so visible in business is lacking in the hospital: each physician is an autonomous entity. Computers can, however, act as a central pool of patient information, providing clinical information to the laboratory and others for better participation in patient care.

Dr. Roy N. Barnett: (representing the College of American Pathologists) I hope the audience was not unduly discouraged by the presentations like those of Dr. Sunderman or Dr. Elveback showing slight differences between a Gaussian curve and true distribution of normal values. From the point of view of clinical practice it is really not vital whether the upper limit of normal blood glucose is 120 or 125 mg per cent, the clinician's diagnostic decision will be influenced more by the clinical impression than by the range of normals given by the laboratory.

Dr. Burns' report to this Conference is actually the report of the Subcommittee of the College of Pathologists on Medical Usefullness. There is no single standard format to meet all the needs of all institutions and all physicians, but these guidelines should be helpful.

Finally, we should examine SNOP which is now successfuly used by many pathologists. It is practical and computer-compatible. This coding system was initially sponsored by the College of American Pathologists and the American Cancer Society. The first edition of SNOP compiled by Dr. Arthur Wells and his committee is a major advance in the field of accurate communication. I propose the participants of this Conference should consider the expanded SNOP as a tool for communication between laboratory and clinical medicine. The use of a term by several clinical disciplines should carry the same meaning. For instance, diabetes mellitus should be used with the same meaning by the clinician describing a disease manifestation, the geneticist, or the laboratory referring to a test result. This could be achieved by a linguistic system like SNOP. In addition, I propose that we all become concerned with the implementation of the recommendations developed during this Conference.

Closing Remarks
by
Conference Chairman: E. R. Gabrieli, M. D.

This Conference was conceived as a task-oriented mental exercise of the leaders in laboratory medicine. The task is to conserve the potential meaning of the laboratory result, to give maximal support to the clinician at the bedside. The discussion following Drs. Melville, Stewart and Barnett shows a clear agreement with regard to SNOP. We all seem to support Dr. Barnett that SNOP should be expanded, made comprehensive for the clinican, semantically distinct, explicit categorization for the communication scientist, and consistent for the computer-oriented medical linguist, like Dr. Pratt. I think I express the unanimous request of this Conference directed to the College of American Pathologists and to the American Society of Clinical Pathologists: SNOP was a

fine start, a solid foundation for information handling.
It is vital to laboratory medicine to have a fully developed
standard language which will sharpen communication
throughout the health field. This will also achieve computer compatibility. Perhaps the most important product
of this Conference is this conclusion. We all urge Drs.
Stewart and Barnett to present this message to our two
organizations. It is an urgent and all important task, and
we feel the College of American Pathologists should proceed with this as rapidly as possible, providing full support to Dr. Wells and his committee.

The topic of this Conference was unorthodox, and
unusual. Although every speaker made an honest effort
to focus on the chosen topic, some of the discussions were
still somewhat quality assurance oriented. The quality
of the laboratory study is, indeed, still very important.
The purpose of this Conference was, however, to focus
the attention of laboratory medicine on interprofessional
communication. At the closing of this Conference, perhaps all we achieved was a hesitating, sketchy outline of
some of the problems, particularly in a man-machine
system. Computers will play an increasing role in clinical medicine and we must prepare ourselves to use this
new tool for communication. Several discussors mentioned in this closing session that this Conference recognized the growing difficulty of communication and defined
the specific problems. Perhaps we could find only the
problems, not their solutions. This shows, however,
that the problems are difficult, and much further time
and effort is required until adequate solutions emerge.
As one of the discussors stated, progress begins with
problem definition, to be followed by problem solving.
The latter is, however, by no means a true elimination
of the problem encountered. All we can hope for is to
reduce this problem, only to find new challenges in this
process of "problem solving". If this is a realistic definition of progress, then I feel this Conference was highly
successful. We certainly appreciate the growing problem

of communication, and we have advanced some possible solutions. This calls for planning another conference, perhaps after 2-3 years of testing those recommendations, to reassess the position of laboratory medicine in the community of clinical medicine.

I would like to thank all speakers for their contributions, and all participants of this Conference for making the discussions of this meeting a valuable learning experience for all of us. The "first" conference on Clinically Oriented Documentation of Laboratory Data is now officially closed.

NO LONGER THE PROPERTY
OF THE
UNIVERSITY OF R. I. LIBRARY